Nutrition and Food Services for Integrated Health Care

A Handbook for Leaders

Rita Jackson, PhD, RD

Adjunct Professor
Nutrition and Dietetics
University of North Florida
Jacksonville, Florida

AN ASPEN PUBLICATION®
Aspen Publishers, Inc.
Gaithersburg, Maryland
1997

Library of Congress Cataloging-in-Publication Data

Jackson, Rita
Nutrition and food services for integrated health care / a
handbook for leaders / Rita Jackson.
p. cm.
Includes bibliographical references and index.
ISBN 0-8342-0760-5
1. Hospitals—Food service—Management.   2. Dietetics.   I. Title.
RA975.5.D5J334   1996
362.1'76—dc20
96-30759
CIP

Orders: (800) 638-8437
Customer Service: (800) 234-1660

About Aspen Publishers • For more than 35 years, Aspen has been a leading
professional publisher in a variety of disciplines. Aspen's vast information resources are available in both print and electronic formats. We are committed to
providing the highest quality information available in the most appropriate format for our customers. Visit Aspen's Internet site for more information resources,
directories, articles, and a searchable version of Aspen's full catalog, including the
most recent publications: **http://www.aspenpub.com**
 Aspen Publishers, Inc. • The hallmark of quality in publishing
Member of the worldwide Wolters Kluwer group

Aspen Publishers, Inc., is not affiliated with
the American Society of Parenteral and Enteral Nutrition.

Editorial Resources: Ruth Bloom
Library of Congress Catalog Card Number: 96-30759
ISBN: 0-8342-0760-5

Printed in the United States of America

1 2 3 4 5

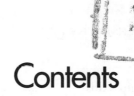

Contents

Contributors

Margo Alexander, MA, RD, DHCFA
Director of Food and Nutrition Services
Mercy Medical Center
Rockville Center, New York

Jacques W. Bloch, CFE, FHCHA
Food Service Consultant
Bronx, New York

Mildred M. Cody, PhD, RD
Associate Professor
Department of Nutrition and Dietetics
Georgia State University
Atlanta, Georgia

Brigid Connolly Sullivan, MA, RD
Director of Food and Nutrition
St. Luke's—Roosevelt Hospital Center
New York, New York

Sylvia Escott-Stump, MA, RD
Director of Dietetic Services
Forbes Nursing Center
Pittsburgh, Pennsylvania

Michele M. Fairchild, MA, RD
Associate Director of Clinical Nutrition
Director of Dietary Services
The University of Iowa Hospital and Clinics
Iowa City, Iowa

Karen R. Greathouse, PhD, RD
Assistant Professor
Western Illinois University
Macomb, Illinois

Mary Gregoire, PhD, RD, LD
Associate Director, Food and Nutrition Services
Rush-Presbyterian–St. Luke's Medical Center
Chicago, Illinois

Laura Guyer, PhD, RD, LD
Associate Professor
Food Science and Human Nutrition
University of Florida
Gainesville, Florida

Rita Jackson, PhD, RD
Food Service and Nutrition Consultant
Editor, *Health Care Food & Nutrition Focus*
MSH/AP4 Director
University of North Florida
Jacksonville, Florida

Dorothy G. King, PhD, RD
Nutrition and Bioethics Consultant
New York, New York

Jimmy R. Lloyd
Director of Food and Nutrition Services
Shands Hospital
University of Florida
Gainesville, Florida

Thomas J. McCann, RD, CDN
Food Service Consultant
Mamaroneck, New York

Mary Frances Nettles, PhD, RD
Assistant Professor
College of Health and Human Services
The University of Southern Mississippi
Hattiesburg, Mississippi

F. Xavier Pi-Sunyer, MD
Director of the Obesity Research Center
Chief of Endocrinology, Diabetes, and Nutrition
St. Luke's–Roosevelt Hospital Center
New York, New York

Ruby P. Puckett, MA, RD, LD
Food Service Management Consultant
Gainesville, Florida

C. Nick Wilson, PhD, FACHE
Associate Professor
Department of Health Science
College of Health
University of North Florida
Jacksonville, Florida

Foreword

Nutrition and Food Services for Integrated Health Care is extremely timely. It challenges professionals in nutrition and food service to look forward to the new century. Rita Jackson is to be congratulated in her effort to move a rather stodgy discipline to think in modern terms.

Health care is changing swiftly in this country. The paradigms that served us even very recently are no longer useful. We need to radicalize our thinking so as to be able to prepare for the changes that are upon us. In the recent past, the hospital and nursing home, that is, institutions, were the center of our gravity. We could be content to sit in an institutionalized setting and look at our umbilicus and our small world, unmindful of what occurred beyond our walls. This is no longer true. The hospital and the nursing home are dwindling in importance. Doctors admit fewer and fewer patients to hospitals and treat more of them at home. There is a decided effort to keep older people at home and with relatives so as to decrease the cost that the aged bring to society. The thrust is to think in integrated systems that overlap in a seamless web, providing care in a manner that is less costly and more effective. The emphasis is on the patients or the clients, and how best to care for them for the least cost.

How does this affect professionals in the nutrition and food service industry? Nutrition services will be required to leap into this new world. A food service director will no longer be responsible for one hospital at one site with a familiar set of employees. The director may be in charge of a group of hospitals, nursing homes, home care services, community services, and the like. Dietitians have to think that much of their work, previously done in an institutional site, may in the future be done in neighborhood clinics, home care settings, and even at the work place.

It is incumbent on nutrition and food service professionals to begin to train their successors with a much wider view of what the industry is about. From the traditional health care model we need to move to a much wider vision. We need to be aware that nutritionists of the future will have to be more malleable, more knowledgeable, and better able to work collaboratively with other health professionals in the new marketplace.

There are important areas where nutrition professionals have not paid much attention in the past but which they will need to highlight in the future. One is patients' rights and professional responsibility. Gone are the days when patients were told what to do and how to behave, no questions tolerated. Another is outcomes assessment. Health and wellness are strongly connected to nutrition. The results of our actions as professionals make an enormous impact on people's lives. We have not assessed this adequately in the past, but we will have to in the future. As competition increases, an emphasis on the quality of the services we provide will become increasingly important. Not only regulatory agencies, but consumers themselves are becoming much more conscious of quality as an element that they can assess and critique. The quality of food and nutrition services includes purchasing strategy, cooking skills and techniques, presentation, safety, and nutrition therapy. All are important and will be assessed.

Finally, we are in an era of cost-cutting. This means a strong emphasis on productivity of the work force which, in turn, requires adequate training of employees, strong motivation for quality work, and intelligent monitoring of performance.

It is important for nutritionists and food service directors to prepare to perform in the new playing field. I believe that you will find this book very helpful in beginning to look ahead. Dr. Jackson has chosen the contributors well. They are leaders in their field, they are knowledgeable, and they wish to help you. Take their advice. Look to the future!

—F. Xavier Pi-Sunyer, MD
Director of the Obesity Research Center
Chief of Endocrinology, Diabetes, and Nutrition
St. Luke's—Roosevelt Hospital Center
New York, New York

Preface

Market forces are radically influencing the health care system in the United States. Although most of the current trends have been apparent for more than two decades, few practitioners actually expected the turbulent changes that are occurring during the health care revolution of the 1990s. It is now perfectly clear to everyone that consumers want improved quality and more "user-friendly" services from a unified delivery system that operates efficiently along the continuum of care with less duplication of effort and lower overall costs. Although the distant future is never completely predictable, the next several years are likely to reveal the traditional health care model finally being cast aside in lieu of an alternative paradigm. Many options are now being tested in the industry. The most promising one of all is the *integrated health care delivery system*, for reasons that are fully detailed in the first section of this book, along with the leadership and management skills that are needed to succeed in this new health care environment.

The impact of today's total restructuring of the health care system on the leaders in food service and nutrition care has been, and will continue to be, greater than any other they have experienced in their entire careers. Drastic changes are needed in the patterns of professional practice, the way staff are organized and managed, the types of skills required, the way care is coordinated among various payers and providers, and the relationships between individuals who provide and those who receive care.

This book is designed to help professionals in a variety of health care settings successfully make the transition to integrated health care. Because the concept of integration represents a *coming together* of all health care components from a previously segmented industry, this topic applies not only to practitioners in the acute care industry but also to those in long-term care, rehabilitative care, ambulatory care, mental health, and community services. The book is meant to be a guide for seasoned professionals to use as they prepare for expanded roles in the integrated health care delivery systems of the future.

Part I of this book, *The Shift toward Integrated Health Care*, provides a broad vision of the industry. Readers will see that the current times of change offer many more opportunities than the stagnant times of the past. Chapter 1, *Industry Trends*, describes the forces that have brought about the current restructuring efforts in the health care industry, and identifies specific trends that will enable practitioners to prepare themselves for the future. In Chapter 2, *Leadership for Quality*, Margo Alexander illustrates how true leaders will be expected to adapt and capitalize on every opportunity. They will balance the lessons of the past with creativity and continuous learning to develop and communicate a vision of success to their followers. Chapter 3, *Management Strategies*, provides practical tools for managing food and nutrition services. Brigid Connolly Sullivan offers many tips for reengineering and restructuring the traditional systems while emphasizing those which are most applicable in the integrated health care setting. There are many lessons from the past that apply perfectly well to the future. Although each and every strategy needs to be questioned and evaluated, it would not be wise to arbitrarily discard all former techniques. Therefore, the most applicable methods are emphasized. Many sample forms, illustrations, and case studies are provided by these and the remaining chapter authors.

Part II focuses on *Nutrition Care*. In Chapter 4, *Managing Nutrition Services*, Sylvia Escott-Stump describes the need for strong management of this component of patient care. She describes the role of the clinical nutrition manager and how this person can effectively plan, direct, and coordinate nutrition care function. In the following chapter on *Outcome-Based Nutrition Education*, Laura Guyer presents a comprehensive view of patient education, a topic which is being stressed now more than ever so preventive health care can become a reality. Chapter 6, *Patients' Rights: Case Study of Medical Nutrition Care*, deals with the legal dilemmas faced by dietitians today. In it, Dorothy King presents two vignettes that illustrate a variety of different ethical and legal concerns. Finally, Chapter 7, *Cost Containment and Revenue Enhancement*, covers the major challenge for dietitians. Michele Fairchild offers many suggestions for inpatient and outpatient programs so dietitians will be able to more successfully cost justify their services in the future.

Management of Food Services is presented in Part III of this book, and the topics in this section progress from purchasing through meal delivery. In Chapter 8, Thomas McCann and Jacques Bloch suggest many alternative approaches for purchasing with helpful forms and illustrations that can be adapted for use. *Alternative Food Production Systems* are covered next in Chapter 9 by Mary Gregoire and Mary Frances Nettles. Tried and tested methods are discussed along with new and promising ones that can help professionals meet the challenges that lie ahead. Karen Greathouse and Mary Gregoire then offer *Options in Meal Assembly, Delivery, and Service*, in Chapter 10. Food service managers are expected to make many decisions in each of these topics and all of the authors provide a comprehensive review from a practical point of view. Chapter 11 covers *Current Issues in Food Safety*. In it, Mildred Cody describes HACCP concepts that apply to all types of food service systems. Suggestions for employee and patient education are described as well. Finally, Chapter 12 focuses on *Revenue-Generating Opportunities* for commercial food services in the health care system. Jimmy Lloyd proposes a model for marketing food services, and offers guidelines for using situational and value analyses techniques.

Part IV, *Preparing for Future Challenges*, will enable professionals to continuously improve productivity and quality of care while staying in step with the future trends in the industry. In Chapter 13, Ruby Puckett and Rita Jackson present *A Systems Approach to Productivity*. Methods for measuring, monitoring, and improving productivity are proposed. The next chapter on *Quality Improvement* describes how outcome-based indicators for quality can be designed and utilized so practitioners can stay ahead of their competitors. C. Nick Wilson then focuses on the future in Chapter 15, *The Changing U.S. Health Care System*, with special emphasis on the skills that will be needed in the 21st century.

The idea of integrated health care is not a new one. Some think of it as how it used to be before the 1970s when many physicians worked to improve the health of their patients from "cradle to grave" as they coordinated care with hospitals, long-term care facilities, community programs, and in the home. But, regardless of when and where it began, it is much more feasible now than in the past due to our increased knowledge and technological advancements. After the health care revolution of the 1990s has passed, we shall look back with a sigh of relief to many of the barriers it destroyed. Among them will be the barriers between various disciplines, and those between patients and practitioners; employees and management; health care providers and managers; third party payers and providers; and health care providers in the community and traditional health care institutions. As the air clears toward the end of the century we can expect to see evidence of a new health care delivery system that is based on increased self-responsibility of patients, ease of communication, increased trust, and cooperative sharing, all of which can result in improved quality, increased efficiency, and lower health care costs. With true integration, everyone inside and outside of the health care system benefits because they interact freely to share resources in an effort to improve the health status of Americans, from the beginning to the end of their lives, wherever they may be. This, combined with reasonable costs for health care services, will ultimately contribute to a more sound economy for the country.

—Rita Jackson, PhD, RD

Acknowledgments

First and foremost, recognition is given to the contributors to this book. They were carefully selected based upon their knowledge, foresight, and ability to practice in a wide variety of health care settings, including acute care, long-term care, rehabilitative care, ambulatory care, mental health, community services, and others. They have had experiences in dietetics, food service management, health care administration, education, and research. Some have achieved advanced academic degrees in the field, others learned in the "school of hard knocks," and most of them have benefited from a combination of the two. All of them have in common an immense passion for their work, which is reflected in the chapters they have contributed. The words of Winston Churchill apply well to them all: "Those whose work and pleasures are one, are fortune's favorite children."

Another characteristic common among the contributors is the fact that they are active in the field and experiencing the same changes and industry demands as the readers of this book. In a variety of roles, they are "in the trenches" and dealing with the changes along with everyone else. This has caused them to have both practical insights and realistic views of the industry. As the book's editor, I am well aware of the sacrifices each and every one of them has made to take time from incredibly busy schedules to share with others in this way. Along with the readers of this book, I am grateful that they decided to make this personal commitment and valuable contribution to the profession. Recognition, as well, goes to their family members, students, and employees who supported them in this effort.

Special thanks also go to the staff at Aspen Publishers, Inc. When I was first approached about providing a book for seasoned professionals in the field, I wondered whether this was possible because of the drastic changes occurring in the industry and the vast amount of knowledge that would have to be imparted. I am especially grateful to Michael Brown, who placed this challenge before me, and to Sandy Cannon and Mary Anne Langdon for their patience and support as I coordinated efforts with the many contributors to the book.

This book is dedicated to Harry Vlismas, with whom I had the opportunity to work, and from whom I learned much, in the early 1970s. Right before my very eyes, this creative individual evaluated the most promising systems and equipment in the country and established partnerships with potential suppliers. He then created, built, and managed a central commissary that produced meals for two existing hospitals and one large new nursing home, all of which were under the same ownership but located geographically many miles from each other. The underlying premise for all activities was to "work smarter, not harder" while drastically reducing costs. The system used simple production and assembly techniques that were common to the manufacturing industry. It used the predecessor of the fax for communications as well as cook–chill, advanced plating concepts, and rethermalization of fully plated meals in a conveyor microwave oven, all more than 20 years ago before most people knew what these things were.

Harry Vlismas instilled in his staff a genuine concern for patient satisfaction through continuous training and by always emphasizing sensitivity to the patient who would receive each meal. The focus was food quality through careful purchasing, production, assembly, and delivery controls. Every detail was studied, monitored, and evaluated. With great respect for his employees, he continuously solicited ideas in an effort to seek the best possible working conditions for them and to find the simplest methods that would work the best. As a result, his employees all felt as if they were a part of a successful team. With a sense of humor that never seemed to be exhausted, he overcame problems in a way that brought even more positive outcomes. As a boss, a mentor, a role model, and a friend, this gentleman, who always managed to stay a step ahead of the industry's trends, shall always have my deepest respect.

The Shift toward Integrated Health Care

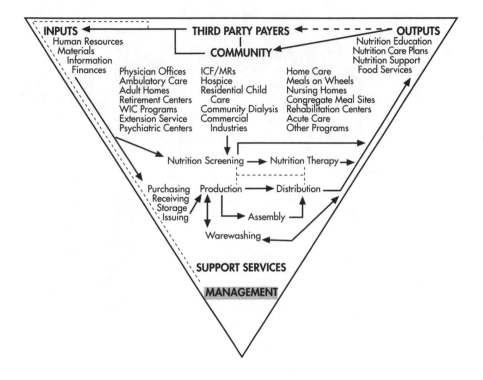

INPUTS
Human Resources
Materials
Information
Finances

THIRD PARTY PAYERS

COMMUNITY

OUTPUTS
Nutrition Education
Nutrition Care Plans
Nutrition Support
Food Services

Physician Offices
Ambulatory Care
Adult Homes
Retirement Centers
WIC Programs
Extension Service
Psychiatric Centers

ICF/MRs
Hospice
Residential Child
 Care
Community Dialysis
Commercial
 Industries

Home Care
Meals on Wheels
Nursing Homes
Congregate Meal Sites
Rehabilitation Centers
Acute Care
Other Programs

Nutrition Screening → Nutrition Therapy →

Purchasing
Receiving
Storage
Issuing

Production → Distribution

Assembly

Warewashing

SUPPORT SERVICES

MANAGEMENT

Industry Trends

Rita Jackson

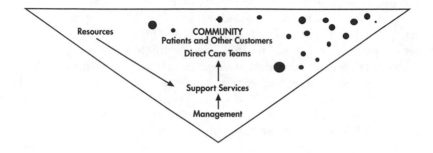

Food service directors and dietitians in the health care industry are currently being faced with major changes. The rules seem to alter daily as the view of an isolated dietary department as a separate and stable entity falls by the wayside. There are new jobs, new titles, new organizational designs, and new ways to manage employees, prepare budgets, purchase foods, assess patients, and serve meals. Many of the old solutions just do not work anymore, no matter how hard practitioners try to do the things they were trained to do.

As the health care system undergoes restructuring, most facilities are adopting the patient-focused approach, which aims to increase flexibility within the organization by using a multiskilled approach, with as much activity as possible occurring directly at the point of care. By 1995, more than half the hospitals in the United States had embraced the patient-focused care initiative (Schiller, 1995). Almost 30% had already implemented patient-focused care, and 15% were in the process of converting. The *Hay 1995 Hospital Compensation Survey* (Farrell & Pagoaga, 1995) included statistics from 885 hospitals in the United States. Of those undergoing work redesign, 94% were creating team processes for the delivery of patient care. Schiller, a well-recognized authority in the field of dietetics, defines patient-focused care as "a reconfiguration of the services a hospital provides for the comfort and convenience of patients." Up until this time, services were primarily designed around the needs of staff instead.

Many organizations are converting to patient-focused care with a broader long-range picture in mind as they realize that, in the future, the hospital will be a much smaller part of the industry. According to Schiller, from 1995 to just after 2000 "the name of the game will be integration." Health care will be focused toward the community in a variety of settings along the continuum of care as preventive, custodial, and acute care services are offered. "When we talk about integration, we are really talking about total health care systems in the business of healthy communities," says Schiller. All health care activities will be integrated and coordinated by interdisciplinary care teams as people move within the network from the beginning to the end of their lives.

Integrated health care systems are global in scope. They refer to much of the larger system, which, according to Schiller, "includes continuums of care that either happen under one roof where a hospital might have a range of services from maternal, pediatric on through subacute care and even long term care in a single institution; or, integrated systems might also mean services provided in a number of different settings under a single sponsorship." This concept is often called seamless health care, which is occurring as hospitals purchase nursing homes, start home care projects, set up satellite clinics, and focus more on healthy communities. Integration of services within facilities among care providers has also been stressed by the Joint Commission on Accreditation of Healthcare Organizations (Joint Commission).

The integrated health care system of the future will most probably consist of a series of networks that disperse themselves over a wide geographic area and extend into sites such as homes, churches, and workplaces (Bergman & Sherer, 1993). Hospitals will no longer be perceived as one large building containing every service imaginable. Ambulatory care centers will replace the typical hospital environment. Initiatives include mergers, networks, closures, and downsizing, all of which will result in thousands of health care practitioners losing their positions through layoffs and attrition. Those who remain will have markedly different jobs. Under these conditions, it is essential that managers in the field keep an open mind, stay flexible, and constantly search for nontraditional solutions from areas outside the realm of traditional health care.

In this chapter, the reasons for the health care revolution of the 1990s are discussed so that readers can understand the need for change in the industry. The nature of change is then presented to show why some are kicking and screaming while others are plunging forward to meet the exciting challenges that await them. Finally, new and promising approaches in the industry are discussed to reveal the different ways that change can benefit everyone when it is headed in the right direction.

THE WORLD IS CHANGING

To understand why drastic changes are occurring in the industry, one just needs to look around at the environment and compare what is seen to "how it used to be." The same things that have influenced the way people live their lives have also affected the health care system. These include changes in the demographics, the information that is readily available, advanced technology that is now at everyone's disposal, and competition in the national and worldwide marketplace. In an effort to serve customers well, one needs to stay abreast of all these trends.

The term *customer* is used here to stress the fact that the health care industry has an enormous potential to serve more than patients. In fact, considering the current trends in the field, one should probably refer to customer-focused health care instead of patient-focused care. Communities are full of people who need varying degrees of preventive, custodial, and acute health care, and there is great potential for nutrition and food service outside the walls of institutions. To limit our market to those requiring traditional hospital or nursing home services not only would restrict the industry but also would widen a gap for underqualified individuals to fill. This, of course, would affect the nation's ability to keep the population as healthy as possible.

There are many different customers who purchase goods and services in the market. To reflect the degree of impact that different types of customers have on an organization, Juran (1989) groups customers into two categories: the *useful* many and the *vital few*. The useful many represent a relatively large number of customers who have a modest impact on the organization. The vital few represent a relatively few customers who have a great impact on the organization. In the hotel industry, for example, the useful many are people who stop and ask for a room while visiting a city or traveling through it. They make individual arrangements for themselves, and each small transaction with them is more or less standardized. The vital few, on the other hand, are the travel agents and conference planners who bring large groups of individuals to the hotel. Each transaction with these customers requires special attention because of the volume of sales it represents.

In health care, the *useful many* are patients who independently select the health care facility they wish to use, and the *vital few* are the third-party payers and the physicians, or *gatekeepers*, who sometimes determine which facility will be used for patients. Table 1–1 shows the different consumer groups that purchase health care in the country. It can be seen that, from 1960 to the present time, private health expenditures have consistently decreased while government expenditures have increased.

More than 70% of total government expenditures for health care go to Medicare and Medicaid programs. They both use managed care organizations and health maintenance organizations (HMOs) more now than ever before (Armstead, Elstein, & Gorman, 1995). Since the inception of the Medicare managed care program under the Tax Equity and Fiscal Responsibility Act of 1982, enrollment of beneficiaries in Medicare managed care contracts has increased. In 1987, there were approximately 1.7 million, and in 1992 there were

Table 1-1 National Health Expenditures (Aggregate Amounts in Billions)

Type of Expenditures	1960 $	1960 %	1980 $	1980 %	1990 $	1990 %	1993 $	1993 %	1994* $	1994* %	1995* $	1995* %
Private												
Consumer out of pocket	13.4	49.5	61.3	24.4	138.3	19.9	157.5	17.8	163.7	17.5	175.2	17.4
Consumer private insurance	5.9	21.8	72.1	28.7	236.9	34.0	296.1	33.5	310.7	33.1	331.3	32.9
Other private	1.3	4.3	12.4	4.9	34.8	5.0	42.8	4.8	43.7	4.7	46.2	4.6
Total private funds	20.5	75.6	145.8	58.1	410.0	58.9	496.4	56.1	518.1	55.2	552.7	54.9
Government												
Federal	2.9	10.7	72.0	28.7	195.8	28.1	280.6	31.7	306.7	32.7	334.1	33.2
State and local	3.7	13.7	33.3	13.3	90.7	13.0	107.3	12.1	113.5	12.1	120.8	12.0
Total government	6.7	24.4	105.3	41.9	286.5	41.1	387.8	43.9	420.2	44.8	454.9	45.1
Total public and private	27.1	100.0	251.1	100.0	696.6	100.0	844.2	100.0	938.3	100.0	1007.6	100.0
Medicare†							154.2	17.4	171.4	18.3	190.0	18.9
Medicaid‡							117.9	13.3	128.5	13.7	138.4	13.7

*Projected amounts.
†Subset of federal funds.
‡Subset of federal, state, and local funds.
Source: Reprinted from the Office of the Actuary, Health Care Finance Administration.

more than 2.0 million. According to Fried (1995), the growth rate in 1993 was 17%, and by 1995 3.7 million individuals were enrolled in managed care. This represented 10% of all Medicare recipients. Testing of new programs in this population is being done conservatively because of the vulnerability of these individuals. Fried (1995) reports that a higher level of patient satisfaction has been found with the managed care arrangements and that the reduction of paperwork has been received favorably by participants.

The number of Medicaid enrollees in managed care contracts has increased much more quickly. In 1980, managed care was virtually unknown in the Medicaid program. As a result of uncontrolled growth of Medicaid expenditures in the 1980s, the states began to pursue managed care as their primary mechanism to restrain costs as they increased access to care for beneficiaries who faced limited numbers of providers available to serve them. By 1990, more than 1.5 million Medicaid enrollees were in managed care programs. Two years later, this figure more than doubled to 3.6 million. A 63% rate of growth occurred between 1993 and 1994, when enrollees passed the 8.0 million mark. Toward the end of 1995, 24% of all Medicaid recipients in the country became enrolled, and Fried (1995) expects that by 1999 the vast majority of Medicaid recipients will be included in managed care arrangements.

These trends have made the Health Care Financing Administration (HCFA) the largest managed care purchaser in the country. Congress has proposed reductions by 2002 in federal spending of $450 billion for Medicare and Medicaid. According to Fried (1995), if this occurs it will be accomplished, in part, by repeal of the nursing home regulations under which nutrition assessments are required for patients in this setting. One promising concept is the medical savings account as an option for seniors. Also called medical individual retirement accounts, these accounts give financial incentives for people to avoid getting health care by motivating them to stay healthy.

Demographics

Shifts in the characteristics of the population affect health care managers on at least three fronts. First, when demographic changes take place, the needs and expectations of current and potential customers change. Second, because the health care system draws employees from the community, the needs and expectations of the work force change as well. Third, the markets from which health care providers obtain equipment, supplies, and income are affected. No matter how hard one may try, one cannot escape changes in the environment.

Juran (1989) stated that customers' needs are a moving target. He encouraged continuous quality management and wrote "We are beset by powerful forces that keep coming over the horizon and are ever changing directions: new technology, market competition, social upheavals, international conflicts. These changing forces create new customers' needs or change the priority given to the existing ones" (Juran, 1989, p. 101).

Everyone learned about *internal* and *external* customers from Juran, the well-known authority in the field of total quality management. Juran wrote that, while trying to focus on customers' needs, one must realize that "the customer is a cast of characters" (Juran, 1989, p. 92). *Internal customers* are those within health care systems who receive the goods and services we provide. They include people such as nurses, who receive nourishments for distribution to patients; members of the medical team, who read and react to dietitians' chart notes; and students, who receive on-site training. Along with other members of the work force these people have a lot to do with how food and nutrition services are perceived. *External customers* include patients, family members, third-party payers, and other individuals or groups that purchase goods or services.

Trends Affecting External Customers

Addressing the topic of outcome assessment, Wilkins (1995) described three types of outcomes to consider: economic outcomes, clinical outcomes, and user satisfaction. He stated that people, in general, make health care decisions based on satisfaction and economic issues because they do not always have the knowledge required to assess clinical outcomes. Gill and Feinstein (1994) reviewed the literature regarding patients' perceptions of quality and the way health care professionals commonly view quality. They concluded "A prime question raised in this review, however, is whether the academic psychometric principles, although perhaps elegant statistically, are satisfactory of the clinical goal of indicating what clinicians and patients perceive as quality-of-life" (Gill & Feinstein, 1994, p. 624). Even when the investigator-specific criteria are fulfilled for measuring quality according to traditional methods, "quality-of-life measurements are aimed at the wrong targets unless individual patients are given the opportunity to express their individual opinions and reactions" (Gill & Feinstein, 1994, p. 624). In addition to focusing on clinical outcomes, Gill and Feinstein challenge practitioners to alter how they measure quality "because quality-of-life, rather than being a mere rating of health status, is actually a uniquely personal perception, representing the way that [individual patients feel] about their health status or nonmedical aspects of their lives" (Gill & Feinstein, 1994, p. 624).

What do external customers want? In general, most want the same thing: value for their dollar in the marketplace. They also expect to be treated at their convenience and in a caring manner with respect, so that their dignity is maintained. If providers fail to offer these things, others will eventually take their place in the highly competitive health care environment of today. It is important to understand that consumers are beginning to have the same expectations when they make their health care purchases as they have while buying other goods and services. For example, when people take their automobile to a shop for repairs, they want an estimate of what it will cost, and they expect that it will be fixed properly at the agreed upon price. In some states, consumer groups have even gone to the extent of demanding legislation, such as the lemon law, to protect their rights when they purchase automobiles.

As time goes on, Americans become more and more demanding in an effort to protect their rights as consumers. They are better educated than in the past and learn much from the media. Consumers have become increasingly knowledgeable about health (including nutrition) and the legal process as well. If their demands are not heard on a local level, they are not afraid to lobby at the state and national levels.

The effects of the consumer movement have already been seen in the health care industry. Many regulations that govern the industry to protect patients' rights have been initiated, such as laws for licensure of health care providers, informed consent, reporting of suspected incidents of patient abuse, ombudsman programs, risk management, environmental safety standards, free access to medical records, and actions to prevent discrimination against persons having certain disabilities and diseases. Stricter controls and inspection of all health care activities have resulted. In addition, through legislation, the government has become a major purchaser of health care services. The data from Table 1–1 show that federal, state, and local governments accounted for only 27% of the nation's health care expenditures in 1960 but for more than 45% in 1995.

In most societies, new laws and increased government regulation normally come about when the people feel they are not being treated fairly. The outcry of the American public reflects dissatisfaction with the cost of health care and the value that people think they are getting for their dollars. Figure 1–1 demonstrates how health care costs continue to rise above and beyond the cost of other products and services purchased by consumers. During the period shown, the Consumer Price Index (CPI) for all items increased from 136.2 to 150.9 (10.8%), whereas the index for medical care alone increased from 177.0 to 217.6 (22.9%). More and more, consumers are now putting others in the position to do bidding for them (e.g., the government, HMOs, and managed care organizations), and this has just begun to curtail costs.

Regarding quality, there seems to be a dichotomy between what the public actually perceives and what many health care providers think they offer. To bridge the gap and reduce costs, the health care industry has attempted to restructure the system. According to Schiller (1995), hospital restructuring is a reconfiguration of departments and patient care teams to implement one or

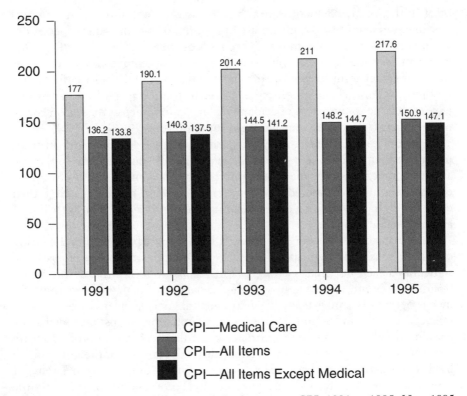

Figure 1–1 Increases in consumers' medical expenses: CPI, 1991 to 1995. *Note:* 1995 figures include first quarter data only. *Source:* Reprinted from the Bureau of Labor Statistics, U.S. Department of Labor.

another piece of patient-focused care: "Basically what is happening is an effort to bring individuals and departments together in an integrated, cooperative, collaborative design in order to reduce some of the problems that have occurred in our former health care systems" (Schiller, 1995).

The concept of restructuring was introduced to the health care field in the late 1980s, but it was not until 1993 that Lathrop organized and presented this topic in his well-known book *Restructuring Health Care: The Patient Focused Paradigm*, which caused the restructuring movement to pick up substantial momentum. By 1994, approximately 30% of U.S. hospitals had patient-focused care initiatives, and another 15% planned to have them in the future. By the end of this century, it is expected that the majority of hospitals will practice patient-focused care. According to Lathrop (1993):

Unfortunately, for the vast majority of the hospitals, the current emphasis on clinical outcomes is probably misguided. The major problems of quality revolve around customer services and process quality rather than the question of whether the vast majority of patients go home with excellent clinical and scientific outcomes. This is not to say that such issues are inappropriate or that we should ignore them. (pp. 7–8)

Lathrop (1993) identified many specific inefficiencies in the health care system that are obvious to patients and contribute to their dissatisfaction. One of these problems is excessive *turnaround time*. Lathrop stated that an average hospital requires about 4 hours to process and deliver simple routine services such as blood work. Another problem he emphasized is *fragmented care*, which contributes to what he called the *continuity of care crisis*. During a 4-day colectomy stay, for example, a patient makes contact with as many as 53 different individuals, not including physicians. Finally, the *sequence and timing of services* are based upon staff convenience rather than patients' desires or preferences.

"We now have the worst of both worlds—high (and increasing) costs, combined with poor service," according to Lathrop (1993, p. 21). He calls for better assessment of patient satisfaction by posing questions about things that make a difference to patients and for major restructuring of the health care system to improve quality and decrease costs. The principles upon which the patient-focused care model is based are decentralization of services, cross-training of staff, simplification of processes, "flattening" of the organizational hierarchy, empowerment of staff, and a collective rather than a departmental focus.

An example of how patient-focused care can reduce costs was reported by Snyder and Lathrop in 1995. Concepts of patient-focused care were implemented in various ways in three hospitals: Mercy Hospital in San Diego, California, St. Mary Medical Center in Long Beach, California, and Spohn South in Corpus Christi, Texas. Capital investments ranged from $1.0 million to $4.5 million. All three hospitals realized positive returns on investment, including an average 8% reduction in cost per case, a 5% reduction in salary costs, and up to a 1-day reduction in length of stay. Employee morale and patient satisfaction also improved.

Data from the largest survey in the industry, which covered 885 hospitals across the country in 1995, showed that 94% of the hospitals that were undergoing work redesign were creating team processes for the delivery of patient care (Farrell & Pagoaga, 1995). New roles for multidisciplinary technical care workers were being established in 64%, and new roles for multidisciplinary patient care workers were being created in 65%.

Addressing the needs of the elderly, Lloyd (1995) cited three national trends that appear to be inevitable: deficit reduction, deregulation, and demolition of power. To reduce deficits, it is expected that federal funds for health care will be cut further. Complex programs such as those initiated under the 1987 Omnibus Budget Reconciliation Act may be curtailed, and power is expected to shift from the federal level to state and local levels. A good portion of health care expenditures covers care for seniors. At the present time, approximately 13% of the American population is older than 65 years, and this, according to Lloyd (1995), is expected to reach 20% by the year 2030. Approximately 5% of elderly citizens are now nursing home residents. The rest are primarily in their homes, and it is becoming increasingly clear that deinstitutionalizing the elderly will not only improve their quality of life but contain health care costs as well.

By far the most impressive demographic trend is the continued increase in the nation's elderly population. This is of special interest to health care professionals in the field of food and nutrition because this group utilizes their services more than any other group. Currently the ratio of men to women is 3:2, but this varies depending upon the specific age group. Because women tend to live longer than men, the ratio changes to 5:2 for the group older than 85 years. At present, 68% of noninstitutionalized seniors live alone. They are mostly women, who currently have three times the chance of being widowed compared with men. Men have their wives to act as caregivers, but women who outlive their husbands often have no one to care for them. Lloyd (1995) also points out that there will be an increased cultural mix in the elderly population of the future.

Income has always been an issue with the elderly because they exist on set incomes. Lloyd (1995) states that fewer seniors were found at the poverty level in the 1980s; now the same number of seniors exist at the poverty level as other adult groups. Specifically, 12% are classified as poor and 8% as nearly poor. The median annual income of male seniors is $15,000, and that for female seniors is $8,000. Those at highest risk for poor nutrition status are elderly women and minority women who live alone. Lloyd (1995) advises that special attention be given to those with poor functional status and those known to need assistance with the normal activities of daily living and instrumental activities of daily living.

Medicare is a federal program that provides hospital and medical insurance for persons age 65 and older, disabled persons younger than 54 who are eligible for Social Security disability payments for more than 2 years, and people with end-stage renal disease from all age groups. Medicare currently represents more than 40% of all government expenditures for health care. Figure 1–2 shows past and future trends in the growth rate of Medicare benefit outlays. It reflects the shift from expensive hospital stays to skilled nursing facility stays in the 1980s and how the growth rate has been, and is expected to be, curtailed.

Trends Affecting Internal Customers

The employees within the organization reflect the same demographic trends as its customers. They are much more intelligent and aware of their rights, and

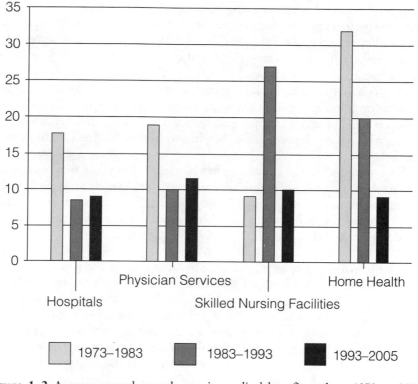

Figure 1–2 Average annual growth rate in medical benefit outlays, 1973 to 2005. *Source:* Data from the Office of National Health Statistics.

they insist that these rights be honored. Like consumers, employees are not afraid to use the legal process to protect their rights. When large groups of employees or potential employees see injustices, or even when the bond of trust is broken between them and their employers, more rules evolve in the system. One recent law that has had a major impact is the 1990 Americans with Disabilities Act, which prohibits discrimination against the disabled or those who are severely ill. Disabled persons, as defined by this Act, include those recovering from substance abuse or from mental or physical impairment, those who are physically impaired (e.g., blind, deaf, mentally retarded, or dyslexic individuals), burn victims, people with acquired immunodeficiency syndrome, and individuals who, by hearsay, are thought to be impaired. In 1986, the Supreme Court ruled that sexual harassment violates Title VII of the Civil Rights Act of 1964 and set regulations to discourage this problem in the workplace.

The Joint Commission has taken a stand on some important issues regarding infection control and human resources. These standards cover topics such as competency, control of epidemiologically significant infections, and situations where the personal beliefs of employees limit their ability to provide high-quality care. For example, the *1996 Accreditation Manual for Hospitals* states "The hospital respects its staff members' cultural values, ethics, and religious beliefs and the impact these may have on patient care. The hospital's process considers whether conflicting cultures, values, ethics, or religious beliefs are sufficient grounds for granting requests not to participate in care" (Joint Commission, 1995, p. 399). The intent of this recommendation is that patient care shall not be jeopardized if employees need to be excused from providing care to practice their beliefs.

The knowledge base of employees has increased along with that of consumers who purchase health care services and insurance. As early as 1959, Drucker first talked about *knowledge worker* and said that by the end of the century knowledge workers will amount to a third or more of the work force. He further defined the knowledge worker as follows (Drucker, 1974):

> The knowledge worker . . . is not productive under the spur of fear; only self-motivation and self-direction can make him productive. He has to be achieving in order to produce at all. The productivity, indeed the social cohesion, of every developed society rests increasingly on the ability to make knowledge work productive and the knowledge worker achieving. This may be the central social problem of the new, the knowledge society. There are no precedents for the management of knowledge work. Knowledge work traditionally has been carried out by individuals working by themselves in small groups. Now knowledge work is carried out in large, complex, managed institutions. The knowledge worker is not even the successor to yesterday's "knowledge professional." He is the successor to yesterday's skilled worker. His status, his function, his contribution, his position in the organization, therefore, still have to be defined. (pp. 176–177)

Because the nature of the worker is changing, many theories of motivation have been developed to increase job satisfaction in an effort to improve quality and productivity of the work force. They are further described in Chapter 2. These efforts are reflected in current trends such as the use of self-directed work teams, cultural diversity programs, competency evaluation, employee recognition programs, and the focus on mentoring skills. Managers are also learning what Drucker (1974) has been saying all along, that employees are indeed "our greatest asset."

In the traditional, pyramid shaped, organizational structures, first line employees and workers are normally listed at the bottom, the place of least importance. This view is changing because managers are starting to realize that these are the people that can make or break an organization. They are the ones that have the most contact with patients, family members, and other consumers; and they have many good solutions to the problems at hand. Yet, in the past, little time and resources has been invested in their development. This concept has become one of the major focal points of restructuring the health care system and can account for many of the trends that are being seen.

In addition to the points made above, employees now approach the job market with different expectations regarding the work hours, salaries, and compensation programs. Americans value their leisure time more now than in the past, and many prefer part time jobs that have equitable benefits, compressed work weeks, and job-sharing abilities. More women are entering the work force, and retired persons with excellent work histories seek jobs for additional income or because they still wish to be productive. These factors, along with the slow employment growth in the health care industry (Table 1–2), have affected the way managers staff their departments today.

Although it can be seen from Table 1–2 that growth actually occurred in employment, hours, and earnings for the private health care industry and that

Table 1–2 Trends for Employment, Hours, and Earnings in the Private Sector*

Employment Indication	1991	1992	1993	1994	1995†	Percentage Growth (Entire Period)
Total employment (in thousands)						
Nonfarm private sector	89,854	89,959	91,889	94,917	95,206	5.96
Health services	8,183	8,490	8,756	9,001	9,145	11.76
Nonsupervisory employment (in thousands)						
Nonfarm private sector	72,650	72,930	74,777	77,476	77,588	6.80
Health services	7,276	7,546	7,770	7,974	8,096	11.27
Average weekly hours						
Nonfarm private sector	33.8	34.3	34.6	34.4	34.3	1.48
Health services	32.4	32.5	32.7	32.6	32.8	1.02
Average hourly earnings						
Nonfarm private sector	10.32	10.57	10.83	11.12	11.36	10.01
Health services	10.96	11.39	11.78	12.10	12.36	12.77

*Excludes all health-related establishments run by governments.
†Data for 1995 include only the first quarter.
Source: Reprinted from the Bureau of Labor Statistics, *Employment and Earnings*, 1995, U.S. Government Printing Office, U.S. Department of Labor.

this growth surpassed that for other nonfarm private industries, growth in the hospital segment has slowed considerably compared with previous years. In 1994, growth in the entire health care industry dropped temporarily below that of other private industries for the first time since 1985. There are, of course, different trends within the health care industry as a whole. Figure 1–3 shows that, although the category including all private health care establishments showed growth in employment by 11.76% during the period illustrated, home health care experienced the most extensive increases (71.8%), followed by nursing homes (11.9%) and then hospitals (3.8%). Private hospitals have been the most slowly growing segment of the industry. Interestingly enough, however, both hospitals and nursing homes had greater increases in supervisory person-

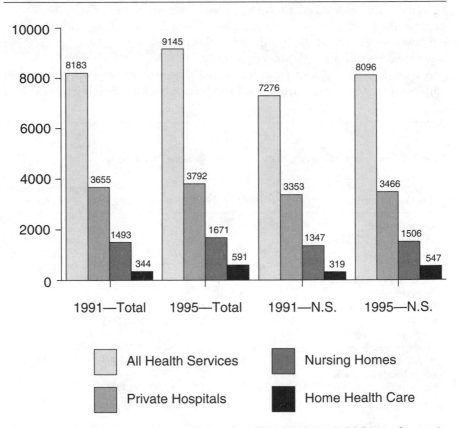

Figure 1–3 Health care employment: Total and nonsupervisory (N.S.) employees (in thousands). *Note:* 1995 figures include only first quarter data. *Source:* Reprinted from the Bureau of Labor Statistics, U.S. Department of Labor.

nel during this period; no substantial differences in the supervisory and non-supervisory groups were found in home health care.

With regard to average weekly hours, differences were also experienced in the various segments. The entire health care industry experienced a slight increase over the same period (1.0%). The highest growth rate was seen in home health care (10.0%), with 28.7 average weekly hours at the end of the period. Hospitals increased by 2.1% and nursing homes by 0.9%. Home health also led the group in increases in average hourly earnings, showing $10.84 per hour at the end of the period after an increase of 15.6% over the entire period. Hospital salaries increased by 15.1% during the same time to $14.80 per hour, and nursing homes showed the lowest ending rate ($8.70 per hour) after a 13.4% increase. The employment trends reflect attempts to find a solution to rising hospital costs. There is tremendous growth in employment for home health care, slow increases for hospitals in the private sector, and substantial decreases for hospitals in the government sector, as can be seen in Table 1–3.

The *Hay 1995 Hospital Compensation Survey* (Farrell & Pagoaga, 1995) included statistics for more than 361,000 professional employees from 885 hospitals in the United States. The survey showed that base salaries and total cash compensation for professionals were continuing to rise, but at a slower rate than in the past. Average 1995 base salaries plus total cash compensation were found to be $188,500 for chief executive officers and administrators, $141,000 for chief operating officers, $116,800 for chief financial officers, $100,100 for top patient care executives, $81,000 for top human resources executives, $79,500 for top management information systems executives, and $79,200 for heads of planning and development. Between 1994 and 1995, total cash income (base salaries plus compensations) increased by 4.6% for all positions. Increases varied for different professional groups, with chief executive officers and other

Table 1–3 Employment Trends for Hospitals (in Thousands)

Type of Hospital	1991	1992	1993	1994	1995*	Percentage Growth (Entire Period)
All hospitals	4,958	5,068	5,100	5,089	5,100	+2.86
Private hospitals	3,655	3,750	3,779	3,774	3,792	+2.75
Federal hospitals	234	235	234	233	229	−2.13
State hospitals	417	419	414	405	399	−4.31
Local hospitals	653	655	673	676	680	+4.13

*Data for 1995 include only the first quarter.
Source: Reprinted from the Bureau of Labor Statistics, *Employment and Earnings,* 1995, U.S. Government Printing Office, U.S. Department of Labor.

executives receiving the greatest increases (10.4% and 8.2%, respectively). Average increases reported for other positions were 6.4% for department heads, 3.5% for nurses, and 2.9% for other professional and technical employees. Nonsupervisory employees in private hospitals realized a 3.5% increase in hourly rates (from $13.70 to $14.18) during the same period (Sensenig, Heffler, & Donham, 1995).

Annual incentive programs were found to be the most frequent method for rewarding hospital executives. Health care management companies were found to use them the most (73%), followed by for-profit hospitals (67%) and not-for-profit hospitals (58%). High-performing hospitals were found to use incentive and bonus compensation programs more than low-performing hospitals. Other types of incentive plans that were found to be prevalent were group incentives (30%), discretionary bonuses (26%), gainsharing (13%), profit sharing (6%), key contributor plans (6%), and skill-based pay (6%). Another finding was that incentive programs are being used considerably less often for employees below the managerial level. Only 10% of professional and technical employees, 9% of nonexempt employees, and 6% of nurses were found to be eligible for individual incentives. Hospitals, though, were found to be moving steadily from traditional pay programs that focus on individual jobs to strategies that emphasize performance and teamwork. One out of every three hospitals surveyed has plans to create team incentive programs in the future.

How do these trends in health care employment affect employees? Many workers who are able to keep up with the facts know that hospitals are experiencing hard times, but they still have difficulty dealing with the disparity in salaries, raises, and compensation programs noted above. As hospitals continue to downsize and/or restructure, employees need to feel a sense of equity and trust that the changes are being made for an honorable purpose and that everyone will be treated fairly in the process. If not, the industry may achieve its short-term goals but will suffer high turnover rates and other long-term consequences that could possibly affect the quality and cost of care.

There are different schools of thought regarding exactly how restructuring should occur. Practices range from outright downsizing, whereby department heads receive a reduced budget and are expected to cut costs in any way they can, to total involvement by administration in efforts to redesign the entire system. The trend is toward the patient-focused care model, which is more of a systems approach coordinated by administrators and involves reevaluation of all processes with special consideration of the activities that occur across all departments and services. This approach addresses issues such as duplication of effort, reengineering of processes, and a complete rethinking of how things are done to achieve the drastic changes that need to occur. Chapter 3 discusses specific techniques that are being used for organizational redesign.

Needless to say, the impact of restructuring on employees has been great. Few have managed to escape redesign of their jobs, decreased hours, or even layoffs. Brockner et al. (1986), in discussing the effects of layoffs on survivors, state "Many organizations resort to layoffs during periods of financial strain in obvious attempts to reduce personnel costs. Less obvious though perhaps no less important are the likely consequences that layoffs have on the work behavior and attitudes of survivors, those employees who are not laid off" (p. 373). Some typical reactions that occur when employees' coworkers are laid off are guilt, anxiety, relief, and anger, all of which can affect the quality and productivity of their work as well as their longevity on the job.

Brockner et al. (1986) used equity theory to explain the impact of organizational changes. Equity theory predicts that, when layoffs are based on merit, the employees who remain perceive that their better performance justified their status as survivors, so that they do not have to heighten their performance. When layoffs are random, employees improve their work performance to establish themselves and secure their jobs. Brockner et al. (1986) confirmed the equity theory in experiments conducted in a controlled laboratory setting with 145 individuals. They concluded "the rule by which layoff decisions are made is one relevant factor; but there are countless others" (p. 382). The other factors include the degree of interdependence between the laid-off worker and the survivor, the professional or personal similarity between the two people, and whether the survivor can easily find comparable work elsewhere. Another factor is probably the degree of continual support and encouragement that survivors get from their superiors. Further research is needed to determine whether the effects found in this study are sustained over time and whether equity theory is generally applicable to the organizational setting.

As restructuring occurs, it must always aim toward the goals of lowering costs, controlling quality, and establishing an increased sense of trust on the part of consumers and employees of the health care system. When consumers are able to count on consistently good service and value for their dollars, the amount of criticism from the media, the number of laws regulating the industry, and the overall perception of health care quality will change. Along the same lines, when workers are treated fairly and consistently, they are more apt to trust their employers and enforce the values of the organization. Regarding the importance of trust in an organization, Drucker (1992) said:

> The final requirement of effective leadership is to earn trust. Otherwise there won't be any followers—and the only definition of a leader is someone who has followers. To trust a leader, it not necessary to like him. Nor is it necessary to agree with him. Trust is the conviction that the leader means what he says. It is a belief in something very old fash-

ioned, called "integrity." A leader's professed beliefs must be congru-
ent, or at least compatible. Effective leadership—and again this is very
old wisdom—is not based on being clever; it is based primarily on being consistent. (p. 122)

Trends Affecting the Marketplace

A major trend in the health care industry has been toward group purchasing
and prime vendor contracts. One survey covered 50 suppliers in the nation that
had contracts with 10,941 independent and system hospitals representing 1.6
million acute care beds, 6,686 nursing homes, and other sites (Scott, 1993). It
was found that the volume of goods and services purchased through group contracts increased by 14% in 1992 alone. The 10 largest suppliers reported data
that accounted for more than 80% of the total volume. This represented a 5%
increase from the previous year. In addition, there is an apparent trend for suppliers of health care products to merge with each other.

For the future, it is expected that actual group purchasing memberships will
probably shrink because many health care networks are finding that they can
negotiate contracts just as well without group involvement. According to Bill
Elliott, the senior vice president of supply-chain management for the Voluntary Hospital Association, "The traditional role that group purchasing organizations have played—serving as a broker and leveraging volume—will become
less important. We're moving to an enabler role—giving networks the tools to
do what they want" (Scott, 1993, p. 52). Because the health care industry is so
large, suppliers are altering their methods to meet need. Many of the other
trends in purchasing are covered in Chapter 8; they include *just in time* purchasing and partnerships with suppliers that help the industry find better ways to
control costs while quality is maintained.

Regarding the foods that are purchased, there has been an ongoing trend
toward the use of convenience foods to help contain labor costs. This reflects
the general consumer trend whereby the public is purchasing more convenience foods and eating more meals outside the home. The market provides a
great variety of special diet foods that attempt to meet quality standards and the
therapeutic needs of patients. Designer foods and branding are popular trends,
and many hospitals have contracted with fast food companies to open storefronts for food service targeted at employees and guests of the hospital.

During recent years, the CPI has not risen as much for food as it has for other
consumer items. For example, between 1991 and 1994, the CPI for food and
beverages increased by a total of 8.1% (average, 2.0% per year), whereas the
CPI for all consumer items excluding medical care increased by 10.9%. The
same trend, but to a much lesser extent, occurred in the producer price index

for this period. An overall increase of 2.7% occurred in the producer price index for food, and a 2.9% increase was seen for all finished consumer goods. Although actual employee salaries were not reported, the Bureau of Labor Statistics' average hourly earnings for nonsupervisory hospital workers showed an overall increase of 10.6% (average, 3.4% per year) during this same period. For dietitians it is known that the rate of increase was substantially higher. For example, from 1990 to 1991, the estimated mean salary for clinical dietitians rose by 6.1%, from $28,000 to $30,700, and for dietitians in management practice it rose by 14.8%, from $33,700 to $38,700 (Kornblum, 1993).

Because rising hospital costs are a major source of criticism today, trends in hospital dietary departments are worth studying. The actual cost and number of full-time equivalents (FTEs) for individual hospital departments have been monitored by the American Hospital Association for more than 25 years as a part of its Hospital Administration Services (HAS) program. General trends from more than 500 hospitals of various sizes are shown in Table 1–4, from the HAS MONITREND reports as analyzed by Cromwell and Butrica in 1995. It can be seen in Table 1–4 that dietary costs represent a small percentage of total operating expenses and FTEs in hospitals and that this percentage has declined over time. In 1980, dietary services accounted for 5.4% of total hospital expenses and 6.4% of total direct hospital expenses. By 1992, these percentages decreased to 2.8% and 3.4%, respectively, even though the cost of dietary services increased by 59.0% over the same period. During the same time frame, overall hospital costs increased by 210%, and total direct hospital expenses increased by 199%.

Table 1–4 Trends in Annual Hospital Costs and FTEs

Economic Indicator	1980	1983	1988	1992
Total hospital costs per adjusted discharge*	$1,532	$2,365	$3,552	$4,755
Total hospital direct costs per adjusted discharge*	$1,299	$1,978	$2,873	$3,883
Costs for dietary services per adjusted discharge*	$83	$109	$123	$132
Average FTEs per hospital	425.6	472.7	524.7	663.2
Average dietary FTEs	31.2	32.9	31.7	35.6

*Inpatient discharges adjusted upward to include outpatient activity.
Source: Reprinted with permission from J. Cromwell and B. Butrica, Hospital Department Cost and Employment Increases: 1980–1992, *Health Care Financing Review*, Vol. 17, No. 1, pp. 147–165, © 1995.

The majority of the cost increases occurred before 1983, the year in which diagnosis-related groups (DRGs) were implemented. Since that time, increases in dietary costs slowed down to an average of 2% per year. Between 1983 and 1988, total FTEs decreased for dietary services by an average of 0.7% per year, whereas total hospital FTEs increased by 2.1% per year. In fact, this was the only department that experienced a decrease during that period. Since that time, the annual growth in FTEs has averaged 2.9%, which is still below the average for the total hospital and all other departments except plant operation and maintenance, which showed an average of 2.8%.

It is apparent from the data reported above that many directors of food and nutrition services in hospitals have done well to contain costs since the DRGs were implemented in 1983 despite the inflation rate for food and increases in employee hourly wages. Their costs represent a small part of the hospital's total expenditures, and yet the services they perform have a great impact on the perceived quality of patient care.

The Information Explosion

Consumers are faced with overwhelming amounts of health information today from the media. They are exposed to wellness programs in the workplace and spend a tremendous amount of money in efforts to improve themselves by joining health clubs, going to classes, and buying books, journals, health foods, and home remedies. Health care professionals have not escaped this trend, and both groups have been influenced by it.

Consumer Response to Increased Information about Health

Life expectancy at birth now exceeds 74 years of age. It was 47 years in 1900. Despite the fact that there has been a decrease in heart disease since the 1950s, it is the leading cause of death in the nation. Heart disease as well as cancer, stroke, and diabetes mellitus, the second, third, and seventh leading causes of death, respectively, are all related to diet. The major health problems are often linked with excessive behaviors. For example, there is currently an epidemic of obesity in the nation. Between 1960 and 1980, one quarter of Americans were obese (20% or more above their desirable body weight). Since 1980, that number has increased to one third for adults. After examining data from four separate national surveys, Kuczmarski, Flegal, Campbell, and Johnson (1994) stated:

> Overweight is associated with a host of adverse health outcomes and places a severe burden on the U.S. health care system. In 1986, the economic costs of illness associated with overweight were estimated to be in excess of $39 billion. Overweight is also a condition known to be

resistant to intervention. Nevertheless, federal health authorities have targeted a reduction in the prevalence of overweight as a national health objective to be achieved by the year 2000. (p. 205)

Obesity is still increasing for adults and children. PiSunyer (1995) states "The imperative is to prevent weight gain, not to try to lose it after it has accumulated. However, alerting the public to this has been difficult. Decreasing food intake and increasing activity seems to be an easy formula, yet it is proving extremely difficult to implement" (p. 238). Despite the incredible amount of information about and general knowledge of nutrition, Morreale and Schwartz (1995) concur: "The results of the 1993 Survey of American Dietary Habits suggest that Americans are at a crossroads when it comes to nutrition. Public awareness of the importance of nutrition continues to grow and intensify, but action to improve the diet has stalled" (p. 307). Their research showed an increase in the gap between consumers' attitudes and actual behaviors. This reflects the age-old problem of people who want to be healthy but lack the motivation to incorporate healthy practices in their everyday life.

One positive result from the explosion of research and literature on health is that Americans have learned that many causes of heart disease, cancer, and stroke as well as the complications of diabetes can be prevented. This concept, coupled with trends toward uncontrollably high costs for "after the fact" treatment of disease, has caused consumers and professionals alike to refocus on prevention as the only realistic solution to both problems. To cross over into the business of disease prevention, professionals need to come out of institutions and work more closely and effectively with people in the community. It is clear that more work is needed to encourage behaviors that result in an overall healthier population from childhood on.

Many strides have already been made in this effort. Food labeling and nutrition education as a part of school and community-based programs are good examples. One need only watch television or visit a bookstore, however, to see that people are exposed to fraudulant schemes and much misinformation about the topic of nutrition. The biggest challenge for dietitians is to counteract misinformation with effective nutrition education that does not instill a fear of food or promote short-lived, obsessive behaviors in the population but rather convinces people that moderate amounts of the right food coupled with routine exercise can result in better health throughout their lives. In this effort, alliances with other professionals and organizations are essential.

One consumer survey by Frank J. Corbett, Inc. (1991) showed that 95% of consumers identify physicians as being highly influential sources of nutrition information and that a domino effect occurs. Of the respondents, 94% said that they are somewhat or extremely likely to pass information gained from a physician along to other people. Other sources of nutrition information were nurses (93%), television advertising (32%), and magazine advertising (17%). Market surveys conducted by others support the fact that a large number of consumers obtain nutrition information from physicians (Gallup Organization, 1994; Ruch, 1995). Because physicians generate about 75% of medical costs through their treatment decisions (Kassler, 1994), dietitians can help control health care costs by continuing to stress the benefits of prevention while communicating with them.

Some feel that the lack of responsibility people seem to have regarding their own personal health has been encouraged by the health care industry. Kassler (1994) writes "a society cannot afford to absolve everyone of personal account-ability, even as it tempers judgements with compassion. From a practical van-tage, there simply aren't sufficient resources" (p. 175). Taking a historical view, she offers an explanation for the inflationary medical expenses since the 1960s:

> Medicine changed when insurers took over the job of paying medical bills. It wasn't that patients suddenly sought access to free care, it was that massive funding to pay for this care was suddenly available. The age of third-party payers unleashed the health industry's entrepreneur-ial zeal. Hospital chains sprouted, medical device companies grew, physicians switched from talking to patients to doing procedures on them. Altruism was no longer the driving force. High technology, with its advances and costs, replaced the more modest achievements of ear-lier days. We got a lot in return, but at a very high price. After 1965, when Congress passed Medicare and Medicaid, health-care costs started to increase at double-digit rates. Health insurers—businesses, government, and insurance companies—eventually balked at the un-foreseen and uncontrolled tab. Each had its own strategy for cost con-tainment, whether that was by shifting costs, cutting fees, or scrutiniz-ing medical decisions. There were endless maneuvers, none of which [was] aimed at controlling system-wide costs. (p. ix)

Kassler (1994) believes that people need to be more responsible for their own health. This can occur if they are at least partially accountable for the cost:

> To shift to greater individual responsibility is not to let society off the hook. The end-stage, hallucinating alcoholic isn't suffering from a cri-sis of willpower. But, at the other end of the scale, the wife-batterer shouldn't be excused as someone suffering—by definition—from men-tal illness. There is a spectrum of destructive behavior, not all of which should be medicalized. (Kassler, 1994, p. 176)

Kassler recommends aggressive public health drives that counteract the negative messages communicated through the media rather than allocating health care dollars to the treatment of individuals.

Professionals' Response to the Growing Body of Knowledge

Professionals in the health care field are also affected by the quickly increasing body of knowledge. How has this trend influenced their practice? The field of nutrition has grown so large that it is ordinarily assumed that one person cannot do it all. As of 1996, there were 27 different dietetic practice groups (DPGs) in the American Dietetic Association (Exhibit 1–1). In addition, there are many other associations in the field, including the American Society for Parenteral and Enteral Nutrition, the American Society for Healthcare Food

Exhibit 1–1 DPGs of The American Dietetic Association

DPG-10	Public Health Nutrition
DPG-11	Gerontological Nutritionists
DPG-12	Dietetics in Developmental and Psychiatric Disorders
DPG-14	Vegetarian Nutrition
DPG-15	Hunger and Malnutrition
DPG-16	Environmental Nutrition
DPG-20	Oncology Nutrition
DPG-21	Renal Practice
DPG-22	Pediatric Nutrition
DPG-23	Diabetes Care and Education
DPG-24	Nutrition Support
DPG-25	Physical Medicine and Rehabilitation
DPG-27	General Clinical Practice
DPG-28	Perinatal Nutrition
DPG-30	Consulting Nutritionists
DPG-31	Consulting Dietitians in Health Care Facilities
DPG-32	Business and Communications
DPG-33	Sports, Cardiovascular, and Wellness
DPG-41	Management in Health Care Systems
DPG-42	School Nutrition Services
DPG-43	College and University Food Service
DPG-44	Clinical Nutrition Management
DPG-45	Technical Practice in Dietetics
DPG-50	Dietetic Educators of Practitioners
DPG-51	Nutrition Educators for Health Professionals
DPG-52	Nutrition Education for the Public
DPG-54	Nutrition Research

Service Administrators, the Dietary Managers Association, Hospital Foodservice Managers, and others, not to mention the numerous societies and federal, state, and local agencies involved in the governance and implementation of food and nutrition programs. This field is not unique in its number of specialties. The same trend has occurred in other health care and management professions.

Just how has specialization in the health care field affected the American public? One positive outcome has been the vast extension of the body of knowledge that is available in each specialty as professionals with similar interests pursue advanced study in their fields. No doubt, great contributions for improved patient treatment have come out of the subspecialty groups. The establishment of standards of care and clinical pathways is perhaps the subspecialties' most valuable role in the managed care environment, where standardization of treatment plans is essential.

Clinical pathways have been defined as collaboratively developed hypotheses that describe what the health care team believes is the best way to manage patients. A survey of 328 hospitals was conducted in 1993 by American Hospital Publishing, Inc. and Medicus Systems Corporation. It also included 38 managed care organizations and physician multispecialty clinics. This survey showed that 62% of the hospitals began their clinical pathway initiative after January 1992, whereas almost half the managed care groups and physician clinics started before that time. For the 202 hospitals reporting data about their pathways, an average of 7.5 clinical pathways had been established to date, and an average of 6.5 were in the process of being developed. The group of managed care organizations averaged more established pathways (10) and the clinics fewer (3). It was also found that no single hospital department was universally responsible for clinical pathways. Rather, ownership was shared among several services: quality improvement (65% of the hospitals), nursing (49%), utilization management (41%), medical director (17%), and risk management (12%). No special designation was made in 24% of the hospitals.

Another benefit of specialization is that it meets the needs of professionals. They feel a part of a special "club," a team whose members are all working toward the same goals as they motivate each other, share ideas, conduct research together, and engage in social activities. This can be a positive factor as long as it does not develop into *turfism*, which is prominent in the industry and only contributes to greater compartmentalization of services. Some of the common signs of turfism in the health care industry as described by Scharf (1995) include each discipline having its own separate agenda instead of all disciplines sharing common goals, misunderstanding others' abilities and intentions instead of having well-coordinated activities, competitive spirit and lack of openness instead of a willingness to cooperate, and lack of trust and respect instead of interdependence. Grindel (1994) advises dietitians to recognize others' expertise, communicate, and learn how to deal with overlapping skills.

Increased specialization in the industry may have other disadvantages. First, it tends to confuse the public. Subspecialty groups issue their own set of recommendations, often utilizing differing terminology and sometimes conflicting content, in answer to the public's simple question: "What should I eat?" All too often, people just remember the "bad" foods that are communicated by the various groups regardless of which disease a message is intended to prevent. The problem of mixed messages is now being properly addressed by some associations that have formed alliances with other groups that have similar goals.

One broad-based initiative that began in 1990 to address the country's health problems was *Healthy People 2000*, which identified national goals to be achieved by the year 2000. More than 300 public and private organizations worked to develop the goals and specific objectives over a period of 3 years. The final report, *Healthy People 2000: National Health Promotion and Disease Prevention Objectives* (Department of Health and Human Services, 1990), included priorities for health promotion, health protection, preventive services, and surveillance (Exhibit 1–2). These objectives were targeted at the major health problems of the population such as coronary heart disease, hypertension, cancer, diabetes, obesity, growth retardation in children, malnutrition in the elderly, anemia, and osteoporosis.

Another attempt to provide a unified approach to voluminous data was the 1993 Food Code, which was revised in 1995 and will continue to be revised every 2 years. In the United States, foodborne illness is a major cause of personal distress, preventable death, and avoidable economic burden. It is estimated that 24 to 81 million people become ill from microorganisms in food, resulting in approximately 10,000 needless deaths each year. The annual cost of foodborne illness is estimated to be between $7.7 and $23 billion. For preschool-age children, older adults in health care facilities, and those with impaired immune systems, foodborne illness is more serious and may be life threatening. For others, it frequently results in discomfort and/or lost time from the job.

Input for the Food Code was initially collected from the industry by the Food and Drug Administration (FDA) to develop the Unicode. Then the models for food services, food vending, and food stores were combined into a single document, and enhanced technical, compliance, and data processing capabilities were added, resulting in the Food Protection Unicode. Input was again received from approximately 150 academic, government, and industry agencies and organizations. This resulted in the final document, which contains standards that are not yet mandatory in the field. According to the FDA (1995):

Exhibit 1–2 Priorities for Healthy People 2000

Health promotion
  1. Physical activity and fitness
  2. Nutrition
  3. Tobacco
  4. Alcohol and other drugs
  5. Family planning
  6. Mental health and mental disorders
  7. Violent and abusive behavior
  8. Educational and community-based programs
Health protection
  9. Unintentional injuries
 10. Occupational safety and health
 11. Environmental health
 12. Food and drug safety
 13. Oral health
Prevention services
 14. Maternal and infant health
 15. Heart disease and stroke
 16. Cancer
 17. Diabetes and chronic disabling conditions
 18. Human immunodeficiency virus infection
 19. Sexually transmitted diseases
 20. Immunization and infectious diseases
 21. Clinical preventive services
Surveillance and data objectives
 22. Surveillance and data systems

Source: Reprinted from *Healthy People 2000: National Health Promotion and Disease Prevention Objectives*, 1990, U.S. Department of Health and Human Services.

The advantages of well-written, scientifically sound, and up-to-date model codes have long been recognized by industry and government officials. Industry conformance with acceptable procedures and practices is far more likely where regulatory officials "speak with one voice" about what is required to protect public health, why it is important, and which alternatives for compliance may be accepted. (p. iv)

Another response to the increasing body of knowledge can be seen from the point of view of health care expenditures. Specialists tend to demand more money for their services because they feel that they have spent increased time in the educational process and have unique skills that are more valuable. This has happened with physicians, and other health care professions have followed in suit. The 1995 Physicians Compensation Survey (Montague & Pitman, 1995), which polled 10,500 physicians, showed that the average income for primary care physicians in practices where less than 50% of their gross revenue was from managed care organizations averaged $108,000 in 1994 and $115,000 in 1995. Specialists in the same type of setting had average earnings of $134,000 in 1994 and $162,000 in 1995. It was also found that primary care physicians in managed care practices still earned more than those in non–managed care practices but that this gap decreased from 27.7% in 1994 to 1.4% in 1995.

National health care statistics show that the expansion of managed care and changes in the Medicare payment system have curtailed the growth of physician service expenditures. As a result of these factors, from 1990 to 1993 physician services experienced the slowest growth rate since the early 1960s (Levit et al., 1994). In 1993, expenditures for physician services reached $171.2 billion, which represented 21.9% of all personal health care expenses in the nation. The American Medical Association began tracking physicians' incomes 14 years ago, and its statistics show the trend continuing. In 1994, for the first time in 14 years, the median pay for all physicians decreased, from $156,000 to $150,000, or 3.8% (Grayson, 1995). In the past, cost-based and fee-for-service payment systems encouraged growth in all medical professions. Between 1970 and 1990, the number of practicing physicians per 100,000 persons increased by 48.4%, from 157 to 233. This ratio is expected to increase to 292 by the year 2010 according to a report from the Robert Wood Johnson Foundation (1994). According to this report:

> There are, however, some common elements that are the tendency to pay physicians by capitation rather than fee for service and a reliance on generalist physicians and other health care practitioners to provide basic services, thereby restricting the use of physician specialists and their technologies. As a result, the staffing of managed care plans differs from the traditional medical care in two important ways: they employ fewer physicians and use a smaller proportion of specialists. (p. 239)

In 1995, the Pew Health Professions Commission reported the number of practicing physicians in the nation to be 600,000. The report stated that there were between 100,000 and 150,000 too many physicians in the United States and that too many were subspecialists. At the present time, more students are applying to medical school than ever before, and statistics from 1993 showed a decline in the percentage of medical students in generalist programs. At that time, 38% were enrolled in the generalist programs, and less than 20% of students who graduated in that year indicated a preference for a generalist career. A 50:50 split between generalist and specialist has been identified as a more desirable plan for the future. Recommendations made by the Pew Health Professions Commission for the medical profession are shown in Exhibit 1–3. Physicians are now being encouraged to take more of a leadership role in the industry by getting involved in administrative functions.

Exhibit 1-3 Recommended Goals for Redirecting Federal Subsidies for Academic Medical Centers

1. Reduce the number of physicians in graduate training positions to 110% of U.S. medical school graduates.
2. Increase enrollment in, broaden the definition of, and enhance the quality of generalist training programs.
3. Disconnect training programs from the service demands of hospitals.
4. Move the bulk of most training programs out of the hospital and into community and ambulatory settings.
5. Protect regional needs within the context of national health care needs.
6. Decrease the number of training programs for medical specialists.
7. Develop and support graduate medical education positions in model delivery systems.

Source: Data from Pew Health Professions Commission. *Shifting the Supply of Our Health Care Workforce,* © 1995, University of California.

Shortages in the field occur primarily in the nursing segment. Some professional organizations have put limits on the number of people who enter the profession. The American Dietetic Association has not done so.

In 1972, the Study Commission on Dietetics reported its findings and recommendations for the profession of dietetics. There were 23,416 members of the American Dietetic Association at the time. The commission encouraged an increase to 38,500 by 1980. Substantial increases were seen after that time, especially between 1976 and 1980. At the beginning of 1996, there were 67,690 members of the association; the number of members had almost tripled. The commission predicted that dietetic practice would be altered in the following six ways:

1. increased differentiation in the roles and functions of dietitians
2. increased specialization of dietitians
3. requirement for new and additional competencies
4. increased delegation of some present tasks and roles to others
5. increased practice in association with other health professionals
6. greater proportion of self-employed dietitians

Recommendations from the 1972 Study Commission on Dietetics paved the way for increased specialization. In 1977, DPGs were established; by 1984, when the study commission next reported, 23 DPGs with more than 26,000 members had been established. The report stated "Specialized practice is here to stay." It had been found that most of the professionals who had become specialists had done so through limitation and concentration of their function in specific settings. This report encouraged continued increases in the number of dietitians in the nation along with certification of specialists. It stated that there is no reason why DPGs should not continue along their present course. The following words of caution regarding specialization were offered:

> It is important to avoid excessive fragmentation and keep the various specialties in the proper relationship to the total field of dietetics. This is possible if the entire process of specialization is coordinated. The dietetic practice groups may be of assistance in maintaining the proper balance. They can help particularly in delineating and defining the specialized areas of practice. It is to their advantage, as well as that of [the American Dietetic Association] as a whole, to see that proper interrelationships are established and maintained. In the growth of speciality practice, it is also important to maintain and support the activities of generalists. As division of practice increases, the need for coordination and supervision also increases. The generalist with a good understanding and perspective becomes a "specialist in breadth." There will be many instances where individual dietitians will have to handle many of the aspects of specialized practice because of the shortage of personnel and resources or because of the location and setting of the practice. Such individuals should not be regarded as inferior in their function, nor should they be less well compensated than the specialists and subspecialists. (Study Commission, 1984, p. 71)

With the advent of patient-focused care, resources and people are being organized around patients rather than specialized departments and disciplines. Everyone has broader job responsibilities, and fewer highly specialized jobs exist. The focus in acute care is changing from compartmentalization and specialization to "multiskilling" and cross-training for workers and professionals alike. Integrated health networks of the future will aim to deliver seamless care in a variety of community settings. Flexible practitioners with general backgrounds covering a wide spectrum of practice may be best equipped to coordinate effective and efficient food and nutrition programs for the variety of community services they will offer. This is not to say, though, that we should ignore specialty services when they are indicated for positive clinical outcomes.

According to Lathrop (1993), "Staff specialization is the personal extension of the evolution of compartmentalization" (p. 40). Lathrop identifies *compartmentalization* as a major contributor to poor quality and high costs in the health care industry. In his opinion, it has come about because hospitals have mimicked health care education, where increased specialization throughout the past three decades has resulted in new disciplines in medicine and the allied health professions. Compartmentalization limits communication and cooperation between disciplines, resulting in duplication of effort and poor continuity of care. The typical 500-bed hospital, according to Lathrop, has 350 different job classifications, and 275 of them have fewer than 10 incumbents. One large teaching hospital with approximately 700 beds was reported to have 2,756 employees who were classified into 388 jobs, and 314 of these jobs had fewer than 6 incumbents.

Division of labor, one might recall, was an outgrowth of past management theories. It contributed to multiple-level, labor-intensive organizational structures that are now being redesigned, and it was very much a part of the era of unionization of the work force, when attempts were made to increase the number of employees whom labor unions could represent. Division of labor clearly contributes to low productivity and high costs as well as the much criticized "It's not my job" syndrome. Patients and other customers do not care whose job it is, as long as it gets done right by their own definition. Most patients tend to prefer an integrated approach taken by a handful of caring individuals who are able to treat them holistically rather than view them as a bundle of distinct body parts and organs that are treated separately by a multitude of practitioners. As previously noted, health care practitioners are learning that there is a delicate balance between clinical outcomes and patients' perceptions of quality. Gill and Feinstein (1994) compared the traditional ways that health care "experts" view quality with the real needs of patients. They concluded:

> Because quality of life is a uniquely personal perception, denoting the way that individual patients feel about their health status and/or nonmedical aspects of their lives, most measurements of quality of life in the medical literature seem to aim at the wrong target. Quality of life can be suitably measured only by determining the opinions of patients and by supplementing (or replacing) the instruments developed by "experts." (p. 619)

Technology

Many of the positive changes in health care would have never happened without advancements in technology. As food service directors and dietitians seek solutions in the future, they will learn that many more alternatives resulting from technological advances are available to decrease costs and improve the quality of care. Historically, some of the most important initial steps were taken in government-sponsored programs. Much of the initial experimentation with microwave frequencies to cook food, for example, were completed under federal sponsorship at Natick Laboratories in Massachusetts. The Space Program set the pace for advancements in food technology as well as hazard analysis critical control points (HACCP), which have recently been implemented in the industry.

By far, the most influential event in institutional food production and service occurred just over 20 years ago, when the new Walter Reed Army Medical Center first opened its doors. At that time, its system was considered one of the most technologically sophisticated ones in the country. There was a bank of computerized cooking equipment from which products were taken and automatically portioned before they were frozen, well before use on the patient menu. The initial tray delivery system was imported from Germany; meals were loaded onto carts that were programmed to keep certain parts of the trays cold while other parts were rethermalized right on the patient units just before meal delivery. The carts containing the assembled chilled meals were transported automatically by monorail through the interstitial spaces throughout the hospital. Just about every aspect of the service reflected advanced technological methods, including food storage and dishwashing.

Thousands of visitors passed through the doors of the Walter Reed Army Medical Center to see the equipment and processes, which were modeled after state-of-the-art advancements adapted from facilities throughout the world. Some of the technology worked, some if it did not, but the state-of-the-art concepts adapted from our European counterparts certainly paved the way for American manufacturers to create systems that were similar and yet even more improved. This allowed everyone in the United States to benefit from their experiences.

The 1960s also reflected a trend away from decentralized meal assembly, which had previously been accomplished in separate pantries from steam tables transported from a central kitchen where foods were prepared. It was thought that lower food and labor costs would result when employees operated out of one area because supervision was easier and more control of food portioning could occur. Long tray assembly lines were installed for mass assembly of patient trays. In some systems, dietary employees served meals; in others, nursing did this. After centralization, managers began to observe peaks in the demand for labor around meal assembly times and decreased activity between meals.

With the advancements in freezing and chilling of foods adapted from the food processing industry, the next step was to level the workload by implementing "food factories," which aimed at separating food production processes from meal assembly processes. This led to the cook-chill and cook-freeze concepts that are still in place today. Research reported by Nettles and Gregoire in 1993 covered more than 1,800 hospitals across the country. They found conventional food systems to be used in 89.2% of hospitals, cook-chill systems in 6.9%, cook-freeze systems in 0.5%, and combinations of the various types or convenience systems in the remaining 2.4%.

For the labor-intensive task of tray assembly, technological advancements include new layout schemes that reduce the number of worker positions required. The difficult to clean and maintain skate-wheel, roller, and slatted tray conveyors have been replaced with simpler systems. A new type of thin belt, made of Dura-San, that spans the length of the unit has enabled manufacturers to design conveyors that have no cleaning tanks, springs, sockets, links, or mechanical connection devices to worry about. The thin, flexible belts are somewhat elastic and lift easily for cleaning from the top. Food carts can be rolled under some of the new conveyors, which are at eye level; employees face the conveyor, which eliminates 90° body turns with each tray. Slanted overshelves put foods in easy reach.

Chapters 9 and 10 describe food production, assembly, delivery, and service systems in great depth. The most interesting trend in the past several years is that hospitals are now returning to decentralized systems. With patient-focused care, the concentration of employees has shifted back to the bedside, and members of the care team are assuming menu planning and meal service functions again.

Robots are even beginning to show up for material management and tray delivery (Cappa, 1994; Jackson, 1995). They come with rechargeable batteries that last up to 12 hours and can be recharged while the unit is intact. Robots can be programmed in advance and can even use elevators. They can be purchased outright or leased. At Danbury Hospital in Danbury, Connecticut, robots are used for delivery of late trays. Four large or 8 small trays slide into the robot, which is programmed to go directly to patient units. If something obstructs its path, a sensor causes the robot to stop and say "Excuse me, I'm about to pass." For more than a year, robots have served this hospital's needs. Two of them make up to 10 trips per meal, delivering as many as 40 late trays.

Automated pot washing and dishwashing have also acted to curtail labor costs. One new system washes dishes conventionally in one machine while the trays and silverware proceed on a belt to a second machine, which requires no further attention by employees. A magnetic device picks silverware off trays for washing and drops it into bins afterward.

Other trends include better control of energy costs, more efficient equipment, more stringent safety standards, and attempts to minimize valuable space for other revenue-producing services. Automatic dispensing systems for both food and cleaning products also show great promise. They control cost while taking the guesswork out of portioning foods and diluting chemicals. One exciting concept for infection control is the *quick test* for on-site assessment for the presence of bacteria, now being tested in the meat packing and livestock industries. Although the Extension Service of the U.S. Department of Agriculture (1995) states that the implementation of the on-site quick test is still very much in the future, this concept holds the key for quality assessment for food safety and sanitation of the food-handling environment.

By far the most extraordinary technological trend is computerization. It is now possible to automate practically all diet office activities, menu tallying, production scheduling, inventory, and purchasing functions. Cafeteria cash registers network with these processes as well. Menu analysis and printing can be done by computer, and in facilities that have computerized medical records, the diet ordering, screening, assessment, and care planning processes are also frequently on line. There is great promise for interactive computer programs for data collection from patients, education of patients, and training of staff. CD-ROM interactive programs have a variety of applications that can help dietitians save time, especially in the clinic setting. The products have an advantage over video and audio cassettes because they progress at the individual's pace and keep him or her entertained and actively involved in the task at hand.

In the School of Medicine at East Carolina University in Greenville, North Carolina, ambulatory care dietitians collect data on food intake from patients and provide nutrition education using interactive programs that have clever graphic animation, audio messages, and even background music. According to Kolasa (1995), "dietitians are happier; this has freed up their time, and they are now able to perform the more advanced tasks which they were trained to do. . . . The major advantage of this approach is that computer mediated nutrition education decreases boredom on the part of the patient."

According to Biesmeier, approximately 15% of hospitals in the United States are using computerized medical record systems (Jackson, 1995). She further states that dietitians dedicate approximately 32% of their time to documentation. They document in the medical record and frequently write in the nursing Kardex, nutrition Kardex or binder, separate nutrition files, and one or more computer programs. Even within the medical records, Beismeier points out, several locations often require documentation, such as progress notes, flow sheets, clinical pathways, calorie counts, care plans, and discharge planning records. The limitations of traditional documentation systems are familiar to all health care professionals. According to Biesmeier:

> Dietitians have problems with review of their notes by other providers; implementation of their recommendations; follow-up on their own plans or recommendations they make to others; missing data; lack of care protocols; inability to focus on outcomes; inconsistency in the type and amount of information available; documentation not being organized to reflect their decision-making process; and the inability to communicate their care plans to others, especially after patients are discharged. (Jackson, 1995, p. 6)

In addition to these paperwork hassles, time is spent in gathering data from a wide variety of documents. Biesmeier describes the numerous sources of data:

"the medical record itself, bedside records, flow sheets, the nursing Kardex, MARs, preadmission data forms, patients, family members, computer information systems, diet office systems, standards of care and practice, diet manuals, clinical pathways and oral communications with other providers during rounds or casual conversations" (Jackson, 1995, p. 6). Even with all these sources, all the pertinent data are not always available when needed. Biesmeier goes on to state:

> There is a need to evaluate our documentation systems and methods. . . . Due to current trends in the health care field there is less time to do the same or sometimes more work than before. There is more of a focus on interdisciplinary teams and the need for more effective communication. Patient focused care is causing us to want to document at the point of care. And, work redesign and multi-skilling are affecting the work we do and when we do it. (Jackson, 1995, p. 7)

Biesmeier cites other factors that dictate the need for change, such as cost control and the need for outcomes management and research. She also states that dietitians should be able to work more productively while planning nutrition programs for alternative sites, such as nursing homes, home care agencies, and other community-based programs, but that the technology is not yet in place to do this. With the advent of technologically sophisticated computer systems, it is only a matter of time before access to complete medical records and nutrition standards of care will be achieved at the point of care, whether this is at the bedside, in the clinic setting, in community-based programs, or in the home.

Telemedicine is one technological advancement that has recently undergone rapid growth. "Telemedicine is the use of telecommunications technology to provide health care services to people who are at some distance from the provider" (Grigsby, Kaehny, Sandberg, Schlenker, & Shaughnessy, 1995). Even though telemedicine has been tested for nearly 30 years, little information is available regarding its cost and effectiveness. This is probably due to the fact that the HCFA requires that medical services be delivered in person for coverage of physician–patient contacts. To date, the feasibility of telemedicine has been tested in projects using a variety of technologies, including fax, radio, still images via telephone, and interactive television. The National Aeronautics and Space Administration monitored the physiological functioning of astronauts in space with equipment designed by Lockheed. This paved the way for a project for the Papago reservation in Arizona, whereby the feasibility of using advanced technology to bring medical services to remote areas was established. In 1991, the armed services successfully integrated telecommunications with mobile health units in the Persian Gulf, and computed tomography scanners were installed in transportable modular hospital units in the Saudi desert as well. Much of the large-scale research has been conducted by government programs. Grigsby et al. (1995) summarized various applications of telemedicine that have been tested and compared with traditional *face-to-face* methods. Exhibit 1–4 shows selected topics from their report.

Competition

America was built on the free enterprise system, but for the most part, the industry has been an exception to this. Consumers are now demanding a change. In 1983, the DRGs began a trend toward decreases in length of stay and occupancy rates. Hospitals began to compete with each other for patients as they tried to contain costs without sacrificing quality. Between 1980 and 1991, 603 acute care hospitals and 225 specialty care facilities closed. Before this trend began to slow in 1992, an additional 39 hospitals either decreased their services or closed (Bunda, 1993). Before long, alternative payer organizations, particularly managed care organizations and HMOs, sprouted up, guaranteeing their subscribers low-cost health care services.

Managed care organizations rely on primary care physicians to control costs as they manage patient treatment. They also inspire a spirit of competition among providers. Case managers facilitate equitable arrangements between providers and payers to limit unnecessary health care costs. Under capitation,

---

Exhibit 1–4 Selected Topics of Recent Experimentation with Telemedicine

Interactive video for the examination and rating of patients with Parkinson's disease
Microwave transmission of cardiac auscultation using electronic stethoscopes
Telediagnosis for pediatric echocardiography via modem over standard telephone lines
Transmission of electrocardiograms using fax machines and standard telephone lines
Dermatological diagnosis using televised color and black-and-white images taken from slides
Telepsychiatry using telephone, hands-free telephone, and computer-based video conference systems
Otorhinolaryngological diagnosis using interactive television
Transmission of fetal ultrasound
Diagnostic imaging for patient management under disaster situations
In the home health setting, monitoring of lung and heart transplant patients and exercise programs for cardiac rehabilitation patients using various methods
Remote examination and consultation by physicians using clinic televisions and telephones

Source: Data from J. Grigsby, M.M. Kaehny, E.J. Sandberg, M.D. Schlenker, & P.W. Shaughnessy, Effect and effectiveness of telemedicine. *Health Care Financing Review,* © 1995, 17(1), 115–131.

payments to providers are in set amounts (per patient, per day, or per month) for every person covered without regard for the services that may be used. Case managers come with a variety of backgrounds and are found in different settings. Case managers may be independent consultants, own private companies, work out of their home, or be employed by insurance companies, preferred provider organizations (PPOs), HMOs, or federal and state governments. Some are even employed by health care facilities to coordinate contracts with their counterparts on the outside. In 1995, a study covering 1,200 hospitals showed that managed care is succeeding in decreasing costs while providing positive outcomes. It was found that markets with high levels of managed care are experiencing lower hospital costs, reduced lengths of stay, and decreased mortality rates (Joint Commission, 1995).

According to Arkin, "Case managers are advising physicians more and more on products and health care" (Jackson, 1995, p. 6). Their role is to coordinate the most appropriate, timely, and cost-effective health care for their clients, who range from large groups such as insurance companies to individual employers that have contracted for management of their health care programs. Arkin further states "Case managers carefully monitor and control costs on behalf of their clients, and they can refuse unnecessary or uncovered care" (Jackson, 1995, p. 6). She stresses the fact that, above all, case managers are patient advocates, and they are in a position to demand quality health care for their clients.

Arkin goes on to state "The case manager, more than anyone, looks at continuity of care. More now than ever before we must look at the health care system as continuous care from the home to the doctor's office, hospital, rehabilitation, nursing homes, and so on" (Jackson, 1995, p. 6). A case manager's efforts cross traditional boundaries and follow the patient wherever he or she needs to go for care. The importance of nutrition is not universally accepted by case managers. Arkin recommends that dietitians "create an awareness of nutrition and stress 'macro' outcomes such as decreases in length of stay, fewer emergency room cases, and prevention of hospitalization. 'Micro' outcomes are improved weights, control of lipid levels, decreasing medication usage, weaning from artificial feeding, and delaying of dialysis" (Jackson, 1995, p. 6).

In 1994, the American Dietetic Association became engaged in a tremendous lobbying effort to have the services of dietitians included in the proposed health care reform legislation. They competed with all other health care professionals to obtain increased recognition for their services in hopes that the final plan would reflect more equitable reimbursement for their services. Evidence to cost justify nutrition services that were performed by registered dietitians was gathered nationwide by the association's government and legal affairs group. For example, it was shown that the average savings with nutrition intervention for patients with high cholesterol levels was reported to be $2,496 per case and for kidney disease to be $19,039 per case. According to Wright (1994), a representative of the Wexler Group, the firm contracted to assist with this effort, the American Dietetic Association was swept into the politics of health care reform. Along with other special interest groups, the association was unable to realize substantial gains in 1994. Wright predicted that gains would come incrementally, and dietitians were encouraged to pursue activities on the state level.

Large corporations are extremely active in health care reform because a substantial portion of their expense budgets is allocated to health care plans for their employees. Managed care plans such as HMOs, PPOs, and point-of-service plans are now competing for their business, and there is some speculation in the industry that these plans will eventually be bypassed in the future, when employers take direct control of the provider contracting process themselves or control large coalitions to do this for them.

According to Appleby (1995), managed care plans were competitive enough by 1995 to represent 63% of all covered employees in the nation. He quotes David Langness, vice president of the Healthcare Association of Southern California, who said "The biggest news story missed in the last decade has been big business' impact on health care. Employers have had the largest impact on health care costs—not physicians, hospitals, or health plans" (Appleby, 1995, p. 26). Appleby notes that Xerox spends $3 million annually on employee health care and relies on the performance reports from HMO plans to determine where this money will be spent. Xerox also benchmarks with other corporations to compare cost and quality.

Smaller businesses join nationwide coalitions that contract the best possible plans for them. These coalitions are actively involved in comparing the costs and quality of health care for existing and potential providers. In 1993, one such coalition in Houston, Texas, sponsored a study that assessed $2 billion in charges by 33 local hospitals. They found no correlation between product and pricing. An appendectomy, for example, varied as much as 800% between hospitals that were across the street from one another, even when performed by the same physician. The wide variation in quality and pricing caused the coalition to initiate a policy whereby providers agree to share quality data and adhere to a uniform DRG-based fixed pricing schedule. This resulted in the largest amount of community patient data in that state, which subsequently became the basis for conducting outcomes research.

Langness sees the end result of the rise of business coalitions and the other health care initiatives described above as the corporatization of American medicine (Appleby, 1995). Within the next decade, he predicts that the country will only have 5 to 10 health care providers that will be similar in nature to Columbia/HCA.

Acquisitions and mergers in the health care industry are now commonplace, and it is expected that they will continue. This trend will have a tremendous impact on the way food and nutrition services are managed in the future, and it will seriously affect the things that practitioners do. Professionals who want to grow and attain leadership positions in restructured health care systems of the future will have to adapt to nontraditional and expanded roles. As Pinell (1995) states, "We have to be lean and mean to continue to exist. There is a point where the cost and quality curves cross. Know where that is."

How will these trends affect food and nutrition professionals? For one thing, they will have to accept the fact that standardized methods are essential for effective multisystem management and that their own personal skills and creative abilities can be used to contribute to the design of these methods. Educators in the field need to start now by updating themselves and altering their curricula so that future professionals are ready to accept new challenges that will enable them to compete and succeed in the new corporate environment. Multiple skills, effective interdisciplinary communication, and willingness to coordinate efforts with others will be of paramount importance for future achievement. The case study shown in Exhibit 1–5 illustrates just one possible scenario of how the traditional role of a dietitian can be successfully transformed into that of a corporate leader, the type of role that can have a tremendous impact on the quality of patient care.

With large health care systems taking hold of the industry, the picture for food service directors and dietitians will change. Departmental procedures will need to be streamlined further, and practitioners will have to conform to the standards that are set and followed by others in the system. They will, of course, provide input for the new standards, which will require a proactive stance to guarantee quality within their respective facilities. Standardization of menus, recipes, food specifications, and other food and nutrition care processes will occur. Access to large group purchasing plans that offer lower food and supply prices will increase, and when more than one facility in a network are in close geographical proximity, the possibility of food production from a central commissary will exist. Multiunit management roles will increase as one person becomes involved in the operation of several sites; the possibility of multiservice management will also arise, as illustrated in the case study shown in Exhibit 1–4. Outside food service management contractors are already involved in health care networks, and the performance of independent operators is being closely monitored to determine whether contractors might do a better job. Clinical dietitians will most likely provide services at a variety of sites as they monitor and treat patients who progress through the health care continuum.

The Joint Commission has already set standards for health care networks. It is very much involved in comparing quality across hospitals and systems. In

Exhibit 1–5 Adapting to the Corporate Environment: A Case Study

Jane Atwood began working as a patient services manager in the dietary department at Memorial Hospital in Jacksonville, Florida. Just 6 months after working in this capacity, she was offered the position as acting director of food service. As food service director, Atwood succeeded in reducing the number of FTEs from 91 to 74 while decreasing food and supply cost by 7%. The positive attitude of this young, energetic registered dietitian led to her appointment as director of quality resources, where she acted as a quality coach to facilitate the hospital's transition from quality assurance to continuous quality improvement. "I have seen many dietitians do well in this role," says Atwood. She attributes this to "their attention to both detail and process."

Atwood expanded her role to director of hospitality services and quality resources at the facility, which had also expanded and changed its name to Memorial Healthcare System of Jacksonville (MHS) and had grown to a 353-bed acute care hospital that also had a 110-bed rehabilitation center and three satellite outpatient units. Atwood was asked to be a member of the internal transition team making preparations for a potential partnership in 1995 with Columbia/HCA. At that time, all employees faced the possibility of major changes in their work environment. Their biggest concerns were with job security and benefits. With a special sensitivity to their needs, Atwood had frequent open communication sessions to answer any questions employees had. Many of them reported directly to her when she was the director of food service. They would often ask "Will my job be eliminated?" It was explained that everyone would be faced with the same concerns with or without the partnership because of the current economic state of the health care industry. Atwood alleviated much of the stress by saying "we need a partner to ensure future success."

Like many accomplished managers in our field, Atwood continued to be asked to take on more multiservice responsibilities after the merger. She now directs quality resources for the entire facility and hospitality services, which includes food services, linen, and environmental services. Her budget is $7 million, which includes 195 FTEs.

What prepared Atwood to meet these challenges? "Dietetics was a tough curriculum," Atwood claims, recalling her courses and internship at the University of Florida in Gainesville. "All the biochemistry and other science courses taught me how to develop stamina, and this carried over into the professional world." This attribute was refined with experience after she entered the field. "Many people here were willing to give me a chance, and they took a risk in doing this," she states. "As new projects came up, I made it known that I was willing to take on more challenges. This often meant asking for more when I was already busy!"

1990, the Joint Commission announced its *Agenda for Change*. A part of its plan was the ability to offer cross-organizational comparisons of quality across the nation. The plan included an interactive database for monitoring performance trends so that quality could be compared with national norms (Joint Commission, 1994). The program, IMSystem, is now in effect on a voluntary basis, and it is expected to be mandated soon as a requirement for accreditation. In 1994, the Joint Commission announced its hospital performance reporting system, which is available to consumers for the purpose of comparing quality of care offered. In 1996, they also added the National Library of Health Care Indicators.

In this age of uncertainty, the accrediting and licensing agencies have not escaped the competitive climate. For example, the Joint Commission recently struggled with competitors as it lobbied in states such as California, Washington, Florida, Pennsylvania, and Minnesota to have its systems for measuring quality made a part of its state licensing process. Quality measurement is a profitable business today, and the Joint Commission stands to benefit if its IMSystem, network accreditation program, and public quality disclosure methods are adopted in every state.

Some critics feel that the Joint Commission has not yet effectively demonstrated its value in reflecting quality and that the cost of its accreditation process with associated materials is too high, especially for small hospitals. If accrediting agencies continue to be used for this function, it is quite possible that more than one equivalent agency will be deemed acceptable. The state of Washington is already moving in this direction. In some states, it is thought that the extra layer of an accrediting agency between hospitals and the state will delay the process of revising and improving licensing requirements. In Florida and California, state agencies have experimented with their own quality reporting systems in the form of report cards, which provide annual reports for the public reflecting hospitals' success in achieving clinical outcomes.

THE NATURE OF CHANGE

The Japanese culture embraced the concept of total quality management well before it became popular in the United States. Speaking of engineers in Japanese manufacturing plants, Imai (1986) stated that they were often told "There will be no progress if you keep on doing things exactly the same way all of the time." Some cultures, organizations, and people prefer that things stay exactly the same. After all, it is much easier to deal with the known than the unknown. The path of least resistance is attractive. Others thrive on change and know that it leads to even greater contributions and satisfaction at work and in their personal lives.

One of the oldest books in the world, predating even the teachings of Confucius, is the *I Ching* or *Book of Changes* (Greenleaf, 1991). The *I Ching* is primarily concerned with the philosophy of change and looks at the process of living with change as an organic part of human nature instead of perceiving static as good and change as threatening. This, of course, is contrary to many contemporary beliefs. Wilkins (1995), who was inspired by this work, said "it is in constant change and growth alone that life can be grasped at all . . . change is a natural movement, a development that can only reverse itself by going against nature" (p. 173).

The Structure of Change

Changes in society can occur slowly or suddenly. They may happen without even being noticed or so furiously that they destabilize and monopolize the lives of everyone involved. The one thing that all changes have in common is the different way in which people think about the world before and after they occur. Change alters people's perceptions about truth. The mental models or patterns that seemed, in the past, to explain circumstances are suddenly found to be inappropriate as a person moves on to different beliefs that apply much better to the situation at hand. Kuhn (1974) studied the structure of scientific revolutions and identified how major discoveries come about. New paradigms replace the old ones, "and the successive transformation from one paradigm to another via revolution is the usual developmental pattern of mature science" (Kuhn, 1974, p. 12).

Revolutions are a necessary part of the growth of science. They enable (and sometimes force) people to move on to more accurate and orderly ways of perceiving and dealing with the world around them as they abandon old paradigms that no longer fit. It is common that revolutionary change is seen only by those who are affected by it. "To outsiders, they may, like the Balkan revolutions of the early twentieth century, seem normal parts of the developmental process" (Kuhn, 1974, p. 93). Malfunctions in a system often lead to crises, which in turn result in revolutionary changes. Political revolutions occur when malfunctions are not recognized or considered important to the people inside political institutions. Change is forced by those from the outside. "At that point," according to Kuhn, "the society is divided into competing camps or parties, one seeking to defend the old institutional constellation, and the others seeking to institute some new one" (p. 92). These concepts apply to relatively small changes within departments, individual facilities, large health care systems, and the world as a whole.

Gradual Change

As people progress through their everyday work activities, they evaluate each situation and try to apply standards or rules that they have learned. If the existing protocols work without difficulty, they simply go on to the next task at hand. If they perceive some difficulty, they might ignore the anomaly or seek to solve the puzzle. If the anomaly becomes routinely bothersome or keeps them from attaining the desired outcome, they will be motivated even further to come up with new methods to fit the new situation. Sometimes the correction of such problems happens automatically as people adjust to irregularities in their environment.

This is the normal course of adaptation, which is a part of the evolutionary process. In some cases, though, a rule or standard needs to be changed so that it can better deal with anomalies that are discovered. If a solution is found and reflected in the revised standard that governs the work, the bothersome anomaly disappears, and the person returns to his or her normal routine. In the work setting, people react this way to various situations as change occurs gradually without major disruptions to the system. What they are actually doing is learning how to cope better with the environment so that work can continue to result in desirable outcomes. The rules and standards they apply will shift every time they repeat the process and see the world anew. In many instances, there is no set theory or established paradigm that govern their activities, so that changes of this nature do not affect the stability of the organization. Puzzles are worked out, and new policies and procedures are established.

Constant learning and growth depend upon how astute people are at observing such irregularities or anomalies in the system. If they do not notice the need for change or refuse to accept the challenge, the organization cannot grow. Managers need to recognize and act on even the slightest tendencies that might indicate a need for change. Sudden, earthshaking anomalies are easy to spot and demand, by their nature, that immediate changes be made, but subtle trends that occur over time often go unnoticed until it is too late. Senge (1990) cleverly illustrates this point in his parable of the boiled frog:

> If you place a frog in a pot of boiling water, it will immediately try to scramble out. But if you place the frog in room temperature water, and don't scare him, he'll stay put. Now, if the pot sits on a heat source, and if you gradually turn up the temperature, something very interesting happens. As the temperature rises from 70°F to 80°F, the frog will do nothing. In fact, he will show every sign of enjoying himself. As the temperature gradually increases, the frog will become groggier and groggier, until he is unable to climb out of the pot. Though there is nothing restraining him, the frog will sit there and boil. Why? Because the frog's internal apparatus for sensing threats to survival is geared to sudden changes in his environment, not to slow, gradual changes. (p. 22)

Senge (1990) believes that this is similar to what happened to the automobile industry in the United States. In 1962, the top American firms did not consider Japan a threat because the Japanese only held 4% of the market. Within the next 5 years, this share gradually increased to 10%. By 1974, Japanese manufacturing represented 15% of the market, and by the early 1980s it exceeded 20%. By 1989 the figure approached 30%, and the American automobile industry could account for only 60% of the entire market. Senge states "It is not clear whether this particular frog will have the strength to pull itself out of the hot water" (p. 22). He advises managers to slow down their frenetic pace and pay attention to the subtle as well as the dramatic because the gradual processes often pose the greatest threats.

Most of the trends described in the first part of this chapter have not come about suddenly. Some professions just did not notice them, some ignored them, and others were not in the position to do anything about them. The wise and perceptive leaders saw the writing on the wall and were able to survive and succeed because they gradually reacted as the environment changed.

Turbulent Change

The normal course of change begins with the discovery of anomalies or observations that cannot be explained by existing paradigms. According to Kuhn (1974), major scientific revolutions are characterized by "non-cumulative developmental episodes in which an older paradigm is replaced in whole or part by an incompatible new one" (p. 92). This may occur simultaneously in different parts of the world and/or be done by different researchers. Doubt begins to be cast on the traditional ways of thinking if these observers are truly committed to seeking the truth. The traditionalists who are deeply committed to the existing paradigm are often slow to yield, if they yield at all, to new evidence. They may refuse to consider it, shun the "imposters," or offer an endless number of reasons why the newly introduced data, which violate their belief, cannot possibly be correct. Resistance to impending change is commonly reflected in their actions.

As dissatisfaction with the traditional way of thinking gains momentum, scientists find themselves in a crisis situation because they have no theory to explain the anomaly. Many alternative paradigms are posed, and this adds to the confusion. Kuhn (1974) states "Philosophers of science have repeatedly demonstrated that more than one theoretical construction can always be placed upon a given collection of data" (p. 76). It may take years, or even centuries, for people to establish a new paradigm that fits properly. He feels that "crises are a necessary precondition for the emergence of novel theories" (p. 77) and that the existing paradigm cannot be declared invalid until an alternative candidate is available to take its place because "to reject one paradigm without simultaneously substituting another is to reject science itself" (p. 79).

Such revolutions are seldom predicted by people whose ideas are imbedded in the old paradigms. The outlying data are looked at suspiciously, and only those with open minds and foresight are able to see the value of impending change. Others often tend to live by the existing theory even though they know it will be short-lived. This creates a sense of fear, which leads to motivation and finally to change. According to Senge (1990), "Things must get bad enough, or people will not change in any fundamental way" (p. 154). "Bad enough" does not necessarily mean a threat to one's actual survival but rather enough of a crisis to spur what Senge calls creative tension, which leads to a fundamental shift in one's whole posture toward reality.

Thriving on Change

Effective leadership fosters an atmosphere where new ideas are welcomed and sought out as sources for positive change. When mistakes occur, leaders and their followers look at them as wonderful opportunities for growth rather than as insults. "A mistake is an event the full benefit of which has not yet been turned to your advantage" (Senge, 1990, p. 154). Argyris (1990) discusses ways to diagnose defensive postures and overcome them. He contends:

> Organizational defensive routines make it highly likely that individuals, groups, intergroups, and organizations will not detect and correct the errors that are embarrassing and threatening because the fundamental rules are to: (1) bypass the errors and act as if they were not being done, (2) make the bypass undiscussable, and (3) make its undiscussability undiscussable. (p. 42)

Many leaders say they welcome change and team interaction but do little to encourage either on a routine basis. People develop trust when they are free at all times to volunteer their views. Although a halfhearted approach may work with routine issues, when complex issues that are embarrassing or threatening need to be addressed, the "teamness goes to pot" (Argyris, 1990, p. 45). Senge (1990) characterizes ineffective work teams by describing what he calls the myth of the management team:

> All too often teams in business tend to spend their time fighting for turf, avoiding anything that will make them look bad personally, and pretending that everyone is behind the team's collective strategy— maintaining the appearance of a cohesive team. To keep up the image, they seek to squelch disagreement; people with serious reservations avoid stating them publicly, and joint decisions are watered-down compromises reflecting what everyone can live with, or else reflecting one person's view foisted on the group. If there is a disagreement, it's usually expressed in a manner that lays blame, polarizes opinion, and fails to reveal the underlying differences in assumptions and experience in a way that the team as a whole could learn. (p. 24)

If the approach to teamwork is not open and sincere, it is a waste of time for everyone involved. In an atmosphere of trust, people are free to state their ideas and are not afraid of making mistakes even if they are uncertain about what they say. Dr. Jonas Salk, the eminent immunologist who developed the first successful polio vaccine, knew the value of keeping an open mind. He said his experiences underlined the value of looking at any event from more than one point of view and that "being able to see things—and oneself—from only one perspective is limiting" (Salk, 1995, p. 13).

Senge (1990) notes that "school trains us never to admit that we do not know the answer, and most corporations reinforce that lesson by rewarding the people who excel in advocating their views, not inquiring into complex issues" (p. 25). This limits growth in organizations and blocks out any new understandings that might threaten us. Argyris (1990) suggests how this problem can be overcome through team learning by practicing collective inquiry. According to him, most managers find collective inquiry inherently threatening because they think it means that they must yield to the position of others; when people are able to address an issue collectively, however, their individual prejudices are put aside. The word *collective* means a number of persons or things that are considered a group and relate to one another or have something in common. The word *inquire* means to seek an answer; it comes from the Latin word *inquaerere*, "to seek within." When the two words are put together, the meaning is greater than the combination of the parts. Issacs (1994) built further on the concept of collective inquiry, which he feels is sure to improve open dialogue as well as organizations. He says that communication will backfire if channeled into the intent of forcing a decision; it is best to approach dialogue with no specific result in mind but with the intention of developing deeper inquiry, wherever it may lead the group.

Diverse groups of people who drop their guard and learn how to question collectively tend to discover better solutions to the problems at hand. They teach each other how to change, and they thrive on change by constantly seeking out new opportunities for improvement through learning. Therefore, the focus of change is much more than survival. It is growth. Greenleaf (1991) explains this well in terms of how the *I Ching* applies to the turbulent times of today:

> This may suggest our place today, to see ourselves as responsible people at the center of an organic process of change which, at this time, may be strenuous and confused. But what is done will be more than a saving action. It will begin with the struggle to survive. However, if survival alone is the aim, it is not likely to succeed. It will include a conserving role; there is much that is good in what we now have and it should be saved. More important, it will build anew, build something that may not yet be dreamed of. It will be voluntary, and it will raise the spirit. (p. 174)

NEW APPROACHES TO HEALTH CARE

Thus far in this chapter, the trends in the industry have been described and the nature of change has been discussed. Practitioners only need to glance through the trade journals and magazines to get a good sense of the revolution that is underway and how it is affecting people. A total restructuring of the health care system is imminent. There is no doubt that the traditional health care paradigm is obsolete and needs to be replaced. During the 1980s, some tried to fix the traditional model by making minor alterations here and there, but new anomalies kept surfacing and proved that the whole system needs a major overhaul right down to the basic values that govern the way people think.

Figure 1–4 shows the traditional health care structure with its cumbersome number of hierarchical levels and multitude of job titles. It shall soon be a thing of the past. Even the very largest organization, the Roman Catholic Church, which serves 960 million people around the world, has only six levels: Pope, cardinal, archbishop, bishop, priest, and deacon. There is a wide geographical distribution of member churches in all nations, a respect for local cultural differences, a high degree of autonomy and integration within individual commu-

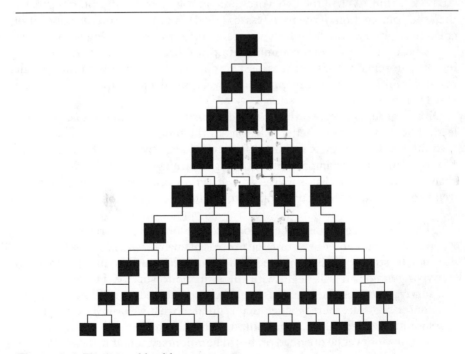

Figure 1–4 Traditional health care structure.

nities, and a limited need for frequent communication with higher levels because the vision and mission are well understood by all. Each church official is trained to take the place of his superior, and each is able to make horizontal moves with little effort. This is not to say that the history of the Catholic Church is free of any signs of revolution, but it is the longest lived organization in the world and is still thriving today. Even with the recent shortage of priests in some areas, deacons and laypersons have been successfully empowered to carry on the mission of the church.

The health care industry is past the point in its revolution of doubting the traditional paradigm. Those who were slow to yield have seen no choice but to face the facts because the evidence is overwhelming. Many groups still resist even the possibility that they may have to change. These people are still being guided by the old theories that are undoubtedly short-lived. Their battle will be the greatest. They will make it difficult, as well, for the teams of positive thinkers who want to move ahead creatively.

As described, many alternative paradigms have been proposed. According to the laws of change, this always adds to the confusion because the revolution will not subside until a new theory is identified and fully tested in a variety of settings. But it is clear at this time that most new models for the future health care system will probably incorporate four major concepts: patient-focused care, integrated health care, the use of self-directed work teams, and quality improvement.

Patient-Focused Care

By looking around the industry and reading the work of Lathrop (1993) and others cited in this chapter, practitioners can learn quickly what is wrong with the health care system from the consumer's point of view. Finding fault is the easy part. The challenge now lies in the next phase: rebuilding the system. At this point in time, the concepts of patient-focused care appear to be most promising, but the term *patient* is limiting with respect to trends in the entire system. Patients are those who are undergoing medical treatment, and future systems will aim to serve more than patients. Remember Juran's words: "Our customer is a cast of characters" (1989, p. 92). All these characters must have a place in the new model if the industry intends to contribute to the health of the nation, and this includes preventive care of people who are not currently sick so that they can be kept that way as long as possible. For a replacement paradigm to work in the future, there is a need to incorporate this concept of prevention by expanding our imaginations outside the walls of traditional institutions such as hospitals and nursing homes.

This is not to say that the basic underlying premise for patient-focused care will not work but rather that it is only a part of a much bigger picture. For example, the incredible growth in the aging population was discussed earlier. Seniors prefer to be in their homes, and it is more cost effective to let them stay there. This explains the fact that home care has been the fastest growing segment of the health care market. The Administration on Aging is responsible for funding community-based nutrition services for older people across the country. As the largest funding agency of its type, it offers services through 57 state units and 650 area agencies. According to Lloyd (1995), in 1994 meals were provided for approximately 2.3 million congregate meal participants and 880 million home-delivered meal participants. Of the total meals served, 47% were home delivered, and 53% were congregate meals. The percentage of home-delivered meals has increased from 10% to 47% in the last 20 years. In addition to the meals served, nutrition intervention is much needed for this population. This large group of consumers, by definition, cannot be considered patients.

One will notice from Figure 1–4 that the traditional organization of the hospital left out patients and other customers entirely. Figure 1–5 shows a likely future model. Patients are a part of the community population. They may be called patients when they are institutionalized, but they spend most of their lives in the role of consumers receiving community-based health care services. In this model, patients are supported by the entire health care system, which meets their needs all the time in whichever community setting they may be.

Integrated Health Care

This leads to the broader concept of integrated health care. The Joint Commission has already applied the concept of integrated care to the hospital setting. One of its standards states "Over time, patients may receive a range of care in multiple settings from multiple providers. For this reason it is important for

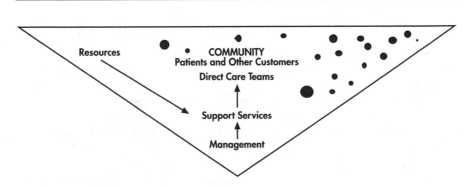

Figure 1–5 Integrated health care model.

a hospital to view the patient care it provides as a part of an integrated system of settings, services, health care practitioners, and care levels that make up a continuum of care" (Joint Commission, 1995, p. 225). The specific processes and activities that need to be coordinated and integrated within the hospital are those that take place before admission, during admission, in the hospital, before discharge, and at discharge.

The Joint Commission defines continuity of care as "a component of patient care quality consisting of the degree to which the care needed by a patient is coordinated among practitioners and across organizations and time" (Joint Commission, 1995, p. 710). Continuity of care is not a new concept. In 1970, the Perloff Report from the Special Committee on the Provision of Health Services of the American Hospital Association identified a community-based regional system as the hub of the health care system (Ackerman, 1992). Two years later, Hannan (1972) encouraged networks to avoid duplication of effort and to reduce costs. He presented the following to the New York Academy of Medicine:

> First we need a rearrangement of our health service structure. Comprehensive care should be provided by interlocking networks starting from the doctor's office—or an outpatient department—to the community hospital, to hospitals for acute care for complicated medical problems, as well as for those specializing in certain areas of disease and, going back down the scale, through the convalescent home, the rehabilitation center, and the nursing home for the aged and chronically ill. There should be a flow of communication and exchange of expertise among these institutions, both horizontally and vertically. And devices must be found to extend the benefits to sparsely populated rural areas as well as those of high population density. (p. 1460)

In the 1990s, trends finally became directed toward vertically integrated regional systems (Ackerman, 1992). Exhibit 1–6 provides a case study of how an integration system that used clinical pathways was recently established for the New York Hospital Council.

Figure 1–5 illustrates the fact that direct care staff members are closest to consumers and provide point-of-care services in centers distributed throughout the community wherever needed. There are no lines in the structure; it is seamless because all services are integrated and a free flow of information to and from consumers occurs routinely. Health care teams can be created as needed to fulfill community needs.

Suppose a new program needed to be established. Appropriate representatives from the health care system would meet with a consumer group to design the new service. They would plan activities, staffing patterns, and budgets and

Exhibit 1–6 Clinical Paths That Span the Continuum of Care: A Case Study

In 1994, the New York Hospital Council set up successful partnerships among 16 highly competitive hospitals and other providers in the northeast region of the state. According to the clinical director, Tina Gerardi, one major goal of this consortium was "to improve patient care management from preadmission through postdischarge" with free-flowing information between hospitals and other providers such as physicians, home care agencies, long-term care agencies, and community centers and by linking quality improvement processes with clinical decision making. Four DRGs were targeted (total hip replacement, laparoscopic cholecystectomy, cardiac chest pain, and cerebrovascular accidents). Hospitals set up clinical pathways and best practice models, all of which contained a nutrition component. Pathways extended from preadmission to home care.

Despite some resistance, the benefits of collaboration were seen immediately. Even before clinical pathways were developed, one hospital reduced the length of stay for cardiac patients by 0.5 days as a result of shared data. Preliminary data showed that 2.5 days had been saved, or $1,500 per case. Both patient and staff satisfaction also improved. The group is now exploring the possibility of having visiting nurses conduct preadmission testing in patients' homes.

Much of the success of this consortium came from widening the communication channels within and among key departments and services and from caregivers having more ready access to collaborative team approaches. Patient-focused teams and care maps or clinical pathways have been found to be useful by this group and many others.

Source: Data from K. Cicone and T. Gerardi, A Regional Approach to the Development of Clinical Paths that Span the Continuum of Care, in *Clinical Paths: Tools for Outcomes Management,* P.L. Spath, ed., pp. 243–265, © 1994, American Hospital Association.

decide how quality and cost would be monitored. Once the new service was satisfactorily implemented, the team consisting of community and health care representatives could dissolve after empowering the new staff to control all activities. Whole systems shared governance would be practiced because the majority of all care decisions would be made at the point of care. Direct computer access to medical records and standards of care would facilitate this process. The planning group might come together again if needed in the future to help with problem solving or to expand the new service, but full authority and responsibility would be delegated to the work group.

Just how do food and nutrition fit into this overall scheme? Figure 1–6 demonstrates how. At the top, one can see the community settings from which the customers come. Under inputs, it can be seen that the community is also the source for human resources, materials, information, and financial support of the health care system. The community centers listed show just some of the programs for which food and nutrition can be provided. Customers are drawn from these programs and enter the system as physicians assess their needs. This process can happen in the acute care facility or at the point of care within the

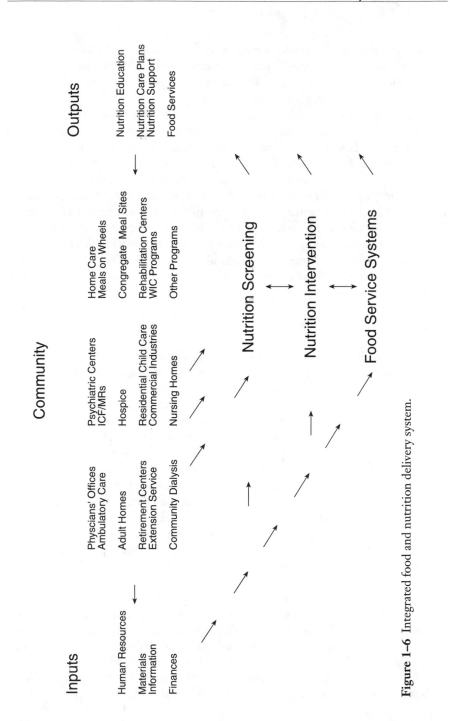

Figure 1–6 Integrated food and nutrition delivery system.

community setting. Nutrition screening is performed, but not necessarily by the nutrition staff. Dietitians' input for development of the screening process is, nevertheless, important. Depending upon the level of risk, nutrition assessment, care plans, and support are provided.

The lower part of the diagram shows the food service system interfacing directly with the nutrition component at the point where meals and supplements are planned. It should be noted that communication occurs throughout the system as individuals provide input, feedback, and referrals to one another. Most of the food service processes probably occur within a central support facility or commissary, which will initially be at the main hospital site. Many commissary operations have fared better when volume production was separated from the daily activities of patient care, so it is possible that entirely different locations for food production and assembly will eventually appear. This model shows a continuous cycle of activities that starts and ends in the community. Although it is impossible to predict the future, the trends in the field appear to be headed in this direction.

Self-Directed Work Teams

The discussion about knowledge workers earlier in this chapter indicated that employees are not only capable of having but need to have more control of their work situation to stay motivated and make substantial contributions that can result in positive outcomes. The organizational structure will be greatly affected by this change. In Figure 1–5, just as the direct care teams support patients and other customers in the community, so does middle and upper level management support employees. There will be fewer numbers and layers of administrative personnel, and some centralization of services will also occur at this level (e.g., food preparation and a central pharmacy), but all direct services will occur in the field. As multiple layers of middle management personnel are peeled away, top level executives will be faced with the reality that first-line supervisors have been trying to explain to them all along: that their success depends upon the direct care and lower echelon employees, who can make or break the institution depending on how well they are treated.

The most successful leaders in the history of the world did not start with extraordinary followers. They took ordinary people and developed them into extraordinary contributors using patience, wisdom, humility, continuous exchange of ideas, and reinforcement. These great leaders saw themselves as servants of their followers and provided motivation along with all the tools necessary to get the job done right. In return for their efforts, they gained the trust and loyalty of their followers. Greenleaf (1991) states "We are in a period of radical transition regarding power, authority, and decision everywhere, and a cloud has settled over all leadership and management in any form. All institutions are affected by these trends and institutional leadership is now quite different from what it was a few years ago. I expect this to continue" (p. 137). Greenleaf describes a more ethical and less manipulative style of leadership. One problem, according to him, is that the words *manipulation* and *management* have a common root (*manus*, "hand"), and both imply shaping others' destinies. Manipulation is not desirable because it implies moving people without their knowing what is going on. When this happens, workers do not accept management as a legitimate power. When employees and managers work together to shape the destiny of an organization, positive outcomes are more likely to occur.

This servant leadership style is contrary to authoritarian styles that have failed in the past. It also varies from *laissez-faire* or permissive styles, where managers lack responsibility and allow employees to control situations fully. Perhaps it is most like participative management, whereby leaders and employees resolve problems jointly in a direct and honest manner. Servant leadership also emphasizes another dimension, however: the responsibility of management to ensure that all the resources necessary for employees to do the job correctly are provided on a consistent and timely basis so that workers can reach the highest level of achievement possible. These resources include the correct raw foods, supplies, equipment, environment, training, schedules, and other necessary information. When workers have all these things at their fingertips, independent work is easily accomplished in a productive manner, and on-the-job stress is diminished. As a result, the manager's role is shifted more toward supporting the worker. Leaders focus more on management of information as they provide and monitor resources to get the job done right. With motivation, empowerment, and provision of proper resources, teams of people require little supervision to get the job done right.

Pinell of the VHA included self-directed work teams in his model for the future. His view of the characteristics of the traditional medical model and the future health care model can be seen in Table 1–5, which compares the two. The traditional medical model focuses on treating acute incidents of illness in an isolated hospital environment that has fragmentation of services. Little, if any, contact is made between previous and future providers of care, and competition exists among individual providers. Under this model, financing and delivery of care are separated. Ownership and control are concentrated in the upper management levels, and success is measured by indicators that focus on the hospital stay.

Tomorrow's health care system will follow the social model, whereby all aspects of health will be addressed for prevention and treatment. People will be held more accountable for their own health in the future, and the concept of continuity of care will act to correct the problem of fragmented services that

Table 1–5 Past and Future Health Care Models

Traditional Medical Model	Future Health Care Model
Goal: Treating incidents of illness	Goal: Managing health
Structure: Fragmented services	Structure: Integrated services along the continuum of care
Competition: Among individual providers	Competition: Among integrated community health networks
Financing and delivery: Separate functions	Financing and delivery: Integrated functions
Ownership and control: Upper management	Ownership and control: Self-directed work teams
Quality measurement: Number of admissions, patient days, length of stay, professional credentials, market share, mission projects	Quality measurement: Covered lives, health status, quality outcomes, community needs, continuum of service, cost effectiveness

Source: Data from M.C. Pinell, *Managed Health Care: Where Are We Now and Where Are We Going.* Presented at the Forum sponsored by the Jacksonville Dietetic Association, 1995.

plagued industry when it followed the medical model. In the future, competition will occur among integrated health care networks, and financing will not be separated from delivery of care. Teams will be empowered to direct the system rather than the system having a vertical structure with decisions being made at higher levels. In the future, success will be measured in different terms. Covered lives will indicate the percentage of the population that participates. Cost effectiveness will reflect the efficiency of the system. Quality will be reflected in the health status of the population that is covered, the quality of patient outcomes along the continuum, and how well the system meets the needs of the community.

Quality Improvement

The roots of total quality management or quality improvement are found in the works of Deming, Juran, and others and in the lessons learned during the 1920s at Bell Laboratories and the Hawthorne Works of the Western Electric Company. Statistical tools for the ongoing evaluation of quality performance, such as Shewhart's control chart, were introduced to analyze variations in quality data. Since that time, the success of Japanese industries, which implemented the concept before Americans, speaks for itself. Much activity in this area has been seen across the United States in the last 15 years. The most recent trend is to convert traditional authoritarian organizations into learning organizations, which have the capability of continuously improving and realizing their potential. In 1990, Senge identified five disciplines that are essential for improvement: systems thinking, shared vision, team learning, expansion of mental models, and personal mastery. The focus is now utilizing people and processes, rather than things, for effective quality improvement. Chapter 14, on quality improvement, includes much more information about current trends in quality management. Methods have become increasingly more sophisticated and will continue to do so, especially with the advent of the computerized medical record, the Joint Commission's IMSystem as previously described, and trends in managed care that encourage cross-organizational comparisons of patient care quality.

In 1989, Laffel and Blumenthal stated that the traditional medical model no longer meets the needs of modern health care providers because of the following limitations: a definition of quality that is too narrow to meet current health care needs, an approach to quality standards that is too static, underemphasis on organizational processes and the contributions of persons other than physicians, and a focus on only some aspects of physicians' performance, such as technical expertise, but not on their ability to utilize a facility's resources effectively to meet patient needs. They established a case for physicians to use industrial quality management science to measure the outcomes of care.

The outcome-oriented approach is also enforced in current regulations, although specific universal indicators have not yet been incorporated in the codes. As indicators are developed, the recommendations offered by Wilkins in 1995 should probably be implemented. He encouraged the use of three major types of measurements: economic, clinical, and user satisfaction.

CONCLUSION

As practitioners plunge ahead to meet the challenges and try to demonstrate more positive outcomes, it is important to realize that, even though the industry is in the midst of a revolution and numerous trends are being seen, many of the old values and techniques have a place in the future, and much can be learned from the past.

In the 19th century, for example, Florence Nightingale, who was one of the most inspiring leaders in health care, recommended standardized patient care in her *Notes on Nursing*, which were originally published in 1859. As early as 1863, she proposed the accumulation of statistical data regarding hospital admissions, recoveries, and discharges. As one reads through her notes, one can see that she was a strong patient advocate and probably the originator of what we now call patient-focused care because she constantly emphasized the basic needs of her patients. Just about every aspect of care in homes and institutions was detailed by her with special emphasis on the care environment, respect for the patient, and education. In those days, patients only routinely saw one person—the nurse—whose work encompassed the tasks that many specialists now perform. The following is an excerpt from her treatise "What Nursing Ought To Be":

> I use the word nursing for want of a better. It has been limited to sig-nify little more than the administration of medicines and the applica-tion of poultices. It ought to signify the proper use of fresh air, light, warmth, cleanliness, quiet, and the proper selection and administration of diet—all at the least expense of the vital power to the patient. (Nightingale, 1969, p. 8)

As the industry moves forward into the 21st century, the pendulum is begin-ning to swing away from the values that created the highly complex and imper-sonal health care system of the present toward integrated care once again.

REFERENCES

Ackerman, F.K. (1992). The movement toward vertically integrated regional health systems. *Healthcare Management Review, 17*(3), 81–88.

Appleby, C. (1995). Healthcare's new heavyweights. *Hospital and Healthcare Networks, 69*(9), 26–34.

Argyris, C. (1990). *Overcoming organizational defenses: Facilitating organization learning.* Boston: Allyn & Bacon.

Armstead, R., Elstein, P., & Gorman, J. (1995). Toward a 21st century quality-measurement sys-tem for managed-care organizations. *Health Care Financing Review, 16*(4), 25–37.

Bergman, R.L., & Sherer, J.F. (1993). A look at health care delivery system in twenty years. *Hospital & Healthcare Networks, 67*(2), 28–31.

Brockner, J., Greenberg, J., Brockner, A., Bortz, J., Davy, J., & Carter, C. (1986). Layoffs, equity theory and work performance. Further evidence of the image of survivor guilt. *Academy of Man-agement Journal, 29*(2), 373–383.

Bunda, D. (1993, June 15). Hospital closing drops for third straight year. *Modern Healthcare,* p. 2.

Burner, S.T., & Waldo, D.R. (1995). National health expenditure projections, 1994–2005. *Health Care Financing Review, 16*(4), 221–242.

Cappa, P. (1994). Outfitting your hospital for the new wave of robots. *Journal of Healthcare Materiel Management, 12*(6).

Cicone K., & Gerardi, T. (1994). A regional approach to the development of clinical paths that span the continuum of care. In P.L. Spath, ed. *Clinical paths: Tools for outcomes management* (pp. 243–265). Chicago: American Hospital Association.

Cromwell, J., & Butrica, B. (1995). Hospital department cost and employment increases: 1980–1992. *Health Care Financing Review, 17*(1), 147–165.

Drucker, P.F. (1974). *Management tasks, responsibilities, practices.* New York: Harper & Row.

Drucker, P.F. (1992). *Managing for the future: The 1990's and beyond.* New York: Truman Talley Books/Plume.

Farrell, J.P., & Pagoaga, J.A. (1995). Making change pay: The 1995 Hay survey. *Hospital & Healthcare Networks, 69*(17), 26–33.

Frank J. Corbett, Inc. (1991). *Consumer market research study.* Chicago: Author.

Fried, B. (1995, October). *Making the case for managed care reimbursement.* Paper presented at the annual meeting of the American Dietetic Association, Chicago, IL.

Gallup Organization. (1994). *How are Americans making food choices?* Lincoln, NE: Author.

Gill, T.M., & Feinstein, A.R. (1994). A critical appraisal of the quality of quality-of-life measurements. *JAMA, 272*(8), 619–626.

Grayson, M.A. (1995). Doctors' incomes are falling. *Hospital & Health Networks, 69*(23), 17.

Greenleaf, R.K. (1991). *Servant leadership—A journey into the nature of legitimate power and greatness.* New York: Paulist Press.

Grigsby, J., Kaehny, M.M., Sandberg, E.J., Schlenker, M.D., & Shaughnessy, P.W. (1995). Effect and effectiveness of telemedicine. *Health Care Financing Review, 17*(1), 115–131.

Grindel, C.G. (1994, October). *Developing successful alliances with other health professionals.* Presented at the 1994 annual meeting of the American Dietetic Association, Orlando, FL.

Hannan, K.H. (1972). Hospitals: Isolated or interdependent? In *The hospital as a community facility.* New York Academy of Medicine, 48(11), 1459–1466.

Imai, M. (1986). *Kaizen, the key to Japan's competitive success.* New York: Random House Business Division.

Issacs, W. (1994). The paradoxes of dialogue design. In P. Senge, A. Kleiner, C. Roberts, R.B. Ross, & B.J. Smith (Eds.), *The fifth discipline fieldbook: Strategies and tools for building a learning organization* (pp. 365–375). New York: Doubleday.

Jackson, R. (1995). What's new in labor saving equipment. *Hospital Food & Nutrition Focus, 11*(8), 7–8.

Joint Commission on Accreditation of Healthcare Organizations. (1990). *The Joint Commission's agenda for change—Stimulating continual improvement in the quality of care.* Oakbrook Terrace, IL: Author.

Joint Commission on Accreditation of Healthcare Organizations. (1994). Joint Commission launches new indicator monitoring system in 1994 [Special issue]. *Joint Commission Perspectives,* 14–15.

Joint Commission on Accreditation of Healthcare Organizations. (1995). *1996 accreditation manual for hospitals.* Oakbrook Terrace, IL: Author.

Juran, J.M. (1989). *Juran on leadership for quality: An executive handbook.* New York: Free Press.

Kassler, J. (1994). *Bitter medicine: Greed and chaos in American health care.* New York: Carol Publishing Group.

Kolasa, K.M. (1995, October). *Incorporating nutrition in objective structured clinical examinations for medical and residency education.* Presented at the annual meeting of the American Dietetic Association, Chicago, IL.

Kornblum, T.H. (1993). Negotiating a higher salary. *Journal of the American Dietetic Association, 93*(2), 142–144.

Kuczmarski, R.J., Flegal, K.M., Campbell, S.M., & Johnson, C.L. (1994). Increasing prevalence of overweight among U.S. adults. *JAMA, 272*(3), 205–211.

Kuhn, T.S. (1974). *The structure of scientific revolutions.* Chicago: University of Chicago Press.

Laffel, G., & Blumenthal, D. (1989). The case for using industrial quality management science in health care organizations. *JAMA, 262*(20), 2869–2873.

Lathrop, J.P. (1993). *Restructuring health care. The patient focused paradigm.* San Francisco: Jossey-Bass.

Levit, K.R., Sensenig, C.A., Cowan, C.A., Lazanby, H.C., McDonnell, P.A., Won, D.K., Sivarajan, L., Stiller, J.M., Donham, C.S., & Stewart, M.S. (1994). National health expenditures, 1993. *Health Care Financing Review, 16*(1), 194–247.

Lloyd, J. (1995, November). *Nutrition across the continuum: Linking home and community nutrition care and services for elders.* Presented at the annual meeting of the American Dietetic Association, Chicago, IL.

Montague, J., & Pitman, H. (1995). Currents (physicians). *Hospital & Health Networks, 69*(23), 13.

Morreale, S.J., & Schwartz, N.E. (1995). Helping Americans eat right: Developing practical and actionable public nutrition education messages based on the ADA survey of American dietary habits. *Journal of the American Dietetic Association, 95*(3), 305–308.

Nettles, M.F., & Gregoire, M.B. (1993). Operational characteristics of hospital foodservice departments with conventional, cook-chill, and cook-freeze systems. *Journal of the American Dietetic Association, 93*(10), 1161–1163.

Nightingale, F. (1969). *Notes on nursing, what it is and what it is not* (rev. ed). New York: Dover. (Original work published 1859)

Pew Health Professions Commission. (1995). *Shifting the supply of our health care workforce.* San Francisco: University of California at San Francisco.

Pinell, M.C. (1995, October). *Managed health care: Where are we now and where are we going.* Presented at the forum sponsored by the Jacksonville Dietetic Association, Jacksonville, FL.

PiSunyer, F.X. (1995). The fattening of America. *JAMA, 272*(3), 238.

Robert Wood Johnson Foundation. (1994). The latest forecast—Managed care collides with physician supply. *JAMA, 272*(3), 239–240.

Ruch, P.R. (1995). Physicians as partners. *Food & Nutrition News, 67*(1), 5–6.

Salk, M. (1995). Dr. Jonas Salk's way to approach . . . and solve . . . problems. *Bottom Line Personal, 16*(15), 13.

Scharf, B. (1995, October). *Sleuthing your way through tribal turf: A field guide for dietetic professionals.* Presented at the annual meeting of the American Dietetic Association, Chicago, IL.

Schiller, M.R. (1995, October). *Hospital restructuring: A challenge for dietetics professionals.* Presented at the annual meeting of the American Dietetic Association, Chicago, IL.

Scott, L. (1993). Buying groups seek compliance. *Modern Healthcare,* pp. 52–61.

Senge, P.M. (1990). *The fifth discipline: The art and practice of the learning organization.* New York: Doubleday Currency.

Sensenig, A.L., Heffler, S.K., & Donham, C.S. (1995). Health care indicators. *Health Care Financing Review, 17*(1), 277–316.

Snyder, J., & Lathrop, J.P. (1995). Cost reduction using patient-focused care concepts. *Managed Care Quarterly, 3*(1), 43–51.

Study Commission on Dietetics. (1972). *The profession of dietetics: The report of the Study Commission on Dietetics.* Chicago: American Dietetic Association.

Study Commission on Dietetics. (1984). *A new look at the profession of dietetics: Report of the Study Commission on Dietetics.* Chicago: American Dietetic Association.

U.S. Department of Agriculture Extension Service. (1995). *E. coli 0157:H7 at a glance.* Washington, DC: Author.

U.S. Department of Health and Human Services. (1990). *Healthy people 2000: National health promotion and disease prevention objectives.*Washington, DC: Author.

U.S. Food and Drug Administration. (1995). *Food code.* Springfield, VA: U.S. Department of Commerce.

Wilkins, R.G. (1995, October). *Outcome assessment: Your role in documenting the value of medical nutrition therapy.* Presented at the annual meeting of the American Dietetic Association, Chicago, IL.

Wright, B. (1994, October). *National health care reform: A report from the nation's capitol.* Presented at the annual meeting of the American Dietetic Association, Chicago, IL.

Leadership for Quality

Margo Alexander

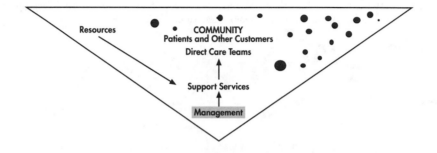

According to the Joint Commission on Accreditation of Healthcare Organizations (Joint Commission), the major goal for leaders in the health care industry is to establish services that respond to community and patient needs (Joint Commission, 1995). Unfortunately, it has been evident that dietetic professionals need to improve their leadership skills to set the pace in providing high-quality food and nutrition services. More than 40 years ago, Rowe addressed this problem as follows: "When the day comes that your executive ability equals your scientific knowledge, your profession will be secure. Until that day, you will be faced with constant and unwelcome challenge" (Dowling & Norton, 1990, p. 1065).

Although some advances have been made, the situation today is somewhat the same. As Barker, Foltz, Arensberg, and Schiller (1994) note, "Pacesetters in the profession have been sounding the leadership alarm for the past fifteen years. Few, however have responded, and a specific approach to dietetics leadership has never been defined" (p. 4).

In an effort to encourage the development of strong leaders in the profession, this chapter describes leadership trends and specific skills that are necessary for success in the present and future. Rather than evaluate and debate the different leadership theories, the focus is *skill development,* so that willing practitioners can alter their behavior while preparing themselves for the inevitable time when the industry will be even less tolerant than it is today of ineffective leaders.

LEADERSHIP TODAY

Most American industries are now stressing the topic of leadership because it is clear that improvements must be seen to remain competitive in the world market. The health care industry is doing the same. Simply stated, good leaders cause organizations to succeed, and poor leaders cause them to fail. Senge (1990) talks about successful leaders:

> Most of the outstanding leaders I have worked with are neither tall nor especially handsome; they are often mediocre public speakers; they do not stand out in a crowd; and they do not mesmerize an attending audience with their brilliance or eloquence. Rather, what distinguishes them is the clarity and persuasiveness of their ideas, the depth of their commitment, and their openness to continually learning more. They do not "have the answer." But they do instill confidence in those around them that, together, "we can learn whatever we need to learn in order to achieve the results we truly desire." (p. 359)

Leaders have an intense awareness of what is happening in the world around them and in their own organizations. "In most companies that fail, there is abundant evidence in advance that the firm is in trouble. This evidence goes unheeded, however, even when individual managers are aware of it. The organization as a whole cannot recognize impending threats, understand the implications of those threats, or come up with alternatives" (Senge, 1990, p. 17).

The Leadership Crisis

Barker et al. (1994) describe various factors that have contributed to the leadership crisis in dietetics. One reason is that rapid changes in society have caused many of the traditional management techniques to become obsolete. Second, there is a nationwide decrease in employees' commitment to work, resulting in decreased productivity in many of our nation's organizations. The third factor is the lack of leader credibility, which is due, in part, to an increasingly active mass media exposing unethical behavior of leaders and criticisms of them by others.

For dietitians, the leadership crisis is compounded by the fact that job satisfaction and salaries are continuing concerns. Barker et al. (1994) cite statistics from the American Dietetic Association's (ADA's) membership survey in 1990, when two thirds of the dietitians did not have departmental budgets under their control, more than one third supervised no employees, and more than half earned $20,000 to $35,000 per year.

The ADA recognizes this problem and has established a special team to lead the association toward more effective integration of the food, food service, and management components. According to Halling and Abbott Hess (1995), several factors during the past three decades have contributed to the current situation in the field. One is that systems theory has been applied in a manner resulting in the concept of management being associated with food service and not nutrition care. Dietitians have tended to dissociate themselves from the management role, not wanting to be known as cooks and believing that they do not have to know how to cook. This has been compounded by the fact that clinical staff often thought that food service department leadership was not strong enough to advocate for them, and a split of some departments into separate food service and clinical units has resulted.

Other reasons include the societal shift from manufacturing to information and technology and the many high-technology advances in clinical nutrition, particularly for enteral and parenteral nutrition. As this occurred, many clinical dietitians dissociated their practice from that of food service while losing their multipurpose, broad-based skills. Actions by the ADA were also cited as contributing factors by Halling and Abbott Hess (1995). Plan IV, for example, decreased courses in foods and management, role delineation studies divided the field into distinct specialties, and registration examinations widened the chasm by having separate sections for nutrition and food systems management. Internships also divided into specialized areas, and the number offering a management emphasis decreased.

Dietitians are now beginning to realize that clinical nutrition must be managed just as food services need to be managed, so that emphasis and research are unfolding in this discipline. One such study by Arensberg, Schiller, Vivian, Johnson, and Strasser (1995) looked at the leadership behavior of 150 clinical nutrition managers as perceived by themselves and their subordinates. Using the transformational leadership model, they found that the dietitians, in general, rated themselves higher in the various leadership categories than their subordinates. In addition, the leadership quality with the lowest scores was *communication*, and that with the highest scores was *respectful leadership*, which reflects one's treatment of others and self in daily interactions. To improve visionary leadership behaviors, especially communication skills, these researchers recommended additional training in colleges and continuing education.

Leadership Defined

Drucker (1992) pointed out "leadership is not by itself good or desirable. Leadership is a means. Leadership to what end is thus a crucial question" (p.

119). The three characteristics he considered important for successful leadership are as follows:

1. The foundation of effective leadership is thinking through the organization's mission, defining it, and establishing it clearly and visibly. The leader sets the goals, sets the priorities, and sets and maintains the standards. He or she makes compromises, of course; indeed, effective leaders are painfully aware that they are not in control of the universe.
2. The leader sees leadership as a responsibility rather than a rank and privilege. Effective leaders are rarely permissive, but when things go wrong (and they always do), they do not blame others. Precisely because effective leaders know that they and no one else are ultimately responsible, they are not afraid of strength in associates and subordinates. Misleaders are; they always go in for purges. An effective leader, on the other hand, wants strong associates. He or she encourages them, pushes them, and indeed glories in them.
3. The effective leader must earn trust. Otherwise, there will be no followers, and the only definition of a leader is someone who has followers. To trust a leader, it is not necessary to like or to agree with him or her. Trust is the conviction that the leader means what he or she says. It is a belief in something very old-fashioned: integrity.

In the past, leaders and followers were not necessarily bound by common goals. Leaders took the initiative and made contact with others for the purpose of exchanging things of value. This type of leadership is called transactional leadership. Transformational leadership, in contrast, results when leaders and followers raise one another to higher levels of motivation and morality. Transformational leadership is discussed further below.

Leaders must first define reality. Department heads and managers of food and nutrition services need to see clearly where they are if they wish to plan and create a viable vision of where they want to be. In directing services, leaders are obligated to provide and maintain momentum. Competent leadership and a strong management team can function synergistically to keep the team focused on recognizable and legitimate goals. This requires sound communication skills, which are most critical in the implementing and coordinating processes. In addition, leaders are responsible for effectiveness and thus must continually seek to improve upon service.

Leadership in Health Care

The Joint Commission has done a superb job in defining the role of leadership for the health care industry, and it provides standards for planning, directing, coordinating, providing, and improving health care services. These functions are further defined in Chapter 3. As previously noted, the Joint Commission identifies the major goal for leaders to be the establishment of health care services that respond to community and patient needs. Leaders are defined as the governing body, the chief executive officer and other senior managers, department heads, elected or appointed leaders of the medical staff and clinical departments, the nurse executive, other senior nursing leaders, and other medical staff members in organizational administrative positions.

Leadership versus Management

There has been some confusion between leaders and managers, especially at middle management levels. Senge's (1990) comments may help clarify the difference. He notes that successful professionals learn continuously as they work because they frequently pause to develop hypotheses, act on their conclusions, and pause again while reflecting on the results of their actions. In other words, they are able to see the big picture and alter their course accordingly.

"Most American managers are too busy running to 'think on their feet,'" according to Senge (1990, p. 304). He characterizes this problem as the "chain gang" model of management, whereby managers view themselves as the boss, the person who sets the speed of the gang. The incessant activity leaves little room for the manager to learn and reflect on the results of the work. Even when this type of manager has time for reflection, experiments show that they simply switch to another strategy and, if that does not work, to another and even to another. Although the strategies change, these managers do not articulate what they hope to achieve, nor do they stop to examine why past alternatives seemed to fail.

Barker et al. (1994) make a similar distinction by stating that, when managers implement change in an organization, it is often planned change, and they function within the existing structure of the organization. Managers make small changes in processes but do not achieve significant organizational gains. "Leaders, on the other hand, are not typically confined by structure. They make changes more readily in organizational cultures and ultimately in the workers themselves. Thus, leaders provide an opportunity for more effective change and significant organizational gains" (Barker et al., 1994, p. 4). It is important to realize that these two concepts are not mutually exclusive and that, in reality, some managers possess leadership skills whereas others do not. The goal, of course, is to increase the number of managers in the profession who exhibit this leadership quality.

Most industries have many managers who can follow routine procedures but few who display exceptional leadership skills. Champy (1996) states "contrary to popular belief a business is built not on numbers—bottom lines, market forces, production quotas—but on ideas and visions of what that business could be, what its managers want it to become" (p. xii).

Nevertheless, according to Champy (1996), "managers at all levels often resist this process of constructing the future" (p. xx). One of the two major reasons for this resistance is that people naturally tend to "keep tapping on the same old drum" and assume that they can manage a business in the same way, day after day, year after year, and still realize success. The second is a fear of the unknown, its potential threats and inevitable risks. Managers who are not afraid to learn and grow refuse to let these factors interfere, and as a result, they assume the higher level leadership roles in their corporations.

An Overview: Past and Present

Professional management, or leadership, in the United States dates back to the early 1900s, when structures were simpler and "the boss" was readily identified. As society and technology expanded, the need for more complex organizational structures developed. Table 2–1 shows the significant changes since that time.

Regarding future leadership trends, Ross (1992) predicts "An age of executive excellence will result from this organizational integration and renewal. Tomorrow's executives will spend more time identifying and rewarding individuals who are risk takers, cultivating innovation and vision rather than merely institutional caretaking" (p. 5).

LEARNING ORGANIZATIONS

The most successful organizations are those that continuously learn and improve. According to Senge (1990), those that "will truly excel in the future will be the organizations that discover how to tap people's commitment and capacity to learn at *all* levels in an organization" (p. xx). Senge identifies five components that are essential to what he calls learning organizations: systems thinking, personal mastery, shared vision, mental models, and team learning.

Incorporation of these five disciplines in the organization's management philosophy will help overcome the learning disabilities that keep many American industries from gaining the competitive edge. "Learning disabilities are tragic in children, especially when they go undetected. They are no less tragic in organizations where they also go largely undetected. . . . Because of them, few corporations live even half as long as a person—most die before they reach the age of forty" (Senge, 1990, p. 18).

Table 2–1 Past and Present Leadership Trends in the Health Care Industry

Years	Era	Description
1910–1935	Initial Structure	Growth of new industries and entrepreneurship, an era of preregulation and high risk. Physicians were individual entrepreneurs; hospitals were free standing and independent.
1935–1955	Productivity Era	A science of *management* began to develop. Units were counted and factories mechanized. Influences of World War II impacted on the delivery of care. The concept of integrated hospitals matured. Individual physicians began focusing on activities of the hospital.
1955–1970	Systems Movement & Management Control	Technology continued to advance and society responded with a new expectation that medicine and the health care system could deliver quality services in limitless quantities. Hospitals began employing management engineers to further operational effectiveness and the concept of division of labor evolved. Organizational charts stressed accountability and the differences between line and staff functions, and planning processes became formalized and structured.
1970–1980	Systems Networking	Group practices and providers began to network to share resources and meet financial constraints. Regulation of the health care industry began to limit decision making flexibility. *For profit* hospital systems began to flourish, *nonprofit* systems adopted corporate structure formats, and *independent* institutions formed new alliances.
1980–1990	The New Competition	This was the era of the shake out and survival of the fittest. High expectations, high technology and high costs were the drivers for change. Health care leaders learned how to "downsize" operations and build management teams capable of rapid decision making. Organizations created tighter internal control mechanisms and began to seek ways to reward risk takers and innovators. The internal conflict in management direction—over whether to increase bureaucratic control or liberate the decision making process—put pressure on the traditional management team and tested the organization's ability to implement crucial change processes.
1990–2000	The Present	Management styles reflect and will continue to reflect a response to economic competition. Management theorists will develop new approaches to help leaders cope in an era that emphasizes the politics of subtraction. Organizations will look for ways to further trim management structures. Top-down bureaucratic control systems are being replaced by highly focused management teams. The art of blending management specialties into highly integrated and independent teams has become even more essential.

Source: Reprinted with permission from A.R. Kovner and A.H. Channing, *Really Trying: A Career Guide for the Health Services Manager,* 2nd Edition, © 1994, Health Administration Press.

Systems Thinking

"Systems thinking is a discipline for seeing wholes. It is a framework for seeing interrelationships rather than things, for seeing patterns of change rather than static 'snapshots'" (Senge, 1990, p. 68). A system is defined as regularly interacting or interdependent group of items (or subsystems) forming a unified whole. This is not a new concept to practitioners in food and nutrition services, but only recently has it been applied to the health care field.

Under the Joint Commission's (1995) recent standards for continuity of care, institutions are now being asked to view quality from patients' point of view. Continuity of care is "a component of patient care quality consisting of the degree to which the care needed by the patient is coordinated among practitioners and across organizations and time" (p. 710). For improved quality and cost effectiveness, continuous care is encouraged, i.e., "care provided over an extended time, in various settings, spanning the illness-to-wellness continuum" (p. 225).

Another illustration of how systems thinking has been incorporated in the health care industry is the use of quality improvement and total quality management principles, which utilize the concept of feedback from external and internal sources to keep the industry abreast of consumer needs and expectations.

Personal Mastery

According to Senge (1990), personal mastery is "the discipline of continually clarifying and deepening our personal vision, of focusing our energies, of developing patience, and of seeing reality objectively" (p. 141). People with a high level of personal mastery are able to realize positive results consistently and approach their lives as an artist would approach a work of art because they are committed to their own life-long learning. Effective management of their personal lives can only spill over into their professional lives and how they affect the lives of those who work with them. People who achieve growth, says Peck (1993), not only enjoy its fruits but give the same fruits to the world.

Personal mastery can be acquired by learning continuously at work, through higher education, or simply by keeping informed of changing trends in the industry. In these fast-paced, frenetic times, practitioners may believe that there are not enough hours in a day or days in a week to spend on enhancing their skills, but this is a serious and dangerous pitfall. According to Nightengale (1986), people have approximately 120 hours of discretionary time each week, assuming that they work the average 40-hour workweek and sleep 8 hours each night. Everyone needs recreation time and time to recharge his or her batteries. Surely, an hour each day or a mere 7 hours each week spent on the development of personal mastery will yield results beyond our wildest expectations and enable us to strengthen our skills.

Techniques for accomplishing personal mastery can be as simple as reading relevant literature during a lunch break or listening to audiocassettes during the drive to and from work. Through this educational process, one finds some of the most extraordinary information of our times from leaders such as Chopra, Blanchard, Haegner, Peck, Covey, and many others.

"Personal mastery goes beyond competence and skills, though it is grounded in competence and skills. It goes beyond spiritual unfolding or opening, although it requires spiritual growth. It means approaching one's life as a creative work, living life from a creative as opposed to reactive viewpoint" (Senge, 1990, p. 141). Two things happen when personal mastery is integrated into one's life. First, it helps one set priorities and clarify what is really important. Second, it enables one to see current reality more clearly. Both help leaders create realistic and attainable goals for themselves and their organizations.

Shared Vision

It is not enough for leaders to have a vision of the future. This vision must be communicated to and shared by all. When employees in any organization hold a shared vision, they succeed. This is not because they have to but because they are motivated to do so. According to Senge (1990), shared vision binds people together around a common identity and sense of destiny. It fosters genuine commitment and enrollment rather than compliance. "In mastering this discipline, leaders learn the counterproductiveness of trying to dictate a vision, no matter how heartfelt" (Senge, 1990, p. 9).

The Joint Commission encourages the same. It requires that leadership provide a collaborative process to develop a mission statement that is reflected in long-range, strategic, and operational plans, service design, resource allocation, and organizational policies. The mission statement is a written expression of the purpose of the organization that usually precedes the formation of goals and objectives. Once determined, the mission statement must be communicated and understood within all levels of the organization so that it can be used effectively as the basis for decision making and setting priorities.

Mental Models

"Mental models are deeply ingrained assumptions, generalizations, or even pictures or images that influence how we understand the world and how we take action" (Senge, 1990, p. 9). In the business setting, inaccurate mental models can be destructive and limiting, especially in cases where changes are essential for survival or success. To manage mental models, the skills of reflection and inquiry are needed. Through reflection, individuals can analyze their thinking processes, become more aware of their tendencies, and understand the way their mental models affect their actions. Through inquiry, others can help uncover the real facts by asking pertinent questions in a nonthreatening manner. This fosters creative thinking and results in discoveries that set the pace for the industry.

Argyris (1990), a long-time student of learning in management teams, teaches the concept of collective inquiry, which is helpful in dispensing with traditional models of behavior. When people approach dialogue with no specific result in mind but only with the intention of developing deeper inquiry, they are more trusting, accepting of others, and able to expose more truths. Argyris states that most managers find collective inquiry inherently threatening because they think it means that they must yield to the position of others. "Advocate your principles, values, and beliefs in a way that invites inquiry into them and encourages other people to do the same" (Argyris, 1990, p. 167).

Team Learning

"When teams are truly learning, not only are they producing extraordinary results but the individual members are growing more rapidly than could have occurred otherwise" (Senge, 1990, p. 10). As more self-directed work teams are used in health care facilities, managers are seeing that, through the process of empowerment, employees are taking on more responsibility for improving quality, increasing productivity, and decreasing costs. In addition, employees benefit because they experience personal and professional growth because they are able to escape from the restrictions of their former, sometimes boring, job descriptions.

Team learning normally does not occur immediately upon formation of the group. There are some growing pains that occur first. Blanchard, Carew, and Parisi-Carew (1990) describe four phases in team development: orientation, dissatisfaction, resolution, and production. These stages are often referred to as forming, storming, norming, and performing.

During the resolution stage, team members begin to develop a sense of trust, mutual support, respect, harmony, and a shared vision. This fosters high morale and a will to perform, and if an effective and resourceful facilitator is involved, growth of the team through learning can occur. "The discipline of team learning starts with 'dialogue,' the capacity of members of a team to suspend assumptions and enter into a genuine 'thinking together'" (Senge, 1990, p. 10). Team leaders must recognize the patterns of defensiveness because, if they go unrecognized, they undermine learning. If defensiveness is "surfaced creatively," it can actually accelerate learning.

MANAGEMENT ROLES

After studying the work of chief executive officers, Mintzberg (1980) identified 10 roles of formal authority that are common to the work of all managers and grouped them into three types: interpersonal, informational, and decisional. Table 2–2 shows how the roles are grouped and how leadership is identified as one of the 10 roles. In an effort to be well rounded and better suited for future management demands, practitioners can use these items as a checklist to determine the roles that they are skilled at performing and those that need improvement.

Interpersonal Roles

According to Mintzberg (1980), the three interpersonal roles focus on relationships. The figurehead role is the one exercised when a manager represents the organization or department at formal events. Examples of tasks associated with this role are official greetings for an outside group, signing certificates or letters, and attending ceremonies as a representative from the organization. The liaison role is important for developing an information system within and outside the organization. Valuable networks and partnerships can be established with suppliers, customers, and other groups when managers are skilled in making, developing, and retaining contacts. The leader role entails tasks such as employee selection, training, motivation, and development. When these tasks are successfully accomplished, followers are more inclined to integrate their personal goals with those of the organization.

Informational Roles

Informational roles relate to the gathering, transmitting, and sharing of data to persons within and outside the organization or department. Mintzberg (1980) states that communication is perhaps the most important part of a manager's job. Monitoring involves selecting the best sources of reliable information while continuously searching for new data that will help the organiza-

---

Table 2–2 Ten Managerial Roles Identified by Mintzberg (1980)

Interpersonal	Informational	Decisional
Figurehead	Monitor	Entrepreneur
Liaison	Disseminator	Disturbance Handler
Leader	Spokesperson	Resource Allocator
		Negotiator

tion progress further. Both formal and informal lines of communication are used for information searches, and unsolicited information is welcomed. The role of disseminator involves reporting information to those who need it within the organization to perform their jobs or make decisions. This can be done in writing, verbally, or through electronic media. As a spokesperson, professionals effectively communicate with others outside their department and communicate messages from the outside to their staff members.

Decisional Roles

Decision making is troublesome to many managers if they have not taken the time to collect necessary information from interpersonal and informational sources. As entrepreneurs, managers voluntarily make decisions about their departments after learning about trends in the field and changes in the environment in which they operate. They take the initiative to move ahead without being asked to do so. Disturbance handlers arise in times of crisis, especially when the causes are beyond their control during situations such as strikes, disasters, and other times when the organization is threatened. Resource allocation involves decisions regarding how and to whom the department's resources will be distributed. This includes tasks such as setting priorities, identifying scope of services, budgeting, and establishing policies that govern the use of resources. The skills of negotiation are essential in organizations that have wide cultural diversity, resistance to change, and complex interdisciplinary communications. Negotiation not only occurs between the manager and employees of the institution but also between managers and customers, suppliers, and community groups.

Crucial Activities

Mintzberg's (1980) 10 managerial roles have been further divided into four role sets (Kovner & Channing, 1994). Table 2–3 illustrates the 30 crucial activities for the successful leader under these four categories. The first, motivating others, is the process of identifying the required skills for improved performance and assisting subordinates in obtaining them. This can be difficult when subordinates are inherited.

Scanning the environment deals with identifying potential weaknesses and strengths, much like SWOT (strengths, weaknesses, opportunities, and threats) analysis. Continuing education and attendance at trade association meetings are also important aspects because networking in these settings provides valuable insights into the successes and failures of one's peers in other organizations.

Negotiating the political terrain is a key element in determining how to accomplish goals within the organizational structure. It involves knowing who the

Table 2–3 Thirty Crucial Activities for the Successful Leader (Kovner & Channing, 1994)

Role Set	Mintzberg's (1980) 10 Managerial Roles	30 Crucial Activities
Motivating others	Figurehead Liaison Leader	1. Recruiting professionals 2. Making decisions regarding professional and managerial salaries 3. Devising work procedures for professionals 4. Devising work procedures for nonprofessionals 5. Promoting and rewarding professionals and managers 6. Conducting employee and management development and training 7. Disciplining professional and managerial employees 8. Motivating and directing immediate subordinates 9. Dealing with personal and interpersonal problems
Scanning the environment	Monitor Disseminator	10. Market research 11. Product research 12. Long-range planning 13. Criteria systems development to control quality 14. Decisions regarding financial and management information systems
Negotiating the political terrain	Spokesperson Negotiator Disturbance handler	15. Conducting public relations 16. Lobbying 17. Conducting labor negotiations 18. Establishing agreements with other institutions 19. Negotiating with powerful external organizations 20. Creating and changing professional job unity 21. Making decisions regarding changes in decision-making and authority structure 22. Influencing decisions of administration or the board 23. Influencing decisions made by the medical staff 24. Arbitrating between internal units and/or other departments
Generating and allocating resources	Entrepreneur Resource allocator	25. Decisions regarding buying procedure 26. Decisions regarding working capital expenses 27. Decisions regarding maintaining building and equipment 28. Decisions regarding charges and prices for services 29. Decisions regarding new construction 30. Decisions regarding general operation

Source: Reprinted with permission from A.R. Kovner and A.H. Channing, *Really Trying: A Career Guide for the Health Services Manager,* 2nd Edition, © 1994, Health Administration Press.

key players are and where the power is so that one can successfully carry the mission forward.

Generating and allocating resources is not a new concept, but in today's climate of shrinking resources it is important to become extremely adept at this process to meet future challenges. Resources include, of course, the financial aspects: operating budget, capital budget, budget monitoring, and staffing. In addition, one needs to become proficient at managing other, less tangible resources, such as time and space.

EMERGING LEADERSHIP THEORIES

In contrast to the hierarchical leadership styles to which we are accustomed, today's successful and emerging styles of leadership are synchronized with the needs and wants of the workplace and the members of the team. Although there are literally hundreds of styles of leadership, we focus here on a selected few that are emerging as the preeminent tools of current and future effectiveness.

Collaborative Leadership

The essence of collaborative leadership is teamwork. Engaging staff members in cooperation and collaboration acts as a motivator in and of itself. Collaborative leaders invite discussion, are willing to adjust the task to fit the needs of the employees, and work with employees to develop cooperative goals (Tjosvold, 1986). This leadership style requires the manager to be engaged in the workplace, have firsthand knowledge of the issues at hand, be familiar with the things that excite and frustrate employees, and have a willingness to share his or her own hopes, feelings, and values without dictating. The leader's function is to help employees accomplish their tasks. According to Tjosvold (1986), the steps for practicing collaborative leadership are as follows:

1. The manager introduces the new project and explains its importance.
2. Employees discuss the project and how it relates to their present work and their own aspirations.
3. The manager and employees develop a team feeling. They know that they will all gain by a successful project and will share its rewards.
4. If necessary, the project is modified so that the team is confident that it can be successful.
5. Tasks are distributed fairly and efficiently; needed resources are allocated.
6. Norms and procedures that encourage managers and employees to discuss problems productively are established.

7. Managers and employees get regular feedback on their group progress and confront inadequate performance.

8. The team members share their rewards and celebrate their common achievement.

Participative Management

This may be one of the most effective contemporary management processes. It begins with a genuine respect for staff members and an appreciation of the unique gifts that each one contributes. Its basic premise is an understanding that each of us, no matter what position we hold in the company, has the same rights and needs to be involved, to understand our mission, to be accountable, and to make a commitment and that relationships count more than structure (DuPree, 1989).

For example, it would seem rather senseless for the hospital chief executive officer to make a decision about the type of dishwashing machine to buy when the food service workers who operate the machine have more knowledge of the pitfalls of equipment failure and more investment in the quality of their daily work routine. Would the department head, as a leader, be committed to the decisions of his or her superiors if he or she was not allowed to have input into the evaluative process? It is clear that successful participative management is built on trust. Trust must work both ways. Put simply, staff will trust in a manager's leadership when the manager trusts in their ability to contribute.

Roving leadership, or "leadership by walking around" as it once was called, is a key element in the day-to-day expression of participative management (DuPree, 1989). Roving leadership demands a great deal of trust and a clear sense of interdependence. A roving leader is someone who is there when needed. Being ready to step in and take action when prompted by urgency, or just being physically present in the work area to see what is going on, is a critical facet of effective leadership.

Servant leadership is somewhat like participative management, but it also emphasizes another dimension—the responsibility of management to ensure that all the resources necessary for employees to do the job correctly are provided on a consistent and timely basis so that workers can reach the highest level of achievement possible. These resources include the correct raw foods, supplies, equipment, environment, training, schedules and other necessary information. When workers have all these things at their fingertips, independent work is easily accomplished in a productive manner while on-the-job stress is diminished. As a result, the manager's role is therefore shifted more toward supporting the worker. Leaders focus more on management of information as they provide and monitor resources to get the job done right (Jackson, 1995b).

Transformational Leadership

This is probably the most difficult style of leadership to achieve, yet it is undoubtedly the most rewarding. The transformational leader pursues a cost–benefit, economic exchange to meet subordinates' current material and psychic needs in return for "contracted" services rendered by the subordinates (DuPree, 1989). The intent is to recognize the existing needs of subordinates and to assist them in elevating to a higher level of need according to a hierarchy of needs (Figure 2–1). Once the primary needs in the hierarchy (physiological and safety) are met, they stop becoming strong motivators, and the need to fulfill the secondary needs (social, esteem, and self-actualization) drives a person to act.

Transformational leaders arouse strengths in subordinates through motivation, so that performance exceeds expectation. This can generally be accomplished in one of the following ways: by raising the level of awareness about the importance and value of desired outcomes and means of achieving them, by encouraging transcendence of self-interests for the interests of the team, or by

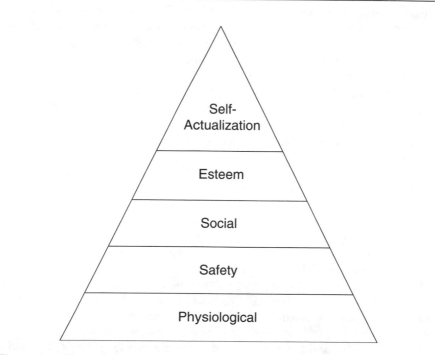

Figure 2–1 Hierarchy of needs.

altering the level of need in the hierarchy or expanding the needs and wants of subordinates. To be an effective transformational leader, the leader must be able to transcend the culture of the organization and visualize the big picture. This style of leadership heightens the aspirations of subordinates, and in doing so it ultimately achieves a higher sense of satisfaction and effectiveness in them.

LEADERSHIP SKILLS

Although management theorists differ with regard to the combination of characteristics that makes exceptional leaders, many specific skills are found repeatedly in the literature. This section describes the most important success criteria for leadership in the field of food and nutrition services.

Communication Skills

Communication is the cornerstone of leadership. In successful organizations, good communication fosters a common bond of interdependence, mutual trust, interlocking contributions, and simple joy (DuPree, 1989). Communication occurs in three forms: written, verbal, and behavioral. It is both a language process and a people process and therefore requires sound interpersonal skills. An effective leader must be able to communicate as a receptive listener, a clear and concise distributor of information, and a spokesperson for his or her department to administration and vice versa.

Communication is influenced by the respective characteristics of the sender and the receiver, such as language, religion, education, culture, life experiences, and work. Understanding between both parties is essential to ensure that the message conveyed is the message received and understood. This requires an effective leader to be understood by, as well as to understand, others.

Written communications, in the form of memoranda, letters, reports, proposals, policies, and justifications, require that the effective leader be skilled in language as well as grammar. Verbal communication is more direct and usually occurs in person-to-person encounters, such as when the leader is instructing employees, conducting meetings, attending business meetings, holding team meetings, and making presentations. Communication through behavior is a bit more complicated and described later in this chapter.

Effective communication depends on two things: how the message was sent, and how the message was received. Feedback, an important component of effective communication, confirms that the message received was indeed the message intended. Some basic rules of communication are shown in Exhibit 2–1.

Byers, Shanklin, and Hoover (1994) describe four basic channels of communication within an organization. *Upward vertical* communication is from subor-

Exhibit 2–1 Tips for Effective Communications

Senders should:
- plan the message and identify the objective sought
- determine the appropriate type of language
- seek to maintain credibility through honesty
- be aware of the message behind the message (i.e., the body language)
- be sensitive to the receiver's perspective
- encourage feedback

Listeners should:
- listen carefully and not interrupt
- consider the sender's perspective
- create a supportive atmosphere for the sender and be aware of body language
- summarize and ask exploratory questions to clarify the message

Both senders and receivers should:
- follow up on a message to ensure that it was sent as intended or received as intended
- avoid the temptation to provide too much information in sending the communication or in getting feedback on it

Source: Data from B.A. Byers, C. W. Shanklin, and L. C. Hoover, *Food Service Manual for Health Care Institutions*, The American Hospital Association, 1994.

dinates to superiors, such as performance or activity reports. When there are several levels between communicators, essential information may be omitted. Successful leaders will acknowledge this and seek accuracy of information as well as avoid depending on lower level staff for essential information. *Downward vertical* communication occurs when superiors communicate with subordinates. This can be for information sharing, issuing directives, and performance evaluations. Most managers believe that they are more effective at this type of communication than they may actually be. A successful leader will examine his or her own patterns of downward communication and work to strengthen any possible weaknesses. *Horizontal* communication is between organizational departments and is essential to ensuring sound interdepartmental cooperation and success. Finally, one of the most informative ways of communication is through the grapevine. This is also referred to as *informal* communication. It is a good means by which to gauge general attitudes and the atmosphere, but if relied upon as a sole source of communication, it can impede a leader's interests. To minimize the potential negative effects of the grapevine, leaders can strive to keep their employees well informed with as much information as possible.

In addition to listening and speaking effectively, leaders benefit when they are proficient in reading skills. Although one would expect that most managers have learned these in grade school, it is amazing how many are deficient in this area. Practitioners are expected to respond to and generate reams of paperwork today, and if these skills are not strong one will surely fall behind. Most colleges and universities provide remedial training in these skills today. Speed reading courses are also advisable, if only to help one get through tons of professional and trade journals each month.

Interdisciplinary Collaboration

More than ever before, it is imperative that managers see the organizational structure without departmental boundaries. When a dissatisfied patient does not return to a facility because he or she perceives the service as uncaring, it does not matter which department was at fault. Interdepartmental communication and cooperation are everyone's responsibility: therefore, everyone is to blame if a system fails.

The Joint Commission actually found the need to include interdisciplinary communication and cooperation in its standards because it found them lacking in many facilities that had poor patient outcomes. Many feel that poor interdisciplinary cooperation stems from the lack of integration of professions in the university setting, where students develop their first impressions of the field. Some attempts have been made to remedy this situation. For example, in the School of Nursing at Baylor University in Dallas, Texas, a new elective entitled "Collaboration in Health Care" has been added. The course is subtitled "Who Are All Those Other People, What Do They Do, and How Can We Do It Better, Together?" McEwen (1994), who works with this program, states:

> In order to adequately answer the current outcry among Americans for dramatic changes in the current system, alterations in traditional health care provision must occur. One component of this change should begin during education of health care providers. Ultimately, cross-discipline courses should be encouraged, at least to some extent. The idea is not to overlap disciplines or to infringe on another discipline's territory, but to enable providers to better understand the variety of roles and practices in order to work together better to deliver higher quality care within a "true" system. (p. 307)

The department with which food and nutrition practitioners interface the most is nursing services. Addressing nursing relations, O'Sullivan Maillet (1993) stated "The team concept of nutrition care needs to be developed. Turf battles have interfered before but, as the roles of nutrition professionals of all levels continue to expand, we must clarify their uniqueness" (p. 45).

Grindel (1994) encourages practitioners to work together to identify how overlapping skills should be used. In her presentation at the 1994 convention of the ADA, she suggested the following:

- Recognize the expertise of others and communicate.
- Help each other by sharing assessment data. Do not bury data in the charts, where it takes too much time to find them.
- Engage in collaborative management of patient symptoms related to nutrition status.
- Make food preference cards accessible to nursing staff, or put them by the bedside because they are an important part of patients' care.
- Use computerized information when available.
- Interface directly with physicians, and be patient if you need to wait for a response.
- Realize that nursing is overloaded, too!

Motivating Employees

"Motivation is the process by which individuals are stimulated to act on their innermost needs, desires, and drives" (Byers et al., 1994, p. 30). Some theories of motivation have been described previously in this chapter, and a hierarchy of needs has been illustrated (see Figure 2–1).

There are many sources in the literature that contain complete descriptions of motivational theories, and this information will not be repeated here. Nevertheless, it is essential for managers to understand that financial rewards are not always necessary because there are many other ways that they can motivate their employees. The way employees are treated and the atmosphere of the workplace are two important factors. Everyone wants to feel a part of a team and be recognized as a special and unique individual. When managers show that they appreciate employees' contributions, regardless of their differences, their subordinates feel as if they are a part of the team. Successful managers recognize and celebrate diversity among employees, and this explains the current trend toward recognizing and respecting cultural differences in the workplace.

"A company's culture cannot be proclaimed or easily manipulated. It consists of the deeply shared values and beliefs of its people, which show up in how the company and its people behave" (Champy, 1996, p. 96). It has been found that, unlike the case of past practices, employees cannot be expected to conform to the corporate culture; rather, appreciation of diversity in the workplace yields more positive outcomes.

Some ways to demonstrate a sensitivity to cultural differences are knowing what holidays staff members celebrate, sharing the meaning of different holidays with others who do not celebrate them, and creating a climate of "us" through the sharing of and caring for each other's values and beliefs. People develop trust in each other only when they think others share or respect their beliefs.

Of course, say Kovner and Channing (1994, p. 63), "people have different ideas about what is important or good." For example, a boss can have tremendous ability and intelligence; be friendly, cheerful, enthusiastic, and witty; and appear open. Yet he or she may also have an enormous ego and be dishonest, hot-tempered, and inconsiderate. This executive might read employees' mail and insist that they never close their office door. In some employees, this might inspire a determination to do only what is specifically requested and to look out for themselves rather than their boss' or the organization's interests. Yet this executive may be successful in meeting the demands of superiors and in attracting and retaining competent staff.

Another boss might be able, friendly, cheerful, open, witty, honest, considerate, intelligent, and calm. If he or she has a big ego, it is concealed in everyday relations. This boss obtains the resources necessary for staff to accomplish their work and is always available to help with a job-related or personal problem. The staff's response may be to do anything this manager asks and to give much higher priority to their boss' concerns and to the organization's. Yet this manager may be perceived by other subordinates and colleagues as cold, ruthless, and insufficiently concerned with the rights of others.

One other common example is when dietitians tend to disbelieve leaders who appear to be financially motivated rather than patient focused. Such distrust must be overcome through behavior and communication with the leader for the department to be managed successfully on the basis of trust.

Demographic characteristics are issues because, no matter how the leader manages, staff members are likely to question whether the leader is "one of us." Therefore, if a manager's socioeconomic, ethnic, and/or religious background is different from that of his or her subordinates, it will be extremely important to create a climate of "togetherness." This can be accomplished first by the leader developing a sensitivity to other cultures and social values.

Leaders vary with regard to their management personalities or personae. According to Kovner and Channing (1994), "Managerial personality is an important aspect of the way managers are perceived, of whether they are trusted. Personality can have a significant impact on managerial effectiveness and survival" (p. 63). Those who present a good example and share power with employees encourage trust while motivating their staff to take on higher levels of responsibility.

Although difficult, successful leaders will be able to see themselves as others do and, without attempting to change their natural tendencies, will become able to adapt to situations with awareness of their own weaknesses and utilization of their natural strengths. Because personality may affect the way subordinates share information, the leader must become adept at eliciting necessary information and feelings from his or her subordinates. This is of paramount importance to effective team building and successful leadership.

Byers et al. (1994) suggest a variety of activities that can motivate employees. They emphasize the importance of designing jobs that are interesting and challenging to each worker and allowing employees to set their own goals within the limits of the department's goals and objectives. Informal rewards, such as praise, can be combined, when appropriate, with formal rewards, such as benefits, salary increases, bonuses, and opportunities for advancement. When performance is not up to par, the positive aspects should continue to be praised while suggestions for improvement are offered; subordinates should not be threatened or punished. One worthwhile strategy is not to criticize people but to explain why certain behavior is not acceptable in terms of patient care or customer satisfaction goals.

Employees need to feel important, so that it is beneficial to encourage, help, and support them in their work. To earn trust, managers should protect employee privacy and confidential information. To demonstrate trust, responsibilities can be delegated. Above all, the work environment, including its layout, equipment, and people, should be responsive to employee needs.

Leading by Example

Modeling the performance standards that are established for subordinates is also a key element for successful leadership. The old adage "Do as I say, not as I do" simply will not produce desired results in the next millennium. Shifts in our society's culture demand that managers behave as they expect others to.

The example that managers set for their subordinates may actually speak louder than their words. If they are viewed as being trusting, then they will be trusted. If they are perceived as being consistent, then they can realistically expect consistency in their subordinates. If the goal of quality patient services is to be realized, managers must exemplify the type of behavior they expect to see in their staff: friendliness, courtesy, and responsiveness to others. When managers do not mirror the behaviors expected in their subordinates, they have failed as successful leaders.

Empowering Teams

The essence of empowerment is the investment of subordinates with authority or legal power so that they can self-manage through intrinsic motivation. In general, empowerment is a positive outcome of the participative style of leadership. Whether given to individuals or to teams, empowerment works well to identify priorities and to resolve conflicts.

Empowerment affords the leader the opportunity to delegate effectively and at the same time provides subordinates with the resources and support to complete the task at hand. It may be given with strictly defined boundaries, or it may be given within loose controls. Every situation may warrant a different type of empowerment. If employees are expected to be responsible for their actions, they need to be empowered with the tools to act appropriately. Properly executed empowerment will naturally lead to a reduction of the management structure.

Through the process of collective inquiry, teams of employees are better able to practice creative thinking and to come up with innovative solutions to the problems at hand. This fosters personal and collective mastery, which encourages the team to think in nontraditional ways and take more risks. New paradigms are established and tested, and these efforts lead to growth in the body of knowledge available for use in the profession. In some cases, revolutionary discoveries are made that affect the way practitioners do things throughout the industry.

Mentoring and Coaching Skills

Traditionally, mentoring has been the process whereby a young person is guided in all aspects of his or her career by a senior, wiser member of the organization. This relationship generally has occurred in a learning context with a continuing one-to-one relationship between an older (more experienced) individual and a younger (less experienced) person.

It is believed that having a mentor and mentee establish goals and objectives will lead to a long-lasting relationship through which the mentee acquires new skills and knowledge. Darling and Schatz (1991) identified six specific areas for guidance:

1. exploring career options
2. choosing a career path and mastering the career role
3. resolving problems or doubts
4. developing skills and knowledge and expanding beyond the present career role
5. developing strategies
6. expanding or broadening abilities

The outcome of effective mentoring is that the mentee develops the ability to direct his or her own career, there is career satisfaction, and the profession is benefited as a result through staff retention, diversification, and effective use of talents.

Blanchard et al. (1990) discuss four styles of leadership that can be selected depending upon the situation and developmental levels of employees. As subordinates progress in motivation and skill, the leadership style can progress from directive to coaching, supportive, and finally delegation. Coaching is an approach whereby the manager provides close supervision while giving and obtaining feedback, explaining decisions, and encouraging progress in a positive manner. "No coach can make a difference unless the player has an intrinsic desire to achieve something. But given that intrinsic desire, a coach can draw out efforts and understanding which the individual might not access as easily on his or her own" (Senge, Kleiner, Roberts, Ross, & Smith, 1994, p. 197). The first task of a coach is to model the desired behavior and to encourage personal mastery in subordinates. While coaching employees, one should first discuss the desired method or behavior and explain its implications for the department, other employees, customers or patients, and the subordinates themselves. Role playing often works well to establish the advantages and disadvantages of different methods or behaviors. Subordinates need to understand clearly the desired goal and expectations, and feedback is an essential component at all stages in the process.

Decision Making

Decision making is the process of evaluating a situation, considering the alternatives, and selecting the one most likely to produce the results desired. This is an essential component of the planning process, and to be successful managers need to make effective and timely decisions on a routine basis. To do this, personal biases must be eliminated and clear objectives determined. Fear of change or risk taking can also be immobilizing road blocks in the decision-making process.

According to Byers et al. (1994), the decision-making process can be broken down into five simple steps:

1. Define the problem or establish objectives.
2. Identify alternative outcomes and solutions.
3. Evaluate the relative values of alternatives.
4. Activate an action plan for implementing the best choice.
5. Follow through, and monitor the issue.

Dr. Jonas Salk, the eminent immunologist who discovered the first polio vaccine in 1955, states that problem solving is greatly enhanced when many points of view are applied:

I could solve problems more easily because I could look at them simultaneously from the viewpoints of subject and object. Through my imagination, I could even project myself in time and bring to realization intentions or imaginings as if they had actually become self-fulfilling prophecies. . . . Being able to see things—and oneself—from only one perspective is limiting. (Salk, 1995, p. 13)

For this reason, it is important to consider empowering teams to make decisions. There are some limitations to this approach. It can be time consuming, and it can be more difficult to ensure that what is agreed to will be carried forward, especially if a strong component of the team has not participated or does not agree with the decision. Nevertheless, team resolution can yield excellent results if appropriate ground rules are followed and team members leave their individual needs outside the door and strive in unselfish ways to solve the problem at hand. Sound team decisions occur only if the result is fair to all members of the team and if there is a fostering of cooperative solutions to problems. A process commonly referred to as brainstorming is quite helpful in team decision making.

When problems are encountered, successful leaders look at them as opportunities for improvement and encourage decisions that will take the organization to a higher operating level. Sometimes this entails taking risks and testing untraditional solutions to the problems at hand. Drucker (1964) noted that some of the major breakthroughs in business have resulted because managers were not afraid to take risks. He classified risks into the following categories:

- risks one must accept because they are built into the nature of the business
- risks one can afford to take
- risks one cannot afford to take
- risks one cannot afford not to take

For successful decision making, Drucker encourages managers to focus on maximizing opportunities rather than minimizing risk and to scrutinize alternatives systematically, individually and with respect to one another. He also advises managers to understand which opportunities and risks fit the immediate and long-range goals of the business.

Many managers find that, when employees are involved in decision making, buy into new solutions, and/or make a commitment to support decisions, success results even when risks are taken. This illustrates the need for routine communication, follow-up, and feedback from subordinates. It is also important to realize that managers can and do make mistakes, some of which are preventable.

For this reason, it is probably wise to implement solutions on a trial basis until everyone is confident that the right decision has been made.

Productive Conflict Resolution

Leaders are frequently called upon to act as a mediator to resolve conflicts between employees. What many fail to see is the benefit of conflict. In openly discussing conflicts, members of teams become more aware of and able to cope with problems. Knowing that others are frustrated and want change helps the team develop incentives to solve the underlying problem (Tjosvold, 1986). Therefore, conflicts help promote organizational growth and change. They draw attention to issues that impede employee motivation and productivity. Productive conflict resolution will strengthen relationships and morale as well as promote personal development.

Conflict resolution is productive when all people believe that the underlying problem is solved and a new solution created; the relationships between employees have been strengthened, and people feel that they can work together more effectively in the future; and the participants believe that their time and resources have been well spent and the effort involved was not too costly. Conflict cannot be avoided. It is a necessary part of sound leadership. When conflict is approached cooperatively, however, the benefits far outweigh the pitfalls. Exhibit 2–2 provides some brief guidelines for productive conflict resolution.

Exhibit 2–2 Guidelines for Productive Conflict Resolution

Realize that if you are not a part of the solution, you may be part of the problem.
Develop a climate in which it is OK to have conflicts.
Attempt to emphasize cooperative goals and dependence.
Use the team approach; everyone benefits from a resolution.
Show others that you understand them and their points of view.
Ask others to show that they understand you.
Identify and set out to solve the underlying reasons for the problem.
Avoid blaming others for the problem.
Do not set out to prove that you are right and others are wrong.
Avoid making others look weak and incompetent.
Be sure not to hold out for a solution that will benefit only yourself.
Refrain from bragging that you outwitted others.
Celebrate the joint successes of the team.

Source: Reprinted with permission from D. Tjosvold, *Working Together To Get Things Done*, p. 118, © 1986 Jossey-Bass Inc., Publishers. First published by Lexington Books. All rights reserved.

Stress Management

According to Senge et al. (1994), the juxtaposition of vision (what we want) and a clear picture of current reality (where we are relative to what we want) generates a positive force that they call creative tension. Creative tension can move a whole organization forward as people accept challenges to manage the tension within themselves and develop new skills that bring them closer to the goal. This type of tension is normally not detrimental.

Successful leaders know how to cope with stress, and some thrive on it. The typical type A personality of yesterday, however, will not be an acceptable role model for successful leaders of the future. Leaders who exhibit signs of stress will be viewed as being out of control and incapable of managing change. Some amount of stress is a normal, acceptable part of life and actually is favorable for variety, stimulation, and challenge. Too much stress is an obvious detriment to successful leadership, however, as well as to our own health. It is believed that stress may play a role in elevated cholesterol levels, hypertension, and weight problems. Learning to manage stress can therefore improve one's overall health and well being, improve one's work performance, and help establish one's credibility as a productive, successful leader.

There is much advice on the market for stress management on audiotape, in written literature, and from health care providers. Obviously, physical exercise, breathing exercises, emotional outlets, and relaxing hobbies play a role. Exhibit 2–3 summarizes some recommendations that are applicable to health care practitioners for taking hold of stress.

A Word on Ethical Conduct

Ethics can be defined as moral principles or a code of right and wrong. Ethics can no longer be perceived as a matter of personal scruples or an individual act of wrongdoing. Typically, unethical organizational practices involve the unspoken or explicit cooperation of others. They often reflect on the values and beliefs that define an organization's culture. Successful leaders are accountable for developing organizational practices that facilitate ethical conduct. Such practices and policies should encompass food service purchasing, financial management, patient care issues, the nutritional quality of recipes, and any matters that affect the integrity of the work performed.

A case in point is Sears, Roebuck & Company, which in 1992 instituted severe minimum sales and work quotas under the threat of transfers and reductions in work hours (Paine, 1994). New organizational pressure was exerted, but management failed to ethically appropriate between unnecessary service and legitimate repairs, and employees were left to their own devices to meet

Exhibit 2–3 Taking Hold of Stress

1. **Recognize what can be changed; accept what cannot.** If a wish could only change things . . . but it can't. And a wish won't bring comfort to an unpleasant situation. Trying to change the unchangeable means continuing to suffer stress. If you can't change a situation, try to accept it.

2. **Break big problems into little ones.** When a task seems unmanageable and over-whelming, break it into smaller, more manageable tasks. If your department must be downsized, focus on one operational area at a time. If you have a deadline for a 50 page report, develop a plan for completing sections of the report. Set a deadline for each section. Step by step, you will finish the report on time.

3. **Eliminate as many stressors as you can.** Certainly you can't get rid of all the stressors in your life, but you can rid yourself of some of them. For example:
   a) To clear the clutter on your desk, throw out unused odds and ends; weed out papers that you no longer use, pass on information that might help subordinates or peers.
   b) Turn off the radio, shut the door, and get rid of annoying or distracting background noise.
   c) Give up 1–2 activities per week to free up some extra time for yourself. Name one or two stressors in your life that you can eliminate. Take time to do this now and save yourself several hours of stress in the future!

4. **Return stress to its rightful owner.** Don't let other people burden you with their problems. If you find you're suffering from someone else's stress, it's time to return the stress to its rightful owner.
   Be direct: Be willing to say "I'm sorry things are not going well for you, but I really can't make it my problem." You don't need to be rude or insensitive, just be straight-forward.
   Be definite: If you don't want to do something, say "no." You might end up negotiating if you don't sound definite.
   Be honest: Returning stress to its rightful owner does not mean avoiding your own responsibilities or unpleasant tasks. Sometimes it helps to distinguish your problems from those that are not really yours. Consider asking the person why he/she asked you to do something. The answer should help you clarify whether the problem or task appropriately belongs to you. If a subordinate is the source of the stress, engage him/her in developing a plan of correction rather than assuming the responsibility yourself.

5. **Avoid predictably stressful situations.** At certain times you have probably placed yourself *voluntarily* in situations that cause stress: long supermarket lines, busy traffic, parties with people you don't like. On the other hand, there may be some stressful situations that you *can* avoid.

6. **Remove yourself from the source of stress.** If you feel stressed as a result of your job or spouse, take a few minutes to get away *physically*. Get up and take a walk, enjoy being alone, refresh yourself, and then go back to face the situation.

7. **Don't overreact.** Reacting dramatically to a situation exaggerates, not relieves, the stress connected with it. Next time you feel like yelling at a colleague or family member, take a few minutes to cool down and consider how the other might be viewing the situation. Then try to discuss your concerns quietly.

Courtesy of The American Red Cross in Greater New York, *Taking Hold of Stress; a fact sheet.*

quotas. When matters became public, management quickly eliminated the quotas and took responsibility for instituting ethical goal-setting systems. Similarly, when a Beech-Nut employee voiced concerns about the purity of its 100% apple juice, he was accused of not being a team player. His manager was afraid to reduce profits by $700,000 and wound up with a $25 million loss in 1987 when a Food and Drug Administration investigation revealed that the company was selling adulterated product.

In the everyday routine of getting work done, people sometimes unconsciously violate the professional code of ethics in blatant or subtle ways. Jackson (1995a) emphasizes the importance for professionals in food and nutrition services to know where to draw the line on gifts from suppliers, especially those that are especially good at using subtle tactics that often lead well-intentioned people to start compromising. Gifts come in many forms that are not included in purchasing agreements, such as books, office supplies, entertainment, the promise of professional contacts, educational opportunities, overly generous samples, and other so-called promotional materials. The best way to handle this problem is for staff members to say politely that it is against their own personal ethics and the facility's policy; if the firm wants to make a donation to the hospital so that patients can benefit from their kind efforts, this would be acceptable (and also a tax-deductible expense for the firm). In this way, a clear message is sent: One wants to avoid risky games that only lead to more compromises and a bad example for others. The word quickly spreads, and the staff become off limits for future attempts.

Charting in medical records also presents ethical concerns. Entries should not be pre- or postdated, and one person should not chart for another or destroy, erase, or change any portion of the record. If an error is made, a single line can be drawn through it with an initial and date. Then the reason is added, such as "charted on wrong patient" or "calculation error." It is also not appropriate to use the chart for showing superiority or criticizing another member of the health care team who does not cooperate, respond, or provide what one feels to be good medical practice. There are other avenues for settling arguments or proving one's point.

In addition, the medical record is hospital property, and information should not be copied or disclosed without permission. Many patients and families have been hurt when they overheard their personal problems being discussed in hospital elevators, hallways, restrooms, and even grocery stores! Confidentiality applies to other things as well. A supplier might ask for the prices of a competitor, or an employee may ask about another's salary or job evaluation. Sharing such information and saying "Don't tell anyone about this" represent a sure clue of poor ethics.

When leaders are honest and trustworthy, they create the possibility of more truth around them. Openness and trust are essential to building ethical behavior in organizations. If a manager discloses confidential information to an employee, it is clear that the manager cannot be trusted with personal and job-related concerns. It is a good idea to discuss policies and issues that lie in ethical gray areas with staff to help them avoid the intent or appearance of any type of compromise.

Many integrity initiatives are really compliance-based initiatives, aimed at ensuring that all regulatory agency requirements are met. For an organization to be truly ethical, integrity must go deeper. Organizations are best served when exemplary behavior is encouraged to prevent damaging misconduct. The hallmarks of effective integrity strategy shown in Exhibit 2–4 are offered as sound measures to ensure integrity (Paine, 1994).

LEADERSHIP SKILLS FOR THE FUTURE

It is expected that health care facilities will continue to downsize, rightsize, and in some cases close. This has been evident since the 1980s. From 1980 to 1991, 603 acute care hospitals and 225 special care facilities closed. The trend continues as lengths of stay and inpatient days continue to decrease and large health care networks take over independently run facilities. As occupancy rates drop, so must health care expenditures. Health care reform, although not as yet enacted, has already had a significant impact on hospital utilization and will continue to do so with increased numbers of managed care programs, and the movement toward outpatient services and ambulatory care settings.

Managers in the field of food service and nutrition care will need to adapt quickly to changes and improve their skills to ensure leadership roles in the future health care industry. The following are suggestions to achieve success in this effort (Beckman, 1991):

Exhibit 2–4 Hallmarks of an Effective Integrity Strategy

The guiding values and commitments make sense and are clearly communicated.

Organizational leaders are personally committed, credible, and willing to take action on the values they espouse.

The espoused values are integrated into the normal channels of management decision making and are reflected in the organization's critical activities.

The organization's systems and structures support and reinforce its values.

Managers throughout the organization have the decision-making skills, knowledge, and competencies needed to make ethically sound decisions on a day-to-day basis.

Source: Adapted and reprinted by permission of *Harvard Business Review*. An excerpt from "Managing for Organizational Integrity" by L. Sharp Paine, Issue 72. © 1994 by the President and Fellows of Harvard College, all rights reserved.

- *Be creative.* Managers will succeed by encouraging innovative staff performance, involving subordinates in decision making, and rewarding them for their contributions.
- *Form teams.* This will foster greater employee satisfaction, personal mastery, empowerment, and more effective problem solving.
- *Be risk takers.* If leaders show that it is acceptable to try nontraditional methods, they will foster ingenuity and resourcefulness on the part of their subordinates.
- *Expect failure.* Sometimes this needs to be stated to subordinates so that they know that creativity cannot be hampered by fear of failure. If one has not failed at anything lately, one is simply not trying enough.
- *Encourage continuous learning.* Practitioners cannot afford to dwell on errors and waste time solving unsolvable problems. Instead, they need to tap employees' commitment and capacity to learn and help them grow from experience so that higher levels of competence and responsibility can be achieved.
- *Communicate effectively.* When leaders improve their written, verbal, and listening skills and use body language and modeling effectively, trust within teams and superior performance are promoted.
- *Symbolize everything.* For example, at McDonald's Corporation, from chief executive officers to managers, everyone spends time working the grill. This not only helps everyone learn how to communicate with staff but also sends a message to every employee that those in management are willing to get their hands dirty.
- *Benchmark.* By comparing performance with that of other operators and finding better methods and systems through sharing of information with colleagues, leaders can see more clearly where they are and plan where they want to be.
- *Walk around.* Instead of hiding behind a desk, leaders need to be visible and involved with the daily activities of their subordinates.

REFERENCES

Arensberg, M.B.F., Schiller, M.R., Vivian, V.M, Johnson, W.A., & Strasser, S. (1995). Transformational leadership of clinical nutrition managers. *Journal of the American Dietetic Association, 96*(1), 39–45.

Argyris, C. (1990). *Overcoming organizational defenses: Facilitating organizational learning.* Boston: Allyn & Bacon.

Barker, A., Foltz, M., Arensberg, M.B.F., & Schiller, M.R. (1994). *Leadership in dietetics: Achieving a vision from the future.* Chicago: American Dietetic Association.

Beckman, J.D. (1991). More tools for the nineties. *Healthcare Forum Journal, 66*, 10.

Blanchard, K., Carew, D., & Parisi-Carew, E. (1990). *The one-minute manager builds high performance teams.* New York: William Morrow.

Byers, B.A., Shanklin, C.W., & Hoover, L.C. (1994). *Food service manual for health care institutions.* Chicago: American Hospital Association.

Champy, J. (1996). *Reengineering management: The mandate for new leadership.* New York: Harper Business.

Darling, L.W., & Schatz, P.E. (1991). Mentoring needs of the dietitian: The mentoring self-management program model. *Journal of the American Dietetic Association, 91*(4), 454–458.

Dowling, R., & Norton, C. (1990). The management component of our profession. *Journal of the American Dietetic Association, 90*(8), 1065–1066.

Drucker, P.F. (1964). *Management for results: Economic tasks and risk-taking decisions.* New York: Harper & Row.

Drucker, P.F. (1992). *Managing for the future: The 1990's and beyond.* New York: Truman Talley Books/Plume.

DuPree, M. (1989). *Leadership as an art.* New York: Dell.

Grindel, C.G. (1994, October). *Developing successful alliances with other health professionals.* Presented at the 1994 annual meeting of the American Dietetic Association, Orlando, FL.

Halling, J.F., & Abbott Hess, M. (1995). Vision vs. reality: ADA members as food/food management experts. *Journal of the American Dietetic Association, 95*(2), 169–170.

Jackson, R. (1995a). Frequent violations of the professional code of ethics. *Hospital Food & Nutrition Focus, 11*(7), 2, 8.

Jackson, R. (1995b). Qualities of an effective leader. *Hospital Food & Nutrition Focus, 12*(1), 2.

Joint Commission on Accreditation of Healthcare Organizations. (1995). *1996 Accreditation manual for hospitals.* Oakbrook Terrace, IL: Author.

Kovner, A.R., & Channing, A.H. (1994). *Really trying: A career guide for the health services manager.* Ann Arbor, MI: Health Administration Press.

McEwen, M. (1994). Promoting interdisciplinary collaboration. *Nursing and Health Care, 15*(6), 305–307.

Mintzberg, H. (1980). *The nature of managerial work.* Englewood Cliffs, NJ: Prentice-Hall.

Nightengale, E. (1986). *Lead the field* (audiocassette). Niles, IL: Nightengale Connant.

O'Sullivan Maillet, J. (1993). Vignettes in dietetic leadership: Dietetic education. In J.D. Gussler (Ed.), *Models of nursing and dietetic leadership: What can we learn from each other?* (pp. 45–46). Columbus, OH: Ross Laboratories.

Paine, L.S. (1994). Managing for organizational integrity. *Harvard Business Review, 72,* 106–117.

Peck, S.M. (1993). *The road less traveled.* New York: Simon & Schuster.

Ross, A. (1992). *Cornerstones of leadership for health services executives.* Ann Arbor, MI: Health Administration Press.

Salk, J. (1995). Dr. Jonas Salk's way to approach...and solve...problems. *Bottom Line Personal, 16*(15), 13–14.

Senge, P.M. (1990). *The fiftth discipline: The art and practice of the learning organization.* New York: Doubleday Currency.

Senge, P.M., Kleiner, A., Roberts, C., Ross, R.B., & Smith, B.J. (1994). *The fifth discipline fieldbook: Strategies and tools for building a learning organization.* New York: Doubleday Currency.

Tjosvold, D. (1986). *Working together to get things done.* New York: Lexington Books.

3

Management Strategies

Brigid Connolly Sullivan

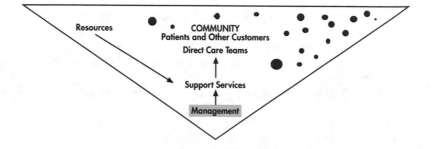

The traditional methods used for deciding how departmental activities are planned, directed, coordinated, and improved have been challenged more in the last decade than ever before. "Nothing is simple anymore. Nothing is stable. The business environment is changing before our eyes, rapidly, radically, perplexingly" (Champy, 1996, p. 9).

In his book *Reengineering Management: The Mandate for New Leadership,* Champy (1996) notes that everything is in question and that the old ways of managing no longer work. The organization charts, the compensation schemes, the hierarchies, the vertical organization, the whole tool kit of command-and-control management techniques no longer work. As a result, he advises that the following measures be taken:

> All operations must be submitted to a thorough critique of their usefulness—of their very existence—in terms of the value they produce for the company—value that must eventually be judged in markets by customers. All employees (including those in all remaining levels of management) must put themselves through a continuous questioning of how their work adds value. And finally (perhaps firstly), if all these radical changes are to come about, there may have to be an equally radical change in the culture of the enterprise. (p. 40)

The major factors that resulted in a need for redesign of the health care system include consumer demands for quality, more intense competition, dwindling financial resources, and the problem of fragmented services, which stimulated the current trend toward patient-focused care.

This chapter discusses the functions of management and presents strategies for redesigning systems that provide nutrition and food services to patients and other customers in the health care setting. It includes three of the four major management functions: planning, directing, and coordinating. The fourth management function, improving, is quite an extensive topic and therefore is addressed separately in Chapter 14. A framework using the four management functions was selected because it is familiar to most practitioners and has been incorporated into the 1996 standards of the Joint Commission on Accreditation of Healthcare Organizations (Joint Commission, 1995).

PLANNING

Planning is defined as determining in advance what should happen (Spears, 1995). The Joint Commission (1995) requires that leaders provide "a collaborative process to develop a mission that is reflected in long-range, strategic, and operational plans; service designs; resource allocation; and organization policies" (p. 275). Furthermore, the Joint Commission's standards state that planning includes defining a mission, a vision, and values and creating the strategic, operational, programmatic, and other plans and policies to achieve the mission and vision. Several tools that are helpful in determining how one should implement the planning process are discussed below.

Levels of Plans

Plans occur at various levels in an organization, and they take different forms. Some are quite general, as in the case of value, vision, and mission statements, which are normally determined at higher levels in an organization. Others are detailed and are most often designed at the supervisory and first-line management levels, as in the case for specific procedures such as those written for avoiding cross-contamination in food preparation areas. Spears (1995) suggests that plans can be ordered as to their number and specificity and that the number of plans required increases with their specificity. Figure 3–1 demonstrates these principles. As the number of plans in each grouping increases, the level decreases, and vice versa.

Values

Many organizations develop a value statement, which is a useful tool for communicating and simplifying the principles that guide employees at all levels. It can be as simple as a catch phrase, such as Ford Motor Company's "Quality is Job One" or Avis' "We're #1." It is important to realize that the values of the organization are best represented when employees are familiar with them and

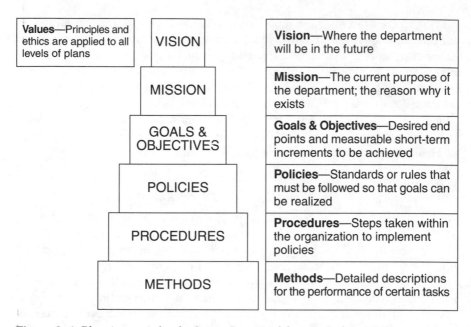

Figure 3–1 Planning at six levels. *Source:* Reprinted from R. Jackson, A Perspective on Planning, *Hospital Food & Nutrition Focus,* Vol. 12, No. 8, p. 8, © 1996, Aspen Publishers, Inc.

reflect them in all plans and decisions that are made. Samples of value statements from two health care institutions are shown in Exhibit 3–1.

Visions

A vision statement is used to identify where the organization is heading and what its priorities are for the future. Developing a vision is essential so that managers and staff can plan how to arrive at the future destination. The concept of shared vision is emphasized in Chapter 2. According to Senge (1990), "The practice of shared vision involves the skills of unearthing shared 'pictures of the future' that foster genuine commitment and enrollment rather than compliance" (p. 9). He stresses how counterproductive it is when managers try to dictate a vision because "people excel and learn not because they are told to but because they want to" (p. 9). Vision statements act to motivate staff, as can be seen in the examples shown in Exhibit 3–2.

Missions

The mission statement is a "public statement that defines the organization's commitment to a quality initiative" (Schiller, 1995, p. 368). As a typical out-

Exhibit 3–1 Sample Value Statements

Value Statement from New York Downtown Hospital

PatientFirst™ — All activities will be aimed at earning and keeping the trust and confidence of our patients, their families, and employees through the provision of quality services.

Teamwork — We will hold ourselves fully accountable for our actions and be honest and ethical in all our dealings. We will have high standards for ourselves and uphold the Hospital's high standards for quality.

Respect for the Individual — We will conduct our activities with patients, staff, families, vendors, community members, and employers with respect for the other person. This includes their ideas and actions.

Teamwork — We will work for New York Downtown Hospital first, our department second. We will support each other's strengths and weaknesses, getting help when necessary.

Value Statement from the VA Medical Center

We are guided by and committed to:
- Supporting Continuous Quality Improvement
- Enhancing Creativity, Curiosity, Investigation, and Innovation
- Ensuring Compassion and Courtesy
- Maintaining Competence through Education, Training, and Development
- Enhancing Timeliness, Efficiency, and Productivity
- Maintaining a High Level of Ethics and Integrity
- Fostering Teamwork
- Encouraging a Supportive Culturally Diverse Work Environment for Patient Care, Education, and Research

Courtesy of New York Downtown Hospital, New York, New York; and Jerry L. Pettis Memorial Veterans' Administration Medical Center, Loma Linda, California.

---

growth of the organization's strategic planning process, mission statements act to identify the organization's purpose, or the reason why it exists. This is normally done through a series of specific statements describing the intended role of the institution. A well-written mission statement will help ensure that all employees share a purpose and common ideals. Sample organizationwide mission statements are given in Exhibit 3–3.

It is important that the department also have a mission statement, so that employees can share a commitment to the department's role within the organization. The departmental mission should reflect the institution's values, visions, and mission while specifying the goods and services that are offered so that the scope of services is clearly understood. In addition, the Joint Commission recommends that the services provided meet the level of care required by patients. Some essential components of the department's mission statement can

Exhibit 3–2 Sample Vision Statements

Vision Statement from New York Downtown Hospital

To be known as a trusted neighbor able to provide a continuum of quality and accessible health care services to our resident community with special emphasis on the Chinese community living throughout the New York metropolitan region.

To be known as well as a center of excellence for ambulatory care, health maintenance, and primary care education for all who work and/or live in Lower Manhattan.

We will realize our vision through community-based facilities, related networks, and our relationship with the New York University Medical Center.

Vision Statement from the VA Medical Center

To be the health care provider of choice in the Inland Empire for veterans through compassionate quality care, education, and research.

To foster a work environment where continuous improvement is encouraged, ideas are shared, achievements are recognized, and teamwork flourishes.

Courtesy of New York Downtown Hospital, New York, New York; and Jerry L. Pettis Memorial Veterans' Administration Medical Center, Loma Linda, California.

---

be found in the following typical statement, which applies to most departments that provide food and nutrition services:

> Our mission is to engage competent staff who work effectively with others within and outside the hospital so that they are able to offer high-quality food and nutrition services by meeting the needs and expectations of the patients, employees, and guests of the facility. Effective nutrition intervention and patient education are offered to inpatients and outpatients. High-quality food services are provided for inpatients, staff, and welcomed visitors.

Goals and Objectives

Goals and objectives determine specific desired outcomes for the future. They are necessary planning tools because they are the basis for departmental operations and are more concrete than mission and vision statements. Goals identify the end points or specific outcomes that one wishes to achieve. For the mission statement shown above, the following are several possible goals:

- Nutrition assessments, treatment plans, and follow-up plans are designed to meet individual needs and expectations of inpatients and outpatients with emphasis on continuity of care.

Exhibit 3–3 Sample Mission Statements

Mission Statement from New York Downtown Hospital

New York Downtown Hospital is a community teaching hospital principally serving the people who live or work in Lower Manhattan.

New York Downtown Hospital offers services and technology appropriate to a community hospital with emphasis on outreach and ambulatory services. New York Downtown Hospital achieves access to specialized services for its patients and community through formal affiliation with an academic medical center.

As a teaching hospital, New York Downtown Hospital will conduct graduate and/or undergraduate educational programs and provide clinical experience for physicians, nurses, and other health professionals.

As a community hospital, New York Downtown Hospital will offer to its patients, medical staff, and employees a caring environment that emphasizes the value of patient dignity and employee and professional pride.

The program and services of New York Downtown Hospital will, within the limits of its resources, respond to the needs of the community.

Mission Statement from the VA Medical Center

To serve veterans by providing quality health care through:
- A well-trained, highly qualified staff who work well together
- A supportive work environment that promotes excellence in patient care, education, and research
- Continuing improvement in all services provided by dedicated, competent staff of empowered employees

Courtesy of New York Downtown Hospital, New York, New York; and Jerry L. Pettis Memorial Veterans' Administration Medical Center, Loma Linda, California.

- Nutrition education acts to improve the health status of inpatients and outpatients.
- Meals and snacks for inpatients are appetizing, are nutritious, adhere to diet prescriptions, meet individual food preferences, and are prepared in a safe and sanitary manner.
- Food services for employees and guests are provided through high-quality cafeteria, catering, and vending programs.
- Continued quality improvement of services occurs through staff motivation, team activities, a conducive work environment, and training for all staff members.

- Leadership and training opportunities for others are offered through liaisons with educational institutions and professional organizations in the community.

Objectives identify the short-term increments that need to be achieved before goals can be reached. They should be written, realistic, and measurable and have assigned target dates for completion. Action plans as well as delineation of responsibilities should accompany the written objectives. It is best if progress is monitored and evaluated periodically. Successful objectives will mirror those of the organization as well. They set the tone for growth, movement, and maximization of departmental operations.

Policies

Policies are statements of rules or standards that staff members need to follow for uniformity and consistency of services. Along with procedure statements, they guide decision making throughout an organization. Policy statements should include the subject, a brief description of purpose, effective date, area of responsibility, review date, accountable person(s), and detailed specific issues and standards.

Policies provide direction for action, thus reducing the amount of managerial decision-making time required for frequently repeated activities. They provide specifications for how to do things and what resources may be allocated, including time. Simply stated, policies are prescribed ways to accomplish an objective (Byers, Shanklin, & Hoover, 1994). They are intended to be distributed to all concerned individuals and made available to all personnel for reference. Policies and procedures should be reviewed routinely in accordance with the codes that govern a particular facility. Many professionals find that this needs to be done at least annually to ensure appropriateness. In addition, it is best to alter the written documents at the time operational changes are made instead of waiting until the end of each year.

One recent trend for the design of policy and procedure manuals in facilities that wish to obtain Joint Commission accreditation is to integrate policies and procedures in a master manual along with other disciplines to demonstrate how everyone works together to meet standards. Before 1995, the Joint Commission separated the majority of food and nutrition standards and put them in the dietetic services section of its accreditation manual. To emphasize the need for integrating patient care, these standards were then dispersed under many different sections, such as assessment of patients, care of patients, education, continuum of care, control of infection, management of human resources, and others.

Creating a policy and procedure manual that reflects the organization of topics used by the Joint Commission is, undoubtedly, a tremendous task. Therefore, some find it helpful simply to cross-reference policies by referring to the policies in manuals from other departments and by identifying the Joint Commission standard code number on each one. Policies can also be indexed separately so that it is easy during accreditation visits to locate how the department complies with specific Joint Commission standards. Regardless of how this is done, it is imperative that an interdisciplinary approach be taken to the planning of policies and procedures when more than one department or service is involved in an aspect of patient care.

Regardless of the location of policies and procedures, certain topics should be considered by practitioners when they develop or revise them. Exhibit 3–4 illustrates these topics. It is important to remember that the policy and procedure manual should be used for more than just demonstrating compliance with health codes. Its primary purpose is to be used as a working tool to identify how organizational and departmental standards are met.

Procedures and Methods

Procedures and methods are lists of how to do what in chronological order. The major difference is that methods are more detailed than procedures. Procedures normally accompany policy statements because they give step-by-step instructions for how things should be done. They give the details of how a policy should be carried out. Exhibit 3–5 shows a policy, procedure, and method for a part of one patient food service goal listed earlier in this chapter.

Types of Planning

The type of planning used at any given time may be mandated by higher administrative levels with control of the planning process delegated from the board of directors or administration. A proactive, successful leader is adept at the planning process and initiates operational and SWOT planning on a regular basis. SWOT planning is a process of identifying departmental *strengths*, *weaknesses*, *opportunities*, and *threats*. It helps identify areas for improvement, new areas for development, and existing strengths that can be utilized. It is a situational diagnosis and can be used to develop short-term objectives and those needed to support the institutional strategy.

As directors become involved in the planning process, it is important for them to remember that health care of the future will be extremely different from what it has been in the past or is now. Apprising one's superiors of ongoing departmental issues will be invaluable in the future for avoiding conflicts with organizational planning. Through a process of regular planning and reporting of departmental issues, the successful leader will ensure that administrators are aware of issues that can interfere with or support the overall strategy or long-range plan. This will

Exhibit 3–4 Suggested Contents for Policy and Procedure Manuals

Introduction
Values, Vision, and Mission
Goals and Objectives
Patient's Bill of Rights
Scope of Services
Organization and Staffing
Organizational Structure
Interdisciplinary Liaisons
Committee Memberships
Attendance Policies
Job Descriptions*
Routine Staffing
Self-directed Work Teams
Daily Job Assignments
Personnel Policies
Recruitment and Selection
Physical Examinations
Performance Appraisals
Orientation Policies
Inservice Training*
Continuing Education
Professional Days
Probational Employees
Paycheck Distribution
Compensatory Time

Holidays and Sick Days
Grievance Procedures
Purchasing, Receiving, Storage, and Inventory
Purchasing Policies
Gifts from Vendors
Receiving Policies
Inventory Procedures
Issuing Policies
Food Specifications*
Supply Specifications*
Food Production
Production Schedules
Production Estimates
Standardized Recipes*
Preparation Methods
Nutrient Conservation
Use of Leftovers
Meal Assembly
Hours of Assembly and Service
Central Tray Assembly
Food Quality Testing
Portion Control
Temperature Controls
Menu Planning
The Cycle Menu*

Menu Substitutions
Menu Distribution
Nutritional Adequacy*
Diet Orders and Patient Food Service
Diet Ordering Policies
Isolation Trays
Discharge Diet Orders
Nourishments/Supplements
Enteral/Parenteral Feedings
Diet Census Records
Diet Rosters
"Hold" Trays
"House" Diets
Patient Kardex
Guest Meals
Services for Special Units
Coronary Care
Dialysis and Transplant
Intensive Care
Open Heart Recovery
Psychiatric Unit
Alcohol/Detox Unit
Obstetrics and Gynecology
Pediatrics

Outpatient Services
Clinic Services
Protocols for Referral
Staffing and Scheduling
Coding
Student Training
Contracts
Rotation Schedule
Insurance Coverage
Role of Preceptors
Infection Control*
HACCP Compliance
Dishwashing/Potwashing
Personal Hygiene
Exterminating
Sanitary Food Handling
Culturing Policies
Employee Health Policies
Special Cleaning
Environmental Standards
Safety and Security
Employee Safety Policies
Risk Management
Material Safety Data Sheets
Unauthorized Possession of Facility's Property
Unauthorized Removal of

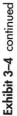

Exhibit 3–4 continued

Facility's Property
Equipment
Maintenance Schedules
Equipment Purchasing
Procedures for Cleaning
Budget/Cost Control
Departmental Budget Plan
Monthly Comparisons
Cost Calculations and
  Formulas

Nutrition Assessments and Care Plans
Nutrition Screening
Assessments and Care
  Plans
Discharge Planning
Patient Education
Patient Care Conferences
Diet Office Procedures
Charting Protocols

Confidentiality
Informed Consent
Drug/Nutrient Interactions
Quality Improvement*
Nutrition Care Indicators
Food Service Indicators
Quality Improvement
  Activity Schedules
Problem-Solving Protocols

Disaster Plan*
Training/Staffing for
  Disasters
Contracts with Vendors
Disaster Stock and Menu
Nonpatient Services
Employee Cafeteria
Catering Policies
Vending Program

*Note: Separate manuals may be used for these policies.
Courtesy of American Nutri-Tech, Amelia Island, Florida.

Exhibit 3–5 Sample Policy, Procedure, and Method

Goal 3:	**Meals** and snacks for inpatients are appetizing, are nutritious, adhere to diet prescriptions, **meet individual food preferences,** and are prepared in a safe and sanitary manner.
Policy:	Patients' individual food preferences are met with the use of selective menus.
Procedures:	1. Selective menus covering three meals for the following day are distributed and collected by patient care associates.
	2. In cases when patients are unable to fill out their menus, the patient care associates help them do so, elicit input from family members, or refer to the dietary Kardex, which lists the foods that patients like and dislike to complete menus for patients.
Methods:	1. By 2:00 p.m. each day, distribute and collect menus on the second and third floors. Bring extra pencils and the diet roster that shows current patients' diets and locations.
	2. Assist patients who are unable to complete menus on their own, and make a note in the Kardex for those patients requiring routine assistance with this task; be sure a list of food preferences is documented.
	3. For patients who are unable to complete menus with assistance, contact family members so that they can make selections for them, and make a note in the Kardex stating this; be sure that a list of food preferences is documented.
	4. If patients and family members are unable to complete menus, consult the Kardex and construct a menu from the food likes and dislikes that are documented. During mealtimes, observe the food intake of these patients for further data regarding food preferences.
	5. The "house" diets are used as a last resort, only after all the above steps have been attempted.
	6. Between 6:00 and 7:00 p.m., identify the patients who have been newly admitted to ensure that they have menu selections for the next day and that food preferences are documented in the Kardex.
	7. In cases when patients are unhappy with the foods they receive, read them the alternatives for the day and place an order for a substitute food immediately.

make it more feasible for departmental goals to be built into long-term organizational goals. Given the fast pace of change in today's environment, there will inevitably be instances when mandates from above require a swift shift in departmental plans. These adjustments can be accomplished easily if the leader establishes a routine and effective planning process. Regularly scheduled planning meetings and brainstorming sessions will foster a sense of team planning with administrators and within the department. Through the development of a planning philosophy within the management team, team members will become more confident in their abilities to adapt readily to change.

Strategic Planning

In general, strategic planning is performed at the level of the board of directors. The chief executive officer (CEO), representing the board, has the responsibility of implementing these plans into the day-to-day activities of the organization. Strategic planning requires the gathering of data; the analysis of the data; development of strategies, goals, and objectives; and implementation of action plans. Market analysis and accurate predictions of future trends in the industry are most essential for both long-term and strategic planning processes.

One key component of effective strategic planning is an ongoing evaluative process with periodic modifications of the plan. The role of food and nutrition managers in the process varies from facility to facility. In the early phases, they are key players in the information gathering process. "Both long range and strategic plans are an integral part of the total planning process and establish the basic framework on which more detailed programming and operational planning can take place" (Spears, 1995, p. 75).

Short- versus Long-Range Planning

Short-range planning normally involves the operational activities that are expected to occur within 1 year or sooner. This includes plans such as budgeting for the next fiscal year and projects that are planned for upcoming weeks or months. It is most often accomplished by first-line managers and department directors. In planning departmental expenditures, it has become increasingly important for managers to realize that income depends upon occupancy rates, which are highly variable; therefore it is best to focus on costs *per patient day* and *per meal served* as opposed to total operating expenses.

Long-range planning refers to periods well over 1 year and as long as 10 years. It requires an assessment of the broad implications of plans for the future and generally requires that one look ahead and predict what one's priorities will be at that time. It may focus on major activities, such as a construction project, or strategic plans. Most often, it is determined by administrators and the board of directors. In many instances, nutrition and food service professionals become involved when they are asked to do feasibility studies when food and nutrition programs will be affected. While doing this, it is essential that they keep in mind the overall mission and vision of the system. Techniques such as market analysis also aid in the process. In actuality, the entire planning process consists of a combination of long-range and short-range planning, with action plans and short-term plans frequently undergoing review and/or revision to model the vision of the future.

Operational Planning

Operational planning is the basis for day-to-day, recurring departmental activities. It is a method of developing accountability and structure for performance within the department. Primarily, operational planning involves the development and enforcement of policies, procedures, and reports. It includes the development of a departmental policy and procedure manual, departmental budgets, and a departmental business plan. SWOT planning is a useful planning tool for developing operational goals and objectives.

DIRECTING

The Joint Commission has standards that judge the ability of leaders to provide organization, direction, and staffing for patient care and support services according to the scope of services offered. Although the function of directing has always been and will continue to be a key function of leadership, it will have a totally different meaning for the leader of tomorrow. Food and nutrition services of the future will divide labor so that work is organized around processes and accomplished by teams of individuals. The meal delivery and nutrition service components will probably be decentralized as patient-focused work teams provide direct patient care. These things will have an immense impact on the facility's organization, direction, and staffing.

Organizational Design

Organizing is "the process of grouping activities, delegating authority to accomplish activities and providing for coordination of relationships, both horizontally and vertically" (Spears, 1995, p. 77). The traditional organizational design for a hospital was described by Zemke and Albrecht (1985): As a facility that is organized and managed by professional specialty—by functions like nursing, housekeeping, security, pharmacy, and so on. No single person or group is really accountable for the overall success and quality of the patient's experience. The traditional organization has always had a CEO, vice presidents, assistant vice presidents, department heads, supervisors, and finally line employees, who in most cases were the least skilled of all although they had direct contact with patients. It had a vertical compartmentalization, whereby authority flowed from the highest to the lowest level of employees. It was defined, organized, and orderly and did not leave much room for flexibility or creativity. Unfortunately, in the traditional organization, more time and dollars were spent in waiting, arranging, and writing things down for patients rather than engaging in more direct patient related activities. One of the problems of this traditional system is that employees lose sight of their primary focus, which is the patient. Managers of the future need to embrace the power of change for a more effective organization.

Organizations have always looked at the bottom line, and they will continue to do so. What leaders are finally realizing, however, is that to improve patient outcomes the patient is the most important commodity. If the bottom line is to stay in the black, then we must be competitive and attract more patients. This concept was illustrated by the Forum Corporation in 1991. Forum conducted research on customer loyalty in the service industry and showed that only 14% of customers no longer patronize businesses as a result of poor quality but that more than two thirds stop as a result of poor customer service as observed in indifferent or unhelpful employees (Schlessinger & Heskett, 1991).

Restructuring

A systems approach applies best to analyzing and restructuring of food and nutrition delivery services. General systems theory was described initially by von Bertalanffy (1951) as it was evident in natural science and was applied to other disciplines by Boulding (1956). It is now widely used to study organizations and processes. According to Jackson (1995):

> A *system* is a set of interrelated and interdependent parts which work together toward a common goal or set of goals. There are political systems, organizational systems, health care systems, and computer systems. Each system has a structure, specific characteristics, inputs, outputs, functions, feedback mechanism, and a set of subsystems which contribute to the whole. (p. 303)

The center of the health care system has finally moved to the patient, so that the first concept for restructuring is to shift emphasis from the needs of staff to the needs of patients. As described in Chapter 1, the future holds further applications for preventive care in the community itself. With integrated health care networks and patient-focused care, services are moved closer to people by means of a multidisciplinary team approach to improve quality. It is common for dietary employees to be deployed to patient units where they come under the jurisdiction of others while providing direct care. This requires alterations not only in organizational design but in the style of management as well, so that staff members are empowered to perform the necessary services at the point of care. Job descriptions will need to change, and there is increased emphasis on training and cross-training of employees.

Currently, the two major trends affecting how we organize are cost containment and patient-focused care. The organizational design in health care systems will be affected significantly because labor costs will continually rise. Organizations will downsize and/or merge, resulting in fewer nonexempt employees and middle management positions. As described in Chapter 1, the new structures that result not only will be more efficient but will focus on patient satisfaction more than in the past.

According to Lumsdon (1994), there are three major areas that one must address when making cost reductions: staff analysis and modifications, changing the process, and reengineering the delivery of care. Integrated health care and restructuring address both financial and quality issues in the field; thus they are key elements for future success. Transition to the new models requires a change from the traditional vertical structure to a horizontal structure, increased integration of provider services, and more focus on the patient. It also requires the development of teams and a change in managerial style from control to empowerment while teams are coordinated, facilitated, trained, and educated (McGinn, 1993).

Just after restructuring concepts were introduced in the field in the late 1980s, major changes quickly occurred. For example, a 1993 human resources survey, which reported on activities in 1,147 hospitals, showed that more than a quarter of the respondents indicated that they were trimming their workforce by as much as 24% (Burda, 1993). According to the American Hospital Association, before Medicare's incorporation of the prospective payment system in 1982, hospitals employed 3.1 million full-time equivalents (FTEs). In 1985, they reduced their workforce to slightly less than 3.0 million, but in 1992 the numbers grew to 3.6 million (Cromwell & Butrica, 1995).

Patient-Focused Care

As the health care system undergoes restructuring, most facilities are adapting the patient-focused care model. The aim of the patient-focused care concept is to have flexibility within the organization by having a multiskilled approach with as much activity as possible occurring directly at the point of care. Many organizations are adapting to this model with a long-term picture in mind as they realize that the entire health care system should integrate services along the continuum of care as well as within individual facilities and departments.

As health care facilities and departments undergo restructuring, traditional job titles, such as *dietary aide*, are being discontinued. This is because tasks, such as distribution of menus and meals, are decentralized and completed by staff members who are based directly on patient units rather than in a central location. These employees may therefore come under the direction of another department, such as nursing or unit services. The new job title may be *patient care associate*, and it would be filled by a person who is cross-trained to perform various tasks, such as distribution and collection of meals, menu processing, cleaning patient rooms, transporting patients, making beds, and stocking supplies. Job titles and approaches tend to vary from site to site. For example, one scenario for hospital restructuring can be seen from the changes that occurred at Central DuPage Hospital, a 358-bed community facility in Winfield, Illinois. This hospital restructured according to the patient-focused care model by incorporating new caregiver positions comprising three categories: patient care technicians, patient service associates, and administrative associates (Burda, 1993).

The typical members of a hospital's patient-focused care team were described by Schiller (1995). The professional member of the team has technical expertise. This is often a nurse with an expanded role, but it could be someone trained from another discipline. The patient service associate is a multiskilled, nonlicensed employee who may be involved in the tasks normally associated with food service, linen, and environmental services. Another team member is the clinical or case manager, who oversees patients and begins discharge planning immediately. Finally, the unit administrator is involved with policies and procedures, patient admission, unit reporting, and other related tasks. It is important to remember that the number of people on the team and the titles for the various positions will vary, but the major concepts of patient-focused care remain fairly constant.

Another example of a hospital restructuring project that incorporated the patient-focused care model at St. Ann's Hospital in Westerville, Ohio, was presented by Kinsel (1995). A three-member care team was developed for each patient unit. It included a registered nurse partner, a multiskilled partner, and a patient service partner. The task of tray passing moved to the units so that it could be performed by the patient service partners. Clinical dietitians were deployed to the units along with other ancillary staff members, such as pharmacists and social workers. The number of managers for food and nutrition services was reduced from seven to one, and the hospital's dietary technician category was eliminated because nutrition screening was included in the patient database.

St. Ann's Hospital started with 72 different departments, which were consolidated into 14 centers. Food and nutrition falls under the Facilities Support Center. The total number of layers in the organization was reduced from seven to four. Middle management was reduced by 50%, and self-directed work teams absorbed much of middle management's former workload. The number of job classifications for food and nutrition was reduced from 15 to 2. The former director of food and nutrition services is now the center leader for outpatient services and is heavily involved in a project to integrate this hospital's services with those of two other hospitals in the area.

Kinsel (1995) notes that high employee turnover rates were experienced during the transition described above. She describes periods of low morale, especially with long-term employees, most of whom were asked to complete self-assessments and applications for new positions in the hospital. Much support of these individuals is needed during a transition of this type. Methods to stream-line processes are also important with labor reduction. Dietitians relied heavily on automated databases and changed to charting by exception to reduce docu-mentation time.

While one is planning to restructure, careful consideration of many factors needs to occur. One must realize that it is a lengthy process, sometimes occur-ring over a 5- or 10-year period. Exhibit 3–6 shows the steps recommended by Henderson and Williams (1991) that can ensure a successful transition. Much work goes into the plan, and the planning team members should not be afraid to involve themselves with the details of the operation. According to the Health Care Advisory Board, "tight management of the patient's entire care regimen is the key to reducing length of stay—the best (most certain) way to reduce oper-ating costs" (Boston & Vestal, 1994, p. 52).

When an institution is restructuring, managers are often challenged to come up with plans and solutions themselves to improve quality and reduce costs. Middlesex Hospital in Middletown, Connecticut, serves as an example of this. In 1994, the managers in this 225-bed hospital were empowered to reduce costs, and they did so by approximately 16% (Lumsdon, 1994). They elimi-nated 45 management and supervisory positions and consolidated these posi-tions into two categories with increased responsibility and more bedside con-tact. One category consisted of patient care technicians, who support registered

---

Exhibit 3–6 Ten Steps for Restructuring Patient Care

1. Set up an action plan/goal and process (time tables, communication networks).
2. Review existing data, such as staffing, productivity, patient and staff satisfaction, morale, and quality.
3. Identify the pilot unit.
4. Communicate and discuss plans with staff.
5. Additional detailed information needs to be gathered and analyzed (regulatory agency requirements, operations, customer and staff perceptions).
6. Discuss findings.
7. Develop an initial diagnosis to change.
8. Develop recommendations and action plans.
9. Review the unit plans with top management.
10. Implement action plans and evaluate.

Source: Reprinted with permission from J.L. Henderson and J.B. Williams. Ten Steps for Restructuring Patient Care, *Healthcare Forum Journal*, July/August 1991, pp. 50–52, © Healthcare Forum Journal.

nurses. The other was patient care associates, who handle food service, house-keeping, and other responsibilities. While hospitals undergo such changes, specific objectives are normally established and time frames assigned. Clouten and Weber (1994) described some of the most important objectives (see Exhibit 3–7). A well-trained, challenged, and empowered staff will result in increases in productivity and patient satisfaction.

Patient Care Centers

According to Schiller (1995), configuring patient units so that patients with similar needs are grouped together is often a part of the restructuring plan. To a certain extent this was done in the past, but it is becoming more common for patients to be grouped into specialties such as cardiac, surgical, renal, and others so that patient care teams can be more efficient in their care duties.

There is a movement in the health care industry to take this concept a bit further by establishing patient care centers or service lines, separate divisions that are somewhat independently managed for each specialty. Lathrop (1993) calls this patient aggregation, the grouping of patients according to their service needs. The term *service lines* can be understood in relation to the concept of product lines, which are commonly used in manufacturing industries. Some people refer to the resulting structure as hospitals within hospitals. In facilities that use this concept, dietitians may be deployed to the various specialties on a

---

Exhibit 3–7 Objectives for Restructuring Efforts

Cross-training of staff so they are able to perform many functions related to patient care.
Empowering of staff to take on responsibility and perform their jobs, thus reducing the management structure.
Deploying ancillary personnel: Patient care units will be staffed with support services.
Deploying services: Electrocardiology, physical therapy, radiology, and respiratory care, for example, may be moved closer to the patient care unit.
Grouping patient populations: Patients requiring similar services can be grouped together for unit efficiencies.
Establishment of work teams: Patient-focused care teams are assigned to specific patient groups.
Critical pathways are customized for standardization of care, quality assurance, and minimizing of patient days.
Minimizing documentation: Techniques such as automation, computerization, and charting by exception save time.
Use of servers: Improve efficiency by containing patient care items at the bedside.

Source: Adapted with permission from the article "Patient Focused Care . . . Playing to Win," from the February, 1994 issue of *Nursing Management*, © Springhouse Corporation.

full- or part-time basis, which puts them under the jurisdiction of the director of these units.

The major advantage of this type of structure is that dietitians have the opportunity to become more integrated into a health care team because they report to the director of the service, who has a commitment to making sure that team members work well together. Second, the plan is helpful in assessing the costs of nutrition therapy for each patient care center. The challenge for dietitians is to cost justify the care they provide in terms of patient care quality and the impact of their work on length of stay and overall health care costs. Sowa (1995) predicted that clinical dietitians in the health care systems of the future would have more advisory or consultant roles instead of acting as unit-based care providers. In essence, this role would be more like that fulfilled by a speech-language pathologist who intervenes for high- or moderate-risk cases, by referral, or at the request of patients.

Multisystem Management

With the creation of integrated health care systems, there are opportunities for food service and nutrition professionals to expand their scope of care and provide their services at new sites within their network. The organizational designs will change accordingly. Integrated systems may combine many services under one roof, or services may be provided in a number of different settings under a single sponsorship. Seamless health care delivery appears to be inevitable.

"One major trend that illustrates the need for reevaluation of the current system, notes Biesemeier (1996), is *whole systems shared governance*, where providers will have increased accountability for the care they give" (Jackson, 1996a, p. 6). Whole systems shared governance is a way to organize health care so that it is structured around populations across the continuum of care. "Decision making is decentralized, and it is made at the point of care" (Jackson, 1996a, p. 6). Under this system, it is expected that 90% of the decisions made will be made at the point of care, that is, in homes, schools, and outpatient centers and at the bedside. With this system, providers will have increased accountability for seeing that outcomes are achieved.

The health care system of the future will require food service and nutrition professionals to expand their roles and responsibilities into the community. Directors of such services will oversee food and nutrition services in a variety of settings that are affiliated with the hospital, including nursing homes, satellite clinics, day care centers, schools, physician offices, home care agencies, and many other units that are on or off site. In many instances, this will require the use of a main commissary, where foods are prepared and shipped to satellite kitchens, and sophisticated medical record systems with databases that can be accessed from the point of care. This concept addresses the age-old problem of duplication of efforts along the continuum of care, which has contributed to escalating health care costs.

Multiservice Management

Multiservice management, sometimes referred to as shared management, is another aspect of organizational change. In the majority of health care organizations it correlates with patient-focused care, but the two need not be implemented together. As hospitals empower employees to be more responsible and accountable, middle managers are finding that job losses often accompany operational improvements. On the other hand, those who are able to see the entire scope of services that will be provided to the patient, have strong communication and leadership skills, and have integrity and the ability to listen will succeed and find themselves responsible for more than food and nutrition services.

To reduce costs, administrators use empowered team members to come up with plans that reduce the number of department heads and provide blended management specialties. For example, the departments of food and nutrition, laundry, and material management can be successfully combined at the managerial level. Having one individual responsible for several departments will lead to standardization, which can result in consistency and a higher quality of services. This may also lead to reduction of costs. The key to success is to focus on management and leadership skills while strengthening human resource abilities.

Many administrators will institute this concept of multiservice management to reduce the number of middle management positions, have decisions made by senior management implemented quickly, and be able to redistribute wages. With the introduction of patient-focused care, coupled with fewer middle managers, the span of control inevitably widens.

Determining Span of Control

Organizing is based on two concepts: span of control and authority. Span of control, sometimes called span of management, is primarily concerned with the number of individuals whom one person can effectively supervise. In general, a wider span of control applies when subordinates do similar and related tasks and are located within close proximity of one another. As the span of control widens, fewer middle management positions will be required. Management may then need supervisors to coach and support staff, rather than control staff, with fewer lines of authority. Employees who are well trained and self-motivated require shorter spans. As responsibilities of the manager increase and the tasks performed become more diverse, the span of control decreases.

When an organization is initially being structured or when it is restructured, the basic concepts of the span of control apply. Spears (1995) recommends that six factors be considered: organizational policies, availability of staff experts, competence of staff, objective standards, nature of the work, and distribution of the workforce. Table 3–1 shows these factors in relationship to decisions that are made for health care systems that are restructuring their organization.

Table 3–1 Restructuring and Span of Control

Factor	Explanation
Organizational policies	When staff are empowered to take on more responsibility, they will be more involved in decision making and policy determination. Once new policies are adapted, it is essential that all staff members understand that they are meant to be universally applied so that goals can be accomplished. Decentralization can lead to chaos if policies are not understood and followed.
Availability of staff experts	To increase span of control, staff experts need to be readily available to act as facilitators, advisors, coaches, and cheerleaders. If not, employees will waste time learning by mistakes and recreating things that are already known by the experts. The roles of experts and patient unit managers need to be clearly defined so that conflicts are avoided and employees are not confused.
Competence of staff	Managers can increase their span of control when employees are competent enough to handle their expanded roles. Cross-training needs to be planned and monitored carefully so that all important concepts are communicated well.
Objective standards	When new procedures are written, they must be clearly defined and illustrated so that employees know exactly what is expected of them. This enables the manager to deal only with the exceptions while avoiding constant supervision of the workforce, which results in the ability to oversee more employees.
Nature of the work	Span of control can increase when subordinates have simplified and uniform jobs. With the change to patient-focused care, individual employees will be performing more tasks than before. Efforts therefore need to be made so that their new tasks are not overwhelming or too complex in nature. In addition, multiservice managers oversee distinctly different departments that are often in different locations, so that a shorter span of control is required.
Distribution of the workforce	With patient-focused care, much of the work is decentralized, and employees are widely dispersed in separate patient units. This would make supervision from a central location difficult and inefficient because a shorter span of control is needed as the number of work sites increases. Therefore, the work of employees is more efficiently monitored by supervisors on the units, who can routinely take input from staff experts.

Source: Reprinted from R. Jackson, How Restructuring Affects Span of Control, *Hospital Food & Nutrition Focus,* Vol. 12, No. 9, p. 8, © 1996, Aspen Publishers, Inc.

Changing Lines of Authority

The traditional organization gave the manager the authority to direct others, to perform job functions, and to take appropriate action. The manager's subordinates would then delegate tasks to their line staff. This part of the organization is known as the vertical division of labor. In the new organization, this vertical structure will no longer be effective. Spears (1995) advises that a horizontal division of labor is more appropriate because the entire focus is that all employees are sharing ideas across departmental lines.

In a restructured organization of average size, the lines of authority will be limited to three or four areas reporting to the director. Classification of employees will be changed, with a universal job title fostering departmental flexibility in utilizing labor resources and integrating services. For the horizontal approach to be effective, training of employees is key, as is the ability to cross-train staff. Each employee must clearly understand the objectives for his or her job function. Policies and procedures will need revision to reflect an increased customer-focused environment rather than one that focuses on the work process. The role of the manager will change to that of a facilitator and coach. We will need to teach people how to increase efficiency and participate in teams. The lines of authority will be simplified, resulting in fewer managerial staff.

Delegation and Empowerment

Delegation is the process of assigning tasks or job activities to specific individuals. For many practitioners in food service and nutrition care, this is one of the hardest things to do. Some feel that if they want it done right, they have to do it themselves. Effective leaders are able to transfer authority and responsibility to their employees, and one critical factor that allows them to do so is the assurance that their staff are competent enough to handle the task successfully.

The way a supervisor perceives his or her subordinates, the amount of work that the supervisor has, and how important his or her decisions are are all predictors of the outcomes of delegation (Leana, 1986). Communication skills are important in the delegation process. Subordinates must clearly understand what their supervisors want them to do and acquire feedback during the conversation to be sure that instructions are understood. Communication with others in the organization is also helpful so that supervisors can support the employee in his or her efforts to complete the task.

To a certain extent, the process of delegation as a management technique is being replaced by empowerment, which is broader in scope. As noted in Chapter 2, empowerment affords the leader the opportunity to delegate effectively while at the same time providing the subordinates with the resources and support to complete the task at hand. It may be given with strictly defined boundaries, or it may be given within loose controls. Regardless of how it is accomplished, subordinates need to feel that the authority for accomplishing a task is in their hands. Power needs to be transferred to them so that they feel trusted and are free to proceed. Along with this transfer of power comes transfer of responsibility for the task being done correctly. Finally, the delegator needs to be sure that the subordinate has all the resources necessary for success so that frustration does not occur. All too often, subordinates are set up for failure because managers hastily delegate a task without providing the necessary tools and time for it to be accomplished.

Part of the restructuring initiative requires that managers change their roles and empower employees to do many of the tasks that they would have normally performed. The emergence of multidepartment management will also necessitate this otherwise difficult transition. If one can delegate responsibility effectively, one will have the necessary time for planning and expanding one's professional role. In delegating, managers need to clarify their expectations in terms of either tasks or results. Staff members will be able to fulfill their tasks only if they understand expectations and are given the appropriate resources.

Empowerment enhances the jobs of employees. It enables staff members to take on a more participatory role and gives them a greater degree of responsibility and autonomy while promoting motivation. There are feared risks in delegating authority: Some are afraid that the job will not get done or that it may be done too well! In either event, the feared outcome makes the manager look incompetent. If managers cannot delegate successfully in the restructured environment, they will risk not fulfilling all their areas of responsibility. If they do not give others more responsibility, then they will not motivate their staff and will thus decrease their own productivity.

Staffing

Staffing involves recruiting, selecting, training, and developing people to meet the goals of the organization. The way health care organizations were staffed in the past has contributed to the problems faced in the industry today, and this has become a major focus in facilities that are being reorganized. In the past 20 to 30 years, food and nutrition care as well as other disciplines have been reorganized into specialty areas. Family practice has been dwindling, and specialists have inundated health care in the areas of orthopedics, surgery, medicine, and so on. This trend has affected the way professionals look at, diagnose, and treat patients. Rather than health care professionals taking a systems approach, patients were dissected into their different needs, which were treated separately.

This problem is called compartmentalization by Lathrop (1993). In the field of dietetics, many institutions suffer this problem even within departments. For example, separate titles have been given to warewashers, tray assemblers, food servers, salad preparers, tray deliverers, and so on. This has encouraged the "that's not my job" syndrome, which limits cooperation and leads to a spirit of disharmony among staff members. To be cost effective, practitioners have learned to look at the various classifications in their departments and to streamline titles to increase flexibility. A worker with a uniform job title who is multiskilled and capable of performing various tasks represents the only way food service and nutrition departments can ensure efficient staffing in the future. In addition, if leaders of the restructured organization are looking at creating quality and improving customer satisfaction, then it is imperative that they look at standardization of routines as well.

The problem of compartmentalization has a direct impact on staffing in terms of how things are done, what is done, and the number of FTEs required. Rising labor costs in the industry acted as the major impetus for restructuring when the trend gained momentum in the early 1990s. At that time, payroll costs were escalating despite previous efforts to control them. For example, from 1987 to 1991, costs per FTE increased by 6% annually for all U.S. hospitals, from $21,938 to $28,305. With such an increase in salaries, one understands why techniques for streamlining staff became important.

Job Redesign and Reengineering

Job redesign is the process of analyzing and reengineering the way work is accomplished in an effort to fit the needs of customers, employees, and ultimately the organization. Juran (1989) describes three basic methods that are used for designing jobs (see Exhibit 3–8). Selection of the most appropriate method depends on the philosophy of management, the reasons for redesign, and the capabilities of employees and managers involved in decisions.

Morell (1995) describes this process as an inside-out change process that aims at improving a particular process to reduce costs and enhance operating performance. "The one objective is to take costs out of the organization without affecting the high quality of care" (p. 66). He stresses that long-term success of the changes will hinge on the ability to articulate a broadly acceptable vision, create a sustainable platform for change, establish meaningful targets, and assume stewardship of the strategy, and ownership of all supporting change processes.

Job redesign begins with job analysis, which is "the process of obtaining information about jobs by determining what the duties and tasks or activities of these jobs are" (Spears, 1995, p. 756). Without a careful analysis of current jobs, the revision and implementation of a new plan would be quite cumbersome and might possibly result in poor job satisfaction. Successful managers do well at placing the right people in the right positions. They look at staffing on a continued basis as it reflects the changing needs of the department, alterations in the organizational structure, resignations, terminations, potential floor closures, and restructuring of the organization. Lumsdon (1994) says that staffing analysis and its resulting adjustments represent the first level of cost reduction. To analyze jobs effectively, managers should refer to the points covered in Exhibit 3–9.

"The typical 500-bed hospital has more than 500 job classes, with an average of only six employees in each class" (Tidkis & Strasen, 1994, p. 38). The more

Exhibit 3–8 Methods of Job Redesign

Job Enrichment

Jobs that are repetitive are converted into jobs of broader scope so that employees can perform a multitude of tasks, are less bored with the work, and become their own internal customers, leading to easier identification of possible deficiencies in the quality of work and its planning. An example of this would be combining all types of cooks into one classification so that they could prepare all the components of a meal and including patient visitation in their job descriptions so that they could realize the outcomes of their work. Job enrichment primarily has a horizontal focus.

Job Enlargement

Employees are assigned multiple functions with more responsibility and control over their jobs. This includes the concept of job enrichment but adds factors such as employee achievement, recognition, growth, and responsibility, and performance of the complete job rather than parts of it is emphasized. An example of this would be to have the same cooks involved in decisions regarding food specifications, issuing, storage, recipe development, and responding to quality improvement results. Job enlargement has a vertical focus.

Self-Supervising Teams

Groups of people who are largely self-supervising decide the work that needs to be performed, who does the work, and how it is done. In addition to the tasks identified for job enlargement, the team also takes on functions such as material purchasing, equipment maintenance, product testing, recordkeeping activities, and implementation of a quality improvement program designed to increase customer satisfaction. The focus is both horizontal and vertical.

Source: Reprinted with the permission of The Free Press, a division of Simon & Schuster from JURAN ON LEADERSHIP FOR QUALITY: An Executive Handbook by J.M. Juran. © 1989 by Juran Institute, Inc.

---

job classifications there are, the more one is likely to find employees who are underutilized and underchallenged, resulting in lower productivity. Therefore, as jobs are analyzed, it is important to determine whether tasks requiring similar skills can be combined into one job classification.

Some institutions hire industrial engineers to determine exactly what employees do; others do it themselves by interviewing employees and supervisors, observation, employee questionnaires or logs, and the like. While doing so, it is important for them to note the amount of time required for each task, the volume of work produced, the times of the day or week it is done, and the competencies required by the worker to perform the task efficiently and successfully. Spears (1995) emphasizes the fact that job analysis should be objective and veri-

Exhibit 3–9 Steps Involved in Job Analysis

1. Focus first on positions that have the best potential for cost savings and/or quality improvement.
2. Become familiar with current performance standards and industrywide standards.
3. Identify tasks and determine their frequency with input from employees and supervisors.
4. Collect data by monitoring the workload for at least 2 weeks to determine:
   - actual frequency of the task performed
   - time required to perform each task
   - competencies required for successful performance
5. Communicate with supervisors and employees who have performed the jobs to get feedback on the data.
6. Involve staff members as a part of the planning committee.

Source: Reprinted from R. Jackson, Job Redesign, *Hospital Food & Nutrition Focus*, Vol. 12, No. 10, p. 8, © 1996, Aspen Publishers, Inc.

fiable. Careful scrutiny of the results of the job analysis can also help managers determine job descriptions, job specifications, and the content and length of training programs. A more detailed task analysis may have to be completed for jobs that are especially complex or unfamiliar to managers. This may involve an actual time and motion study, which identifies the steps required to complete a specific task, the tools used, and the movements made by the employee.

Once job elements and tasks are analyzed, many decisions need to be made. Champy (1996) suggests the following questions to prompt the decisions that have to be made:

- What is this business for?
- What kind of culture do we want?
- How will we do our work?
- What kind of people do we want to work with?

Chase and Aquilano (1992) suggest more specific questions to arrive at the best possible job structure (see Exhibit 3–10).

While redesigning jobs, many practitioners learn that certain tasks can be quickly discontinued because they are obsolete and no longer useful. Some tasks can be deployed to other areas, such as patient care units, because they are most appropriately done at the point of care. Other tasks can be streamlined using new technologies that may accomplish the work faster and with greater accuracy. Also, there may be a need to add new tasks because they are necessary for improving quality or decreasing costs. All decisions that are made should be measured against the overall mission and goals of the organization and depart-

Exhibit 3–10 Factors To Consider in Designing Jobs

WHO:	The mental and physical characteristics of present and future employees
WHAT:	Exactly which tasks will be performed in each job category
WHERE:	The work location that is best for completion of each task
WHEN:	The times, days, and sequence of the work flow for performance of tasks
WHY:	Organizational justification for the job, employee's objectives, and motivation
HOW:	Details of how each task is to be performed, including the resources and tools needed for successful completion

Source: Adapted with permission from R.B. Chase and N.G. Aquilaro, *Production Operations Management, A Life-Cycle Approach*, 7/e BurrRidge, IL, Richard D. Irwin, 1995, p. 437.

ment, and decision makers should always be conscious of the quality of work for employees. Once the job is designed, the new system should be piloted, with ongoing evaluation and adjustments being made as necessary with input from both patients and employees.

The redesign of jobs for facilities using patient-focused care is exemplified by University Medical Center in Tucson, Arizona (Black, 1994). After careful planning, the roles of two members of the patient care team were designed and tested (see Table 3–2). The patient support attendant role was identified as the first step in a career ladder for the medical center's employees to enter and advance to the position of registered nurse. After this position was piloted, it was learned that 75% of the job consisted of housekeeping functions. Because many of the existing environmental services employees did not have a high school education or equivalent, it was determined that the minimal academic requirement for this new consolidated position would be the ability to follow both written and verbal instruction in English. This illustrates how human resource issues need to be considered in job redesign. For this institution, it is feasible that the minimum requirements could be raised in the future and that support could be given to employees for attaining a higher level of education.

Competencies

Competence is the possession of the required skills and knowledge to perform one's duties properly. The Joint Commission (1995) requires the assessment of competency for each individual as part of the performance evaluation process. Leaders in the organization should define the qualifications and performance expectations for all staff members, provide an adequate number of staff members whose qualifications are consistent with their job responsibilities, and ensure that competency is assessed, maintained, demonstrated, and improved continually.

Table 3–2 Redesign of Jobs for Patient-Focused Care at University Medical Center (UMC), Tucson, Arizona

Discipline	Patient Care Technician (Under the Supervision of the Registered Nurse)	Discipline	Patient Support Attendant
Physical therapy	Performs specific rehabilitation-related duties to carry out the patient's therapeutic plan of care	Housekeeping	Performs housekeeping functions properly
Occupational therapy	Performs specific rehabilitation-related duties to carry out the patient's therapeutic plan of care	Transportation	Transports patients, specimens, and medications in a safe and efficient manner
Phlebotomy and clinical laboratory	Obtains and maintains integrity of specimens in accordance with UMC policies and procedures and physician orders	Materials management	Maintains adequate floor stock on a daily basis
Respiratory therapy	Provides selected respiratory care to patients following accepted respiratory care practices, UMC policies and procedures, and physician orders	Dietary	Distributes and assists patients with meals and nutrition
Electrocardiology	Performs electrocardiograms following UMC policies and procedures and physician orders		
Documentation/ reporting	Documents and reports care delivered under the direct supervision of the registered nurse		

Source: Reprinted from R. Black, Patient Care Restructuring and Human Resources, in *Patient-Centered Care: A Model for Restructuring*, M.L. Parsons and C.L. Murdaugh eds., © 1994, Aspen Publishers, Inc.

Some of the tools used to measure staff competencies are audits, pretests, posttests, and job descriptions with specific performance standards indicated adjacent to the job responsibilities, as shown in Figure 3–2. Frequently, the major categories on the performance appraisal form are weighted with regard to the percentage of time employees dedicate to the various tasks. For example, the cooks in the position illustrated spend approximately 60% of their working time performing the duties shown in the first section of the form. At the end of each performance appraisal session, the manager and employee can identify the specific items in need of further development and how improvement can be accomplished. This might entail continuing education on or off the job, more self-discipline on the part of the employee, routine coaching on the part of the manager, or joint efforts to improve the work design to make it easier for the employee to achieve his or her goals.

The purpose of identifying staff competencies has been, and will continue to be, to evaluate performance within the organization. According to the Joint Commission (1995), performance standards should be specific in identifying job competencies. They must be appropriate and meet the needs of the patient population. For example, the skills required for a dietitian serving pediatric patients would be different from those for an adult population. Dietitians serving certain ethnic groups not only will have to know the characteristics of the culture but will need to know how to read, speak, and provide educational materials in another language.

It is helpful to develop competency checklists and written tests and to ensure that these are documented in employees' files. One can set up an ongoing system whereby competency is evaluated, training is provided, and patient care outcomes improve accordingly. Such a system will benefit employees as well. Although appraisals can be used to determine performance and as tools to award salary increases or promotions, employees benefit because they grow as a result of this process and gain substantial job satisfaction, which has a direct effect on the quality of their work life.

Quality of Work Life

According to Kotler (1990), managers can improve the quality of work life by creating a sense of belonging, recognizing employees' successes, contributing to their self-esteem, and empowering them by giving them a sense of control and the ability to live up to their ideals. When managers motivate their employees in these ways, it makes their work more productive, challenging, and satisfying.

Blessing (1986) suggests four ways to do this: by encouraging mastery of skills, autonomy, relationships, and change. Staff need to know that their skills are important. A manager can encourage mastery of skills by making employees aware of their strengths and by allowing and encouraging them to build on these strengths, enabling them to grow. Autonomy is fostered when employees feel in charge of their work. When people feel that they are part of a vision and can grow on the job, they gain a sense of ownership. To create autonomy, managers can be open to the point of view of their subordinates and use their ideas whenever possible. Good relationships and communications between employees and supervisors are key elements in motivating staff to provide excellent service. Performance reviews can be used as a tool when they enhance and develop the assets of the employee.

Development and growth imply change. Successful leaders are able to help each employee identify goals, values, and talents and how these things can be put into practice on the job. This not only motivates the employee but enhances

		Rating and Comments
1	**Follows menus, production sheets, and standardized recipes to determine proper methods, amounts, and portions of food to prepare (60%)**	5 4 3 2 1
	a) Obtains the correct amounts of the right ingredients for food production	
	b) Checks food quality before and after food production, and does not serve foods that are below the standards of quality written on each recipe	
	c) Follows correct procedures listed on standardized recipes for baking, roasting, broiling, steaming, and other cooking activities, and does not prepare foods in advance of the times indicated on production schedules	
	d) Applies the principles of nutrient conservation while producing foods	
	e) Uses batch cookery as indicated in standardized recipes to minimize holding time, and holds foods at the proper temperatures	
	f) Adheres to standardized cooking times, and takes the internal temperatures of foods to determine "doneness"	
	g) Minimizes overproduction and waste, and utilizes leftovers within 24 hours	
	h) Works and operates equipment in a safe manner	
	i) Makes appropriate menu substitutions, and reports problems with food, supplies, or equipment to supervisor immediately	
2	**Follows all safety and sanitation standards (30%)**	
	a) Maintains the Public Health Food Service Sanitation Certificate	
	b) Follows all HACCP guidelines shown on recipes	
	c) Covers, labels, dates, and rotates foods in storage	
	d) Keeps work area clean and orderly, and follows proper cleaning procedures	
	e) Follows the department's standards for personal hygiene and food handling	
	f) Knows and applies all fire and other safety precautions and procedures	
3	**Other job requirements (10%)**	
	a) Routinely provides assistance on the tray assembly or cafeteria line as needed	
	b) Attends all inservice training classes, implements the new techniques that are taught, and participates in training other employees	
	c) Participates in team activities for quality improvement and cost containment	
	d) Willingly performs other duties, and volunteers creative suggestions	
4	Is prompt and reliable and has good work attendance	
5	Maintains good working relationships with other staff members	
6	Follows all the policies and procedures of the organization and department	

Figure 3–2 Performance appraisal for cooks.

the organization. Staff will buy into change and solutions if they are involved in creating them. This enhances job satisfaction. For health care organizations to produce positive changes in the quality of work life, there is a need to focus on the *person–job fit* and to identify the stress-producing aspects of the job, beginning with the smallest unit of organized work.

Henderson and Williams (1991) provide the following tips for improving job satisfaction in restructured organizations. They stress the importance of either maintaining or increasing motivation and job satisfaction, which requires that staff have an understanding of the purpose of the change and the goal and direction underlying the change. This, in turn, will help increase productivity.

- Encourage, wherever possible, effective use of career ladders for advancement opportunities.
- Recognize outstanding individuals through reward programs, employee of the month awards, feedback from patient surveys, and the like.
- Create a department that reduces stress and supports changes by improving the social and managerial aspects of the work environment.
- Use as a basis for selecting, training, performance assessment, and planning those key competencies that distinguish high- from low-performing employees.

Work Scheduling

As individual health care systems reorganize to contain costs and strive to meet the needs of patients rather than the convenience of staff, new designs in work scheduling are needed. As this happens, the nature of the workforce will continue to change. More and more women have been entering the workforce, and labor shortages continue to increase in many areas, increasing the need to incorporate more flexibility into the scheduling process. Olmstead and Smith (1989) theorize that by the turn of the century, managers of human resources not only will need to increase employee productivity but also will need to create structural flexibility. The trend in the health care industry toward the use of multiskilled employees will enable more flexibility, thus creating a more dedicated and committed workforce.

Some of the factors that need to be addressed in planning schedules are as follows: Overtime should be used only when absolutely necessary, schedules should be balanced to avoid understaffing and overstaffing, teamwork will foster a sense of cooperation among employees on the same schedule, and time should be factored in for special projects, such as training and team planning. It also helps to look at scheduling from the viewpoint of employees. They are primarily concerned with off days, schedule flexibility, and standardization of time with their family and friends. Many, especially working mothers, who are on the increase in the work setting, carry the burden of family responsibilities and have special needs that need to be considered. When employees' needs are not met, higher turnover of labor, increased absenteeism, and decreased productivity result.

According to Schlessinger and Heskett (1991), the companies on the cutting edge of family issues have found that giving part-time benefits and using flextime, job sharing, compressed work weeks, parenting leave, and off-site employment (working at home) are just some employment packages that employees find popular; some of these are defined below. Before any new scheduling system is implemented, it is important to learn which plans employees like best, communicate the rationale behind schedule changes, and gain support from employees. When unions are involved, union representatives need to be included as well. Unions naturally benefit by having more employees in a given organization, so that effective partnerships with union representatives are of paramount importance in getting the organization's goals accomplished.

If everyone contributes to and understands schedule changes, the chances for employee acceptance will be greater. In the words of Jerome Rosow, the former president of the Work in America Institute, "new work schedules, when carefully chosen, designed and executed, are among the best investments an employer can make. The cost is small, the risk is low, and the potential return is high. Best of all, they benefit all parties involved" (Olmstead & Smith, 1989, p. 50).

As mentioned above, when considering scheduling options managers should look at part-time retirement, phased retirement, leave time, work sharing, and voluntary reduced work time programs. Other alternatives include the following:

- flextime, which is flexible starting and quitting times as determined within limits set by management
- a compressed work week, 40 hours worked in fewer than 5 days (e.g., 10- to 12- hour shifts)
- part-time employees, with prorated benefits and other rights, such as job security
- job sharing, in which two employees share one full-time job with prorated salary and benefits

In the next decade, there will probably be an increase in part-time workers and an increase in the use of the 12-hour shift in the health care industry. The 12-hour shift, in particular, can be effective if properly implemented because in many instances it will meet the employer's needs, the employee's preferences, and health and safety requirements. For this to be successful, managers will need to incorporate appropriate rest breaks, educate employees on strategies in coping with the 12-hour shift, and have ongoing safety programs. Coleman

(1992) offers some suggestions when 12-hour shifts are being considered (see Exhibit 3–11).

Twelve-hour shifts may not be an alternative for every facility. Instead, benefits may come from the use of part-time employees to have one full-time and one part-time shift each day, which can also create flexibility in scheduling.

Staffing Levels

To ensure that labor costs stay below budgeted amounts, it is best to establish the staffing levels before schedules are planned. This entails determining the exact number of employees in the different job categories who are needed to operate the department. While one is doing so, it is important to realize that staffing requirements may be different at certain times. For example, fewer clerical, store room, and cafeteria workers are normally needed on weekends because of the lower volume of work on these days. A sample plan is shown in Exhibit 3–12 for the food service segment of a 325-bed hospital that averages 75% occupancy, has a moderately active employee cafeteria, and has menu and tray-passing functions done by the staff on patient units.

Based on job and task analysis, one can determine the number of different positions needed each day. In this case, it can be seen that the employee assigned to the store room is not needed on weekends and that there is one fewer dietary associate on the weekend early and late shifts. The simple mathematics at the bottom of Exhibit 3–12 show how the number of FTEs for the department is established. By considering the number of meals produced for patients and cafeteria services and the amount of work employees contribute to each of these functions, manhour allocations can be identified so that the patient and nonpatient cost centers will reflect labor costs. Time studies can also help establish these allocations in cases where separate staff are not used for the two functions.

Once minimum staffing levels are determined, they can be used as the basis for employee schedules. For the example shown, if occupancy rates consistently fall below or above 75%, the number of scheduled hours can be adjusted accordingly. This enables the manager to flex the schedule according to patient days. Along the same line of thinking, if cafeteria or catering volume changes substantially from the norm, scheduling changes can be made as well, and they will be justified by the additional meals served or income for those days in the schedule.

Daily Work Patterns

While planning minimal staffing levels, the manager should be able to justify all hours by identifying the tasks that are accomplished by each employee. *Daily work patterns* are used for this purpose. Determining the content of each daily work pattern consists of arranging the tasks that need to be performed in order

Exhibit 3–11 Suggestions for 12-Hour Shift Scheduling

Maintain costs—If employees work 37.5 hours per week, then it is necessary not to exceed that for a 12-hour shift. Contract language, pay factoring, waivers, and renegotiating of shift differentials may be some of the necessary ways to devise a plan that will maintain costs.

Unplanned vacancies—Come up with a plan in advance to cover vacancies by considering techniques such as on-call employees, built-in relief, or mandatory coverage.

Staffing needs analysis—If the same individuals are repeatedly called in to cover vacancies, this may defeat the purpose of the 12-hour shift schedule. A careful analysis of needs can help prevent such problems.

Check viability—Not every position may lend itself to 12-hours shifts. For example, a manager in a cook-chill operation may only want to implement a 12-hour shift with production or tray assembly staff.

Sick time policies need to be adjusted—Careful planning should result in policies that prevent other workers from financially benefitting when an employee on a 12-hour shift calls in sick (i.e., overtime does not have to be paid).

Vacation and holiday policies need adjustment—Days granted for vacations and holidays will need to be converted to hours. Consider also holidays that can create a pay loss on a 12-hour shift.

Breaks and lunch policies need revision—Base breaks and lunch times on a 12-hour shift after checking for compliance with past practices, facility policies, and union contracts in mind.

Develop a training plan—Prepare staff by developing daily staffing patterns and training them in how to follow them, the master schedules, and the policies that are implemented with the new plan.

Ensure continuity of operations and communications—As the new system is phased in, monitor employee satisfaction, adherence to daily work patterns and schedules, and impact on the provision of food and nutrition services. React quickly to problems by making adjustments to the plan when necessary.

Avoid implementation during union negotiation—Work with union representatives to pilot the plan before it is finalized, and avoid making it an issue during the phases of union negotiation.

Build employee consensus for change—Give employees options. Learn about their needs and expectations, and incorporate these into the plan. Explain the policies regarding pay and coverage, and then work with employees to build the schedule.

Source: Data from M. Coleman, Twelve Hour Shift Schedules: What You Need to Know, *Human Resources Focus*, Vol. 69, pp. 16–17, © 1992.

of importance. For accountability and tracking purposes, this can be done by arranging the responsibilities either on a percentage basis devoted to that task or by actually listing each function and duty within an allocated time frame. Knowing the tasks for each position is extremely important, and the best way to accomplish this is to identify what needs to be done within a given time period and writing down the responsibility for each job function.

Exhibit 3–12 Staffing Levels for Patient and Nonpatient Food Services

Position	Schedule Code	Work Hours	Hours per Day	Requirement for Weekdays	Requirement for Weekends and Holidays	Allocation: Patient Services	Allocation: Nonpatient Services
Certified Dietary Manager	M1	6:00–2:30	8	1	1	70%	30%
Certified Dietary Manager	M2	10:30–7:00	8	1	1	85%	15%
Cook	C1	6:00–2:30	8	1	1	70%	30%
Cook	C2	9:00–5:30	8	1	1	85%	15%
Dietary Associate (Receiving, Storage, Issuing)	SR	6:00–2:30	8	1	0	70%	30%
Dietary Associates (Patient Service)	P1–P4	6:30–3:00	8	4	4	100%	0%
Dietary Associates (Patient Service—Part Time)	P5–P8	3:00–7:00	4	4	4	100%	0%
Dietary Associates (Cafeteria Service)	NP1–NP2	6:30–3:00	8	2	1	0%	100%
Dietary Associates (Cafeteria Service—Part Time)	NP3–NP4	3:00–7:00	4	2	1	0%	100%
Dietary Associate (Potwashing, Utility)	UT1	6:00–2:30	8	1	1	70%	30%
Dietary Associate (Potwashing, Utility—Part Time)	UT2	3:00–7:00	4	1	1	70%	30%
Number of 8-hour employees				12	10		
Number of 4-hour employees				7	6		
Total scheduled hours				124	104		
				× 5 days	× 2 days		
Scheduled hours per week				620	+	208	= 828
FTEs @ 40 hours/week							20.7

Being detailed and explicit as well as coordinating processes are key in developing work patterns. In addition, the input from employees and supervisors is extremely valuable during planning and implementation stages. The design of daily work patterns should be a team effort, with the manager acting as a facilitator. The outcome will be a listing of tasks performed by each individual in the sequence in which they need to be accomplished for the best possible service to patients and other customers, as illustrated in Exhibit 3–13. The listing also acts as a visual reminder of things that must be done to provide high-quality care, such as washing hands and checking menus; with training, employees can use their judgment when other situations require them to do these things.

To determine how much time should be given for certain tasks, job and task analyses can be performed. Managers who are well experienced in departmental operations find that they can normally estimate the time required to complete tasks. Nevertheless, it is important to verify these estimates and allow employees to offer their input while determining time and sequencing standards. The methods of job analysis that have been discussed previously in this chapter are helpful in gathering data for planning work patterns. Before decisions are made, it is also helpful to consider the fact that some employees are quicker than others. Employees normally consider it fair to use average times, somewhere between the time it takes the slowest and quickest workers to perform the tasks. This helps resolve the dilemma. As the plan is piloted, it can be fine tuned and techniques tested to improve efficiency further.

Work patterns can be used as a dual tool, for the supervisor as well as for the employee. They are useful teaching tools, are helpful for orientation of new employees, and ultimately can be used for measuring productivity and job performance. Above all, they encourage *management by exception*, whereby teams of employees go about their daily work responsibilities without the need for someone constantly telling them what to do. Daily work patterns are commonly posted in kitchen areas, and workers understand that they are to accomplish the tasks to the best of their ability. In cases when the prescribed routine cannot be followed, the supervisor is notified and can assist with problem solving as needed. Otherwise, it is assumed that the work is being accomplished as planned. This acts to free up more of the supervisor's time for other duties and makes him or her more productive as well. When the process is used in combination with employees' input for design of the work patterns, workers tend to gain a sense of empowerment and independence as they perform their duties. For those requiring more direction, the written patterns provide direction and structure for work routines.

Exhibit 3–13 shows an example of a daily work pattern for several dietary associates involved in food preparation, tray assembly, and dishwashing tasks. It is common to assign a standard code to each position (P1 through P4 in this

Exhibit 3–13 Sample Daily Work Pattern

	Dietary Associate—P1	Dietary Associate—P2	Dietary Associate—P3	Dietary Associate—P4
6:30	Wash hands and check menu Check and record refrigerator temperatures Make coffee and assemble foods for beverage station	Wash hands and check menu Turn on hot food tables, set up portioning utensils Check and record food temperatures	Wash hands and check menu Set up starter station, get menus, line up carts	Wash hands and check menu Set up station with bread, cereal station, special items
7:00	Operate beverage station	Operate hot food station	Operate starter station	Operate bread/cereal station
7:45	Clean station and return items Cover, label, and date leftovers	Clean station and return items Cover, label, and date leftovers	Clean station and return items Cover, label, and date leftovers	Clean station and return items Cover, label, and date leftovers
8:15	15-Minute break	15-Minute break	15-Minute break	Make up late trays
8:30	Wash hands Prepare foods on cold food production sheet for lunch	Wash hands Set up dish machine, check temperatures and chemicals Wash dishes (loader) Wash/sanitize carts	Wash hands Make up late trays Wash/sanitize tray line Wash dishes (receiver) Wash/sanitize carts	15-Minute break Wash hands Make and deliver nourishments Assist with cold food preparation
11:00	Make coffee and assemble foods for beverage station	Turn on hot food tables, set up portioning utensils Check and record food temperatures	Set up starter station, get menus, line up carts	Set up station with bread, cereal station, special items
11:30	Operate beverage station	Operate hot food station	Operate starter station	Operate bread/cereal station
12:30	Clean station and return items Cover, label, and date leftovers	Clean station and return items Cover, label, and date leftovers	Clean station and return items Cover, label, and date leftovers	Clean station and return items Cover, label, and date leftovers
12:45	45-Minute break	Make & deliver late trays Wash/sanitize line	45-Minute break	45-Minute break

continues

Exhibit 3–13 continued

	Dietary Associate—P1	Dietary Associate—P2	Dietary Associate—P3	Dietary Associate—P4
1:30	Wash hands Set up dish machine, check temperatures and chemicals Wash dishes (loader) Wash/sanitize carts	45-Minute break Wash hands Assist with cold food preparation	Wash hands Prepare foods on cold food production sheet for dinner	Wash hands Wash dishes (receiver) Wash/sanitize carts
3:00	Off duty	Off duty	Off duty	Off duty

example). These codes can be inserted in the employees' weekly schedule, showing them which position they will fill each day. Such a system further demonstrates the principle of managing by exception. Some employees like routine, and they prefer to be assigned to the same position every day. Others get bored easily and like to be rotated from one position to another. Once employees' preferences are known, they can be incorporated on the master schedule for ease in planning.

There are several concepts that apply to the design of daily work patterns, one of which is *variety*. More strenuous physical work can be alternated throughout the day with less physical work. Typically boring tasks can be alternated with creative tasks. Independent work can be alternated with group work, and so on. The concepts of *job enrichment* and *job enlargement* can also be effectively applied. For example, in Exhibit 3–13, it can be seen that employees prepare the foods for their own tray assembly line positions, set up these stations themselves, and clean their areas afterward. Tasks such as dishwashing, which are not the most favorite ones, are shared equally among the employees so that no one has the burden of doing them all the time.

The concept of balancing the workload also applies to distribution of tasks for each position. All employees should have an even distribution of work; one position should not be lighter or easier than another so that employees perceive that they are being treated fairly. Employees' perceptions have much to do with workload distribution; therefore, it is important to make the design of daily work patterns a team effort. In Exhibit 3–12, it can be seen that *overlapping* shifts have been avoided with the use of part-time employees. This increases productivity and may be appropriate after an analysis of peak activity times is completed. Only the manager and cook positions overlap for morning and afternoon shifts because there is enough work required to keep them busy during off-peak hours.

If the concept of *staff development* is incorporated into this process, a career ladder will be available for employees who are interested in growing within the organization. There are three different job categories shown in Exhibit 3–12: dietary manager, cook, and dietary associate. Dietary associates can be cross-trained in each other's positions and in the cook's position. Cooks can be cross-trained to handle the dietary manager position as they attain certification by attending classes in colleges or through correspondence courses. This enables the organization to offer the potential for growth to its employees.

The incorporation of *employees' personal preferences* is another concept that can be successfully applied to job design. When a team approach is taken, employees have the opportunity to express their own choices, the things that make them happier on the job. For example, employees tend to like to take breaks together. This can be accomplished, for the most part, as long as one person stays present in the work area to perform services needed by patients or customers. This concept is illustrated in Exhibit 3–13, where the task of covering kitchen activities while others take their breaks is rotated from one position to another. Another way to implement the concept of choice is to involve employees in deciding who will fill the various roles each day. Some people like to do the same things every day, and others like to follow a different work pattern from day to day. The master schedule shown in Exhibit 3–14 shows how work assignments can be varied based on employees' personal preferences.

Another important concept to apply while one is planning daily work patterns pertains to the *menu plan*. Patient and cafeteria menus are the *blueprints* for work distribution. They determine the amount and kind of food that need to be produced and, in effect, the work done by each employee. They even determine the number of dishes and pots that have to be washed. Wise managers are able to consider the menu while planning daily work patterns, and they are also able to structure their menus to meet the staffing ratios that are available. Careful menu planning is essential in balancing the workload from meal to meal and day to day so that peaks and valleys do not occur in employees' routines.

Finally, the concept of *flexibility* needs to be incorporated into daily work patterns. Employees who work in teams are expected to help each other willingly when necessary and not to use the daily pattern to dictate their every action. The patterns are only guidelines for the day's events. Exceptions will always occur in the daily routine, and a team effort works best to overcome disruptions in the system.

Master Schedules

Master rotating menus help managers save time; master rotating schedules do the same. Master schedules list employees' names, job titles, and work hours with a repeated pattern of days off for a 2-, 3-, or 4-week period. The purpose of

Exhibit 3–14 Biweekly Food Service Employee Schedule

	Sun	Mon	Tues	Wed	Thur	Fri	Sat	Sun	Mon	Tues	Wed	Thur	Fri	Sat
Dietary Manager FT	M1	M1	M1	M1	M1	M1		M2	M1	M1	M1	M1	M2	M1
Dietary Manager FT	M2	M2	M2	M2	M2		M2	M1	M2		M2	M2		
Dietary Manager FT	M2					M2	M1	M1						M2
Cook FT	C1		M1	C1	C1	C1			C1	C1	C1	C1	C1	C1
Cook FT		C2	C2	C2	C2	C2	C2	C2		M2	C2	C2	C2	
Cook FT	C2	C1	C1			M2	C1	C1	C2	C2			M1	C2
Dietary Associate FT	P1		P1	P1	P1	C2			P1	P1	P1	P1	C1	P1
Dietary Associate FT	P2	P2		P2	P2	P2			P2	P2	P2	P2	C1	P2
Dietary Associate FT		P3	P3	P3	P3		P3	P3	P3	P3	P3	P3	P3	
Dietary Associate FT		P4	P4	P4	P4	P4	P4	P4	P4		P4	P4	P4	
Dietary Associate FT	P1	P1	P2	P4	P2	P3	P1	P1	P3	P2	P4	P2	P1	P2
Dietary Associate FT	NP1	NP1	NP1	NP1	NP1	NP1	NP1	NP1	NP1	NP1	NP1	NP1	NP2	NP1
Dietary Associate FT		NP2	NP2	NP2	NP2				NP2	NP2	NP2	NP2	NP2	
Dietary Associate FT	SR	SR	SR	SR	SR	SR			SR	SR	SR	SR	SR	
Dietary Associate FT	UT1	UT1	UT1	UT1	UT1	UT1			UT1	UT1	UT1	UT1	UT1	UT1
Dietary Associate FT	P4	UT1	NP1	SR		NP2	NP1	NP1		NP2	SR	NP2	NP1	P4
Dietary Associate PT	P5		P5	P5	P5	P5	P2	P2	P5	P5	P5			P5
Dietary Associate PT	P6		P6	P6	P6	P6			P6	P6	P6	P7	P6	P6
Dietary Associate PT		P7	P7	P7	P7		P7	P7	P8	P7	P7	P7	P7	
Dietary Associate PT		P8	P8	P8	P8	P8	P8	P8	P8	P8	P8	P8	P8	
Dietary Associate PT	NP3	NP3	NP3	NP3	NP3	NP3			NP3	NP3	NP3	NP3		NP3
Dietary Associate PT		NP4	NP4	NP4	NP4	NP4	NP4	NP4	NP4	NP4	NP4	NP4	NP4	

continues

Exhibit 3–14 continued

	Sun	Mon	Tues	Wed	Thur	Fri	Sat	Sun	Mon	Tues	Wed	Thur	Fri	Sat
Dietary Associate PT	P7	P6			P8	P1	P5	P5	NP4			P6	P2	P7
Dietary Associate PT	P3	P5	NP3			P7	P6	P6	P7	NP4			P5	P3
Dietary Associate PT	P8	UT2	UT2			NP4	UT1	UT1	UT2	UT2			NP3	P8
Dietary Associate PT	UT2			UT2	UT2	UT2	UT2	UT2			UT2	UT2	UT2	UT2
8 hour employees	10	12	12	12	12	12	10	10	12	12	12	12	12	10
4 hour employees	6	7	7	7	7	7	6	6	7	7	7	7	7	6
Total scheduled hours	104	124	124	124	124	124	104	104	124	124	124	124	124	104
Scheduled hours/week							828							828
FTEs (@ 40 hrs/wk)							20.7							20.7

the master schedule is to systematize the scheduling process while ensuring that adequate coverage is provided. Computerization of schedules can also be used to increase efficiency and reduce the time required for schedule preparation.

Exhibit 3–14 shows a biweekly master schedule for the same department described previously. The codes shown on the schedule correspond with job assignments specified in the daily work pattern (see Exhibit 3–12). By using this method of scheduling along with daily work patterns, employees know automatically what tasks they need to complete each day, thus avoiding the need for constant supervision.

The steps involved in completing a master schedule include the following (of course, the specific parameters used for scheduling depend upon the payroll period and policies of a given organization):

1. Determine the minimum staff needed to get the job done.
2. List all employee names, hours of work, and job titles in the left column of the schedule.
3. Include alternate weekends off for all employees, where appropriate.
4. Ensure that employees work no more than 5 consecutive days without a day off.
5. When employees work on a weekend, make sure they are off 1 day before the Saturday they work and 1 day after the Sunday they work.
6. Relief or part-time employees should be scheduled when full-time employees are off.
7. Balance the schedule by counting the total number of employees in each job category for each day. Make sure that daily yields correspond with the daily staffing pattern.

Employees can be involved successfully in planning master schedules. The days they prefer to have off can be accommodated as long as proper operation of the department is not jeopardized. Some employees prefer to have weekends off, and others prefer to have weekdays off to do their shopping or spend their leisure time while everyone else is working. These things will not be known unless employees provide input in the scheduling process. In the example shown in Exhibit 3–14, most employees are able to have every other weekend off, and when this is not possible the same two consecutive weekdays are granted each week to provide a dependable routine for workers.

The concepts of staff development and cross-training are also reflected in the sample schedule. For example, cooks take turns in covering the dietary manager position from time to time, and dietary associates take turns covering the cook position. This enables the organization to meet several objectives. It ensures adequate coverage of duties for vacations and emergency situations when relief is needed. It gives employees the opportunity to test out their skills at a higher level, the level they may ultimately wish to achieve. It also provides a more global perspective for employees because when they walk in someone else's shoes they have a better understanding of the system and how people can work together to improve services. In many settings, this type of system would require payment of employees at the higher level, but most managers feel that the benefits they reap are worth the small investment. In unionized facilities, care must be taken to ensure that these types of incentives are in line with union contracts.

In the sample schedule, it can also be seen that dietary associates are rotated in the various job functions and according to their preference. Those who prefer to follow a certain job pattern routinely can do so as long as they are adequately cross-trained in the others. When employees' preferences conflict, it is common to use seniority as the basis for decision making.

Flexible Scheduling

The concept of *flexible scheduling* has been practiced in the restaurant, hotel, and other highly competitive industries for years. Managers in those setting know that, to succeed in business, they must balance variations in income with variations in expenditures. Many people in the health care industry are just now learning how to do this. They are also learning that some expenses that were previously assumed to be fixed are not really set in stone as such and that these expenses need to be reconsidered as potential targets for cost reduction.

Flexible scheduling is the process whereby the number of scheduled work hours is set to conform to the expected outputs of the department. One example already described for Exhibit 3–12 is how fewer employees are scheduled in the cafeteria on weekends because the sales volume is lower on these days. The same principle can apply to patient services. For patient food service employees, it is advisable to increase and decrease scheduled work hours based on patient days so that the number of manhours per patient day remains constant. In some settings, the number of manhours per meal served might also need to be considered.

For the clinical staff, this type of scheduling may be a bit more complex because a set rate for income to the organization for clinical nutrition services is often difficult to identify. One might consider the model used by the nursing staff because it normally takes into account patient turnover rates and the concept of acuity levels. By using techniques of task and job analyses, one can define the average amount of time for various nutrition services that are routinely performed and from this identify the average time required for each new admission. Table 3–3 provides an example of time estimates for the various clinical tasks. It has incorporated data from DeHoog (1985), Dietetic Staffing Commit-

Table 3-3 Sample Time Allocations for Patient Care Activities

Activity	Basic (Moderate risk)	Comprehensive (High risk)
Nutrition screening	5 minutes	10 minutes
Assessment and care planning (data collection, chart review, developing plan and charting)	45 minutes	60 minutes
Consultation with team members	15 minutes	15 minutes
Follow-up or discharge referral	15 minutes	30 minutes
Nutrition education	30 minutes	45 minutes
3-Day nutrient intake analysis	45 minutes	45 minutes

Source: Reprinted from S.H. Laramee, Monitoring Productivity of the Clinical Staff, *Hospital Food & Nutrition Focus,* Vol. 11, No. 10, pp. 4–5, © 1995, Aspen Publishers, Inc.

tee (1982), Gates Smith, Konkle, and Semen (1991), Grant and DeHoog (1991), and McManners and Barina (1984). Essential time spent in other activities can be built into the final ratio to determine the number of manhours per patient day, patient admission, or adjusted patient admission.

Before flexible scheduling is attempted for food service or clinical staff, it is important to undertake the steps recommended for job redesign. This enables managers to discontinue obsolete tasks and prioritize the activities that are essential for high-quality service. The next step is to be sure that cross-training occurs so that, if the daily staffing pattern needs to be collapsed, the remaining employees can perform all the tasks that are essential to maintain quality. After this is done, the points or thresholds at which staffing should be increased or decreased can be identified. For example, the staffing level for food service personnel in the 325-bed hospital illustrated in Exhibit 3–12 is based upon a 75% occupancy level (244 patients per day). If average occupancy is reduced and sustained at 70%, this might trigger reassessment of the current staffing level, and the employee schedule would reflect this reduction. Because a 7% decrease in patient days had occurred (from 244 to 228), the daily staffing level for patient activities would have to be decreased by the same percentage, and hours for employees assigned to patient activities would be affected accordingly. This would result in a decrease by 7.3 work hours on weekends and 8.7 hours on weekdays.

At this point, one would have to determine the source of the reductions, that is, exactly which positions would have to be altered. If cafeteria volume had not changed, it would be logical to focus on the employees with greater time allocations to patient services and not to alter the hours dedicated to nonpatient functions. With input from the staff, an alternative schedule could be determined to implement various options depending upon the extent of reduction in patient days. For example, one or more of the following scenarios could occur:

- Change the hours of position P4 to cover lunch and dinner instead of breakfast and lunch, while letting others (UT1 or SR) assist during breakfast. Position P8 could be discontinued to save 4 hours (3%) per day.
- Collapse positions P1 through P4 into three positions, and P5 through P8 also into three positions, while allowing cooks and other workers (UT1, UT2, and SR) to serve hot foods on tray line as necessary to save 12 hours (10%) per day.
- Discontinue the SR position, and have dietary managers perform their tasks with assistance from cooks and other employees to save 8 hours (6%) on each weekday.

Greater cooperation is achieved when staff members and union representatives are involved in setting the strategy for flexible scheduling. An important issue that needs to be addressed is reaction time, that is, just how soon after the changes in occupancy occur should the staffing level change. Large departments, such as nursing, may flex from day to day to maintain adequate levels. They may have a pool of per diem employees who can be scheduled on a day-to-day basis to meet the need. Smaller departments probably need a longer reaction time, especially when per diem workers are not available. When flexible staffing is incorporated, these departments would obviously benefit from the use of part-time employees and shorter scheduling periods, especially if patient days are found to be highly variable.

It is imperative that managers work with administrators to set up a plan that is best for patients, employees, and the organization. A 1-week reaction time may work well as long as part-time employees are hired with the understanding that flexible staffing may affect their hours. In addition, acceptable benefit programs need to be available to keep these employees motivated to continue their employment during periods of low occupancy.

One advantage of having a flexible staffing plan is that the department is able to cope well when employees unexpectedly fail to report to work. If predetermined options such as those suggested above are established as back-up systems, one can avoid overtime and the need to call in relief personnel. For essential positions, many managers find it helpful to establish a telephone tree, whereby employees automatically call certain part-time employees to cover for them as soon as they know of their inability to report to work. A follow-up call to the department can then be made to inform the manager of the situation and arrangements for coverage.

Human Resource Issues

Drucker stated "You cannot manage workers, unless you realize that the workplace is something for people. And your biggest problem and your biggest opportunity is that you integrate physical and inanimate objectives" (Beckham, 1991, p. 66). It is clear that successful directors of food and nutrition services in the year 2000 and beyond will be much more sensitive to the management of human resources. With shortages of unskilled workers, proficiency in creating departments that attract and retain staff will be necessary. Those who feel that they are deficient in this area might consider retraining so that they acquire the expertise to "tune" the people who really make a difference: their staff.

The 1996 Joint Commission (1995) standards state that leaders "create a culture that fosters self-development and continued learning to support the organization's mission" (p. 381). When this is done, it promotes an environment that motivates staff to contribute to the organizational goal and fosters employee satisfaction and productivity. Spears (1995) states that human resource management signifies the extension of the traditional requirements for managing people effectively. In earlier times, it simply represented the efforts, by teams, to produce products. In the new or reengineered organization, according to Spears, communications will be multidirectional, employees will be more involved in decision making, autonomous work teams will play a greater role, cross-functional training will be necessary, performance evaluation will incorporate team goals, financial and group rewards will become more important, peers will have increased involvement in the selection process, and horizontal career paths will be emphasized more. It is also expected that human resource policies will be able to reflect quality and customer service issues in addition to having measurable results.

It is the responsibility of managers to provide employees with the tools needed to perform their jobs and to assess and develop their skills on an ongoing basis. It is also their responsibility to show employees that they are honest, inspiring, and competent and really care about their personal development. Only then will staff members feel a strong sense of team spirit, feel committed to the organization, and see their values as consistent with those of the organization. If managers work with their employees and constantly update their skills, then they will anticipate change. When staff members are made a part of that vision, then they will take on the responsibility of contributing to the growth of an organization. Careful selection, orientation, and training are critical for these things to occur. Readers are referred to Chapter 14 for discussion of these topics.

INTEGRATING AND COORDINATING SERVICES

According to Stichler (1994), integration is "the process of organizing activities internal to the system to perform the functions of the system" (p. 48). With fewer supervisory and managerial staff available in the restructured organization, it will be key that the whole is equal to the sum of the parts and that staff never lose sight of the goals and objectives of the department. This will require that the manager carefully coordinate all the activities involved, not only within the department but also interdepartmentally. While managers are attempting to integrate services, it is necessary to demonstrate effective communications, clear objectives and goals, and appropriate action plans to reach these goals. The vision of the organization should always be the focus, and this requires constant reinforcement. Leaders of the new organization will need to have frequent meetings with staff to review the goals and to provide support for those with changing roles.

Integrating services can be considered a developmental process. Stichler (1994) describes the following stages in its progression:

1. competition, as staff become territorial to protect their turf
2. cooperation, as staff then start sharing ideas
3. coordination, as staff focus on tasks that are related to the goal
4. collaboration, as staff gain trust and a working relationship
5. integration, the final step, when staff have worked through the other stages

Integration of services will require a great deal of time and effort on the part of the leaders of the future. Stichler (1994) emphasizes the fact that integration will require time, be relationship based, and be highly dependent on trust within the group. In the words of Henry Ford, "Coming together is a beginning, keeping together is a process, working together is success" (Stichler, 1994, p. 53).

Implementing self-directed work teams and patient-focused care is a good beginning. Ensuring that managers act as facilitators offering continued support will keep it together.

Integrated Health Care Systems

Integrated health care systems were described earlier in this chapter. These systems show great promise for the industry because they combine the efforts of everyone concerned with health care in the community. A wonderful example of how leaders in food and nutrition care can expand their roles into the community can be seen at Gundersen Lutheran Medical Center in La Crosse, Wisconsin. This 180-bed facility employs 17 dietitians, who spend most of their time providing nutrition services in the outpatient clinics and various community settings. Their 500 Club™ is a program whereby dietitians work with chefs to develop meals that do not exceed 500 calories. Consumers look for these meals at restaurants, grocery stores, convenience stores, and universities. Consultation is provided for nursing homes, school systems, wellness centers, colleges, and grocery stores. Dietitians even teach nutrition on television in their *One Minute Morsel* program, which they produce at the medical center.

Interdisciplinary Coordination

Whether professionals find themselves working in large health care systems or independent institutions, there is a need to coordinate efforts with other members of the health care team. Grindel (1994) urged dietitians to "recognize the expertise of others and communicate." She encouraged practitioners to work together to identify how overlapping skills should be used and suggested that nurses and dietitians help each other by sharing assessment data, not burying them in charts where it takes too much time to find them. Other suggestions for dietitians are to engage in collaborative management of patient symptoms related to nutrition status and to interface directly with physicians and be patient if they need to wait for responses to their recommendations. Most important, while dealing with the nursing staff, dietitians need to realize that they are overloaded, too (Grindel, 1994).

Personal mastery is key to establishing good relationships with others in the health care setting. PiSunyer states "The most important thing is for dietitians to be knowledgeable in the rationale behind the changing of an order. This makes them more self-confident and articulate in presenting reasons for a change. Then the physician will be more likely to follow their recommendation" (Jackson, 1995, p. 7). He believes that when dietitians are well informed they can be more effective in changing a physician's mind. Direct communication with physicians is advised as well: "It is a mistake to use nurses as medians for communications from the dietitian to the physician. They are also very busy and have a different point of view. Messages often get lost in the translation" (Jackson, 1995, p. 7). Dietitians should approach physicians directly because they know the changes they would like to see and the rationale behind their recommendations and can answer any questions that the physician may have. Another suggestion offered by PiSunyer is not to make chart notes too lengthy because others may not have time to read them all. He encourages dietitians to sharpen their writing skills and communicate in a well-organized, brief, and concise manner while providing the rationale for why patients will benefit from any changes that are recommended.

One good way that interdisciplinary teams can work together to cut costs and increase quality is by using critical paths. The department of nursing at New England Medical Center Hospitals in Boston, Massachusetts, was one of the first to introduce critical paths as a management tool based upon standards of care for particular diagnoses. The critical path used was somewhat of a shorthand or diagrammatic method that included nursing diagnoses, achievable clinical outcomes within the length of time allotted by the diagnosis-related groups, intermediate goals with estimated dates for each outcome, and nursing/physician interventions to facilitate progress toward each goal. Variances from the plan were evaluated to identify problems in the system, and this ultimately led to improved care and lower costs.

Critical paths have more recently evolved into more of an interdisciplinary approach. Nutrition care is included in the critical pathways at Mt. Clemens General Hospital in Mt. Carmel, Michigan. The pathways were tested for congestive heart failure patients to determine whether improved patient outcomes would occur, and dramatic results were seen. The control group, consisting of 389 patients who were treated using traditional methods, had an average length of stay of 7.8 days, whereas the clinical path group, consisting of 65 patients, had an average length of stay of 5.1 days. The readmission rates for the two groups averaged 23.9% and 16.9%, respectively, showing the long-term benefits of this integrated practice. A sample of this pathway is provided in Chapter 4.

At the Jerry L. Pettis Veterans' Administration Medical Center in Loma Linda, California, an integrated system for initial patient assessment was implemented to replace the traditional fragmented design, which involved separate screening by many departments. An interdisciplinary team developed a new method to minimize redundancy, make assessment information more easily accessible to all providers of care, and reduce paperwork. By comparing the former and revised models (see Figures 3–3 and 3–4), one can easily see how increased efficiency can result from interdisciplinary coordination of activities.

Intradepartmental Coordination

Before professionals even try to improve relationships with persons outside the department, it is essential that strong, trusting bonds exist within. Often, conflict occurs between food service and clinical staff, which is detrimental to the department and to the organization as a whole. A balance must be achieved between these two components of the department if patients are to be served in an effective and efficient manner. Neither aspect is more important than the other, and to achieve the goal of high-quality food services and nutrition care both must be valued equally in the mind of the person leading the department as well as his or her followers.

In cases where the food service component predominates, dietitians often lack resources, support, and motivation to perform nutrition assessments and develop effective care plans for patients. On the other hand, when the clinical nutrition component predominates, aspects involving the purchasing, production, and management of employees engaged in these processes are often weak.

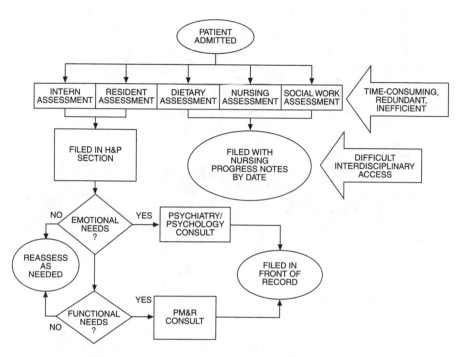

Figure 3–3 Traditional patient screening system. Courtesy of Jerry L. Pettis Veterans' Administration Medical Center, Loma Linda, California.

When this happens, dietitians are unable to meet the nutritional needs of patients, who must receive tasty meals that conform to their food preferences and diet prescriptions so that they are able to improve their health status. A good lesson can be learned from Arrucci, an orchestra conductor:

> My job is to shape and mold the musicians so they are unified in tempo. Each one comes with their talents, the skills they have mastered through hard work and practice. The singers must work together. The musicians on strings must coordinate their bowing first with others in their section, and then blend in with the other sections, the woodwinds, percussion, and brass. They must work as a team, so to speak. Professional musicians are very serious people for the most part. Their individual personality normally has no effect on outcomes because it is the strength of their skills that really makes the difference. When a conductor leads musicians, it's up to this person to see that all players produce the same emotion with their instruments so the parts of the music build together simulta-

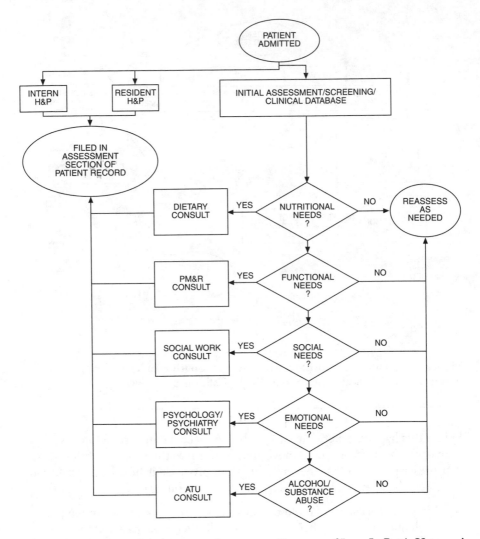

Figure 3–4 Integrated patient screening system. Courtesy of Jerry L. Pettis Veterans' Administration Medical Center, Loma Linda, California.

neously. Each and every instrument has equal importance. For example, the bass does not get to play the melody but since it has the lowest sound it provides the foundation for all the others and there is no depth without it. At times certain instruments must take the spotlight. Musicians learn when their part is to be prominent as they take on the melody, and when to be soft as harmony and provide background for other instruments.With so many skilled musicians, just what is the exact role of the conductor? The conductor is the only one with foresight, and this person knows the ultimate outcome well enough to lead the orchestra to success (Jackson, 1996b, p. 2).

REFERENCES

Beckham, J.D. (1991). More tools for the nineties. *Healthcare Forum Journal, 34*(4), 63–66.

Black, R. (1994). Patient care restructuring and human resources. In M.L. Parsons & C.L. Murdaugh (Eds.), *Patient-centered care: A model for restructuring* (pp. 181–200). Gaithersburg, MD: Aspen.

Blessing, B. (1986, October). The muscles behind the smiles. *Training Magazine*, p. 52.

Boston, C., & Vestal, K.W. (1994). Work transformation. *Hospital & Health Networks, 68*(7), 52.

Boulding, K.E. (1956). General systems theory—The skeleton of science. *Management Science, 2*(3), 197–208.

Burda, D. (1993, December 20). Cutting down. *Modern Healthcare*, pp. 49–58.

Byers, B.A., Shanklin, C.W., & Hoover, L.C. (1994). *Food service manual for health care institutions.* Chicago: American Hospital Association.

Champy, J. (1996). *Reengineering management: The mandate for new leadership.* New York: Harper Business.

Chase, R.B., & Aquilano, N.G. (1992). *Production operations management, a life-cycle approach.* Homewood, NJ: Irwin.

Clouten, K., & Weber, R. (1994). Patient focused care ... Playing to win. *Nursing Management, 25*(2), 34–36.

Coleman, M. (1992). Twelve hour shift schedules: What you need to know. *Human Resources Focus, 69*, 16–17.

Cromwell, J., & Butrica, B. (1995). Hospital department cost and employment increases: 1982–1992. *Healthcare Finance Review, 17*(1), 147–165.

DeHoog, S. (1985). Identifying patients at nutrition risk and determining clinical productivity: Essentials for an effective nutrition care program. *Journal of the American Dietetic Association, 85*, 1620–1622.

Dietetic Staffing Committee. (1982). *Clinical Dietetic Staffing Kit.* Chicago: American Dietetic Association.

Gates Smith, K., Konkle, K.R., & Semen, M. (1991). Charging for hospital-based nutrition services. In M.K. Fox (Ed.), *Reimbursement and insurance coverage for nutrition services* (pp. 35–60). Chicago: American Dietetic Association.

Grant, A., & DeHoog, S. (1991). *Nutrition assessment and support.* Seattle: Authors.

Grindel, C.G. (1994, October). *Developing successful alliances with other health professionals.* Presented at the 1994 annual meeting of the American Dietetic Association, Orlando, FL.

Henderson, J.L., & Williams, J.B. (1991). Ten steps for restructuring patient care. *Healthcare Forum Journal, 34*(4), 50–55.

Jackson, R. (1995). Making effective dietary recommendations. *Hospital Food & Nutrition Focus*, *11*(10), 7–8.

Jackson, R. (1996a). Computerized medical records. A look at the future. *Hospital Food & Nutrition Focus*, *12*(8), 6–7.

Jackson, R. (1996b). Conducting hospital business. *Hospital Food & Nutrition Focus*, *12*(4), 2.

Joint Commission on Accreditation of Healthcare Organizations. (1995). *1996 Accreditation manual for hospitals*. Oakbrook Terrace, IL: Author.

Juran, J.M. (1989). *Juran on leadership for quality. An executive handbook*. New York: Free Press.

Kinsel, K.K. (1995, November). *Hospital restructuring: A challenge for dietetic professionals*. Presented at the annual meeting of the American Dietetic Association, Chicago, IL.

Kotler, J.P. (1990). What leaders really do. *Harvard Business Review*, *68*(11), 103–110.

Lathrop, J.P. (1993). *Restructuring health care. The patient focused paradigm*. San Francisco: Jossey-Bass.

Leana, C.R. (1986). Predictors and consequences of delegation. *Academy of Management Journal*, *29*, 754–774.

Lumsdon, K. (1994). Want to save millions. *Hospital & Health Networks*, *68*(21), 24–32.

McGinn, N. (1993). Patient centered care: Opportunities for health care professionals to work together. *Dietetic Currents*, *20*(3), 2–4.

McManners, M.H., & Barina, S.A. (1984). Productivity in clinical dietetics. *Journal of the American Dietetic Association*, *84*, 1035–1041.

Morell, J.C. (1995). Turn your focus outside-in. *Hospital & Health Networks*, *69*(23), 66.

Olmstead, B., & Smith, S. (1989). Flex for success. *Personnel*, *66*, 50–55.

Schiller, M.R. (1995, November). *Hospital restructuring: A challenge for dietetic professionals*. Presented at the annual meeting of the American Dietetic Association, Chicago, IL.

Schlessinger, L.A., & Heskett, J.L. (1991). The service-driven service company. *Harvard Business Review*, *69*, 71–81.

Senge, P.M. (1990). *The fifth discipline: The art and practice of the learning organization*. New York: Doubleday Currency.

Sowa, D.C. (1995). *Launching a clinical nutrition practice model for the 21st century*. Presented at the 1995 annual meeting of the American Dietetic Association, Chicago, IL.

Spears, M.C. (1995). *Foodservice organizations: A managerial and systems approach*. Englewood Cliffs, NJ: Prentice Hall.

Stichler, J.F. (1994). System development and integration in healthcare. *Journal of Nursing Administration*, *24*(10), 48–53.

Tidkis, F., & Strasen, L. (1994, September). Patient focused care units improve service and financial outcomes. *Healthcare Financial Management*, pp. 38–44.

von Bertalanffy, L. (1951). General systems theory: A new approach to the unity of science. *Human Biology*, *23*(12), 303–361.

Zemke, R., & Albrecht, K. (1985). *Service America*. Homewood, IL: Dow Jones Irwin.

Focus on Nutrition Care

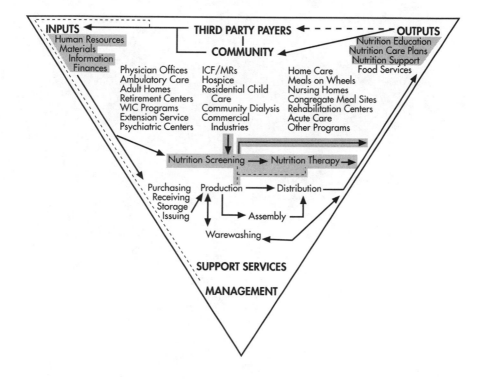

INPUTS
Human Resources
Materials
Information
Finances

THIRD PARTY PAYERS

COMMUNITY

OUTPUTS
Nutrition Education
Nutrition Care Plans
Nutrition Support
Food Services

Physician Offices
Ambulatory Care
Adult Homes
Retirement Centers
WIC Programs
Extension Service
Psychiatric Centers

ICF/MRs
Hospice
Residential Child
  Care
Community Dialysis
Commercial
  Industries

Home Care
Meals on Wheels
Nursing Homes
Congregate Meal Sites
Rehabilitation Centers
Acute Care
Other Programs

Nutrition Screening → Nutrition Therapy

Purchasing
Receiving
Storage
Issuing

Production → Distribution

Assembly

Warewashing

SUPPORT SERVICES

MANAGEMENT

Managing Nutrition Services

Sylvia Escott-Stump

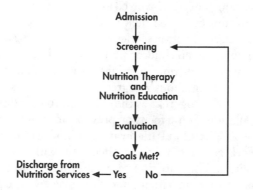

Under the standards of the Joint Commission on Accreditation of Healthcare Organizations (Joint Commission) and other regulatory bodies, the quality of nutrition care is reviewed and evaluated. During the recent years of the Joint Commission's *agenda for change*, direct patient care has been the focus. Important functions have been identified as critically influential to outcomes. Timely and effective use of resources, through multidisciplinary teams, has been the goal. From screening, assessment, and reassessment of needs, development of a nutrition care plan in cooperation with other disciplines, ordering of medical nutrition therapy, communication and preparation of these orders, and monitoring the process to continuous improvement of the nutrition care process, managing quality and productivity is essential.

In dietetic services departments, whether acute care, long-term care, ambulatory, or home care, the nutritional care staff plan, administer, and evaluate services that are rendered to patients or clients. These services are generally administered under the auspices of a clinical nutrition manager, who is a registered dietitian, often with a master's degree in the field. In larger facilities, there may be several administrative layers of clinical management, including associate and assistant directors above the chief clinical dietitian or clinical nutrition manager. In smaller facilities or in nursing homes, the department director may fulfill these functions personally, may delegate some tasks to the staff clinical dietitians, or may hire an outside consulting dietitian for these services. In home care, the dietitians are sometimes consultants or clinicians who must manage time and services effectively to provide excellent care.

For community nutrition services, dietitians or community nutritionists, or professionals with more general backgrounds such as home economists, assume responsibility for nutrition programs. Their focus is the overall health of community members. They design and administer local and federal programs that focus primarily on prevention. They are involved in the surveillance of the population to identify high-risk groups that need their services. These practitioners work in a variety of settings, such as extension services; programs for the aging; school lunch programs; women, infants, and children programs; and others. They educate and guide the population and sometimes administer food programs.

The most exciting thing about integrated health care is that it enables all these professions to come together as they attempt to coordinate their services to benefit the population. Some focus on prevention, and others focus on clinical treatment. The quality of nutrition care and food service will depend upon their ability to work cooperatively and effectively with each other and those from other disciplines. The nutrition care staff must maintain high standards and reliable output so that the patients and clients receive the proper services in a timely manner. In the past, the management function was focused primarily on the food service activities, but dietitians are starting to realize that nutrition care services require careful planning, directing, coordinating, and improving as well. This chapter focuses on these functions, with special attention given to coordinating and evaluating components for nutrition care activities.

ROLE OF THE CLINICAL NUTRITION MANAGER

In the acute care setting, clinical nutrition managers are responsible for developing systems that successfully meet the nutritional needs of patients. Foltz, Schiller, and Ryan (1993) reviewed nutrition screening protocols and assessment procedures used by 388 dietitians in the field and advised dietitians to take more of a leadership role by assuming greater responsibilities for these activities:

> Our study indicates widespread lack of self-confidence or awareness among dietitians that they are ultimately responsible for nutrition screening and assessment policies in their institutions. A relatively large number indicated that physicians, administrators, pharmacists, nurses, or even social workers had greater influence than dietitians did over nutrition assessment procedures and policies. This view suggests a lack of accountability and leadership in an area that is distinctly within the dietitian's scope of practice. (p. 1394)

Their research indicated that nearly all institutions (90.2%) had a protocol for nutrition screening for patients but that only 61.2% of the hospitals actually practiced nutrition screening for all patients who were admitted. In addition, it was found that the majority of the hospitals had protocols for nutrition assessment (84.0%). Variation was found in how patients were selected for assessments. Assessments were performed for all patients in 10.6% of the hospitals, for those at nutrition risk at 66.8%, for nutrition support patients at 54.1%, and for patients referred by physicians at 56.5%. After learning about the specific practices followed at the various facilities, the researchers noted "There appears to be widespread confusion and inconsistency in assessment practices" (Foltz et al., 1993, p. 1395).

The Joint Commission has recently set more detailed standards for screening and assessment for all heath care facilities, and the Omnibus Budget Reconciliation Act of 1987 (OBRA) regulations have provided specific standards for long-term care. Yet these guidelines do leave room for variation among practice settings, and there is a continuing need for dietitians to establish standard protocols for the nutrition care of patients. Many efforts have been made to develop practice guidelines.

In the community setting, many large-scale studies have shown the need for improvement in the health of the American population. A high-priority need set forth in the *Healthy People 2000* report (U.S. Department of Health and Human Services, 1990) was the need for an improved surveillance and data system to support the improvement of nutrition in the nation. According to this report, the National Nutrition Monitoring System should include the following:

- people in hospitals, nursing homes, convalescent centers, and institutions such as those for the developmentally disabled
- physically, mentally, and developmentally disabled individuals in community settings
- children in child care facilities
- native Americans on reservations
- the old and very old living independently
- people in correctional facilities
- the homeless

This report also stated "Attainment of *Healthy People 2000* objectives will depend substantially on educational and community-based programs to promote health and prevent disease" (U.S. Department of Health and Human Services, 1990, p. 250). In addition, it encouraged "national health promotion and disease prevention through increased access to clinical preventive services" (p. 530). According to the U.S. Department of Health and Human Services, clinical preventive services refer to immunization programs, screening for early detection of disease or risk factors, and patient counseling; those services are delivered to individuals in the health care setting. This chapter focuses on the management of clinical preventive services.

PLANNING

Successful clinical nutrition managers of the future will have the leadership skills necessary to ensure proper nutrition care for patients and other customers. They will use a systems approach to develop necessary assignments within nutritional care. As described in Chapter 3, the following six levels of planning need to occur; they are listed in order of their specificity, and further definition of their characteristics is given in Chapter 3:

1. vision
2. mission
3. goals and objectives
4. policies
5. procedures
6. methods

The mission statements, goals, and objectives of nutrition care will be integrated with those of the organization. A mission-based process can be used so that quality management is reflected and a customer-oriented focus is taken whenever possible. O'Rourke and Bader (1993) presented a model that shows how the mission of an organization relates to quality management. Figure 4–1 illustrates how the mission, vision, and goals relate to quality outcomes, processes, value, and satisfaction. This figure also identifies how results of quality measurement are incorporated into the routine reporting system so that future plans can reflect the needs of customers. Chapter 3 includes statements from the hospital setting. Figure 4–2 shows statements from the long-term care setting.

As mission statements, goals, and objectives are identified, it is important to keep the scope of services in mind. The scope of services for food and nutrition departments typically includes meals and snacks for patients, nutrition therapy and education, food services for employees and guests, catering for special events, and other responsibilities that the department assumes. This concept is particularly helpful if restructuring or reengineering initiatives are expected or in progress within the organization. It is helpful to clinical nutrition managers further to define nutrition therapy and education services provided for external customers (patients and other customers) and internal customers (employees within the facility).

The following list can be used as a guide for determining the typical responsibilities of the nutrition care staff. It does not preclude other assignments but rather highlights patient-focused care. The extent of the various assignments will, of course, vary by setting (e.g., acute care versus home care):

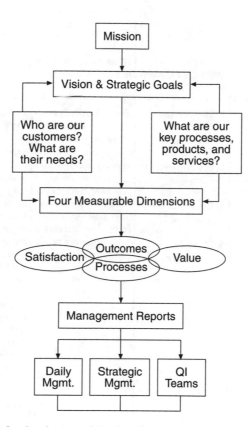

Figure 4–1 Process for developing a board quality and performance report. *Source:* Reprinted with permission from L.M. O'Rourke and B.S. Bader, A Process for Developing a Board Quality and Performance Report, *The Quality Letter,* March, 1993, p. 9.

- processing diet prescriptions and referrals from physicians, nurses, and other team members
- analysis of nutrient or calorie intakes
- food production estimates from patient menus
- monitoring standardized recipes and products for nutrient content or potential allergies
- screening for nutritional risk factors
- assigning priority levels for patient care
- modifying menus according to physician orders and patient preferences, allergies, and religion

MISSION	VALUES	VISION	STRATEGIC GOALS
Why We Exist	What We Believe In	What We Are Striving to Become in the Next Five Years	Major Initiatives Spanning the Next Three to Five Years
Forbes Health System declares its primary mission to be the provision of affordable, quality, personalized services to meet the health-related needs of the western Pennsylvania area. **Mission and Strategic Direction** Forbes Health System will be the provider of choice in eastern suburban Allegheny and western Westmoreland Counties, serving as the principal point of access for area residents to an integrated, regional network of competitively priced, effectively delivered, high value health care services.	1. Innovation 2. Teamwork 3. Responsiveness to Customers 4. Respect for Every Individual 5. Strong Financial Performance	Forbes Health System strives to become a fully integrated and coordinated healthcare system which provides comprehensive programs and services of the highest quality and most reasonable cost (value) to meet the total healthcare needs of the communities it serves.	1. Expand on ambulatory and pre- and post-care by organizationally, program-matically, and economically aligning with our physicians to improve accessibility and manage episodes of care across delivery settings. This focus will be supported by organizational and cultural changes to support our vision. 2. Make our services more affordable by managing resources effectively and efficiently and concentrating on improving our clinical and operating processes. 3. Develop partnerships with key constituents—businesses, communities, insurers and other providers—to identify and fill service/function gaps. 4. Develop outcome measurement and monitoring systems to assess and improve system quality. 5. Maintain a motivated and well-educated work force.

Figure 4–2 Forbes Health System. Courtesy of Forbes Nursing Center, Pittsburgh, Pennsylvania.

- nutritional assessments and timely reassessments
- patient or family education and counseling
- nutrition advisement on potential food–drug interactions or consequences
- nutrition interventions for oral, enteral, and parenteral nutrition modalities (may or may not include writing/updating prescriptions)
- implementing care according to practice guidelines, clinical pathways, care maps, or other facility standards

- monitoring patient outcomes as a result of interventions
- follow-up consultation to monitor patient outcomes
- documentation of nutrition services
- discharge planning for nutrition services in other settings

Policies and procedures are derived from the department's goals and objectives. For clinical nutrition services, Exhibit 4–1 can be used as a guide for organizing the table of contents for the nutritional policy manual. It was developed for use in the long-term care setting, but the concept of delineating specific

---

Exhibit 4–1 Policies and Procedures: Table of Contents for Nutrition Care Services

1. Diet orders and nutrition care
2. Approved diet manual and liberalized geriatric diets for long-term care
3. Therapeutic diets and seasoning packets
4. Resident preference form
5. New admission dietary handout
6. Assistive eating devices and feeding program
7. Nutrition status
8. Documentation of nutrition assessment
9. Anthropometric measurements
10. Resident plan of care
11. Hydration
12. Skin integrity and pressure sores
13. Enteral tube feedings
14. Preparation of mixed tube feedings
15. Enteral formulary
16. Between-meal feedings
17. Tray identification system
18. Nutrition committee
19. Menu processing and editing
20. Nutrition Kardex system
21. Calorie count
22. Authorization for charting in medical records
23. Fluid-restricted diets
24. Dietitian's communications with physicians
25. Use of thickening agents and dysphagia
26. Alcoholic beverages
27. Freedom from restraints
28. Resident discharge
29. Joint Commission and state surveys

Courtesy of Forbes Nursing Center, Pittsburgh, Pennsylvania.

policies and procedures applies to all settings. The next step is to develop a policy for each key performance expectation.

While writing policies and procedures, the clinical nutrition manager must remember to coordinate activities with other disciplines so that the expectations of team members are the same. As noted in Chapter 3, some facilities may set up their manuals in an interdisciplinary fashion to reflect the format and sequencing found in the Joint Commission standards. Cross-referencing policies with these standards and the policy numbers from the manuals of other departments can also be considered. The policy and procedures for enteral tube feedings is shown in Exhibit 4–2. Notice how the disciplines involved in this process are identified.

DIRECTING

The Joint Commission has standards that require leaders to organize, direct, and staff their respective departments in accordance with the scope of services offered. To do this, clinical nutrition managers need to set standards for the methods and specific tasks that employees need to carry out so that procedures can be followed.

Job Design

It is important to identify the tasks and methods that staff members use to fulfill their responsibilities. This provides guidance and ensures optimal accountability. It also provides the basis for performance appraisal. Unlike the majority of food service activities, which follow a routine daily schedule, many clinical procedures vary from day to day, so that daily work patterns are sometimes hard to establish, especially for the professional staff. Exhibit 4–3 shows which members of the clinical nutrition team are responsible for each task. For these allocations to be made, competency levels need to be identified and included in employee job descriptions.

The positions used in Exhibit 4–3 are for the registered dietitian, dietetic technician, and dietary clerk. With the advent of patient-focused care, these tasks may be assigned to individuals with other titles; but it is important that new employees be trained properly.

The principles of job analysis and design presented in Chapter 3 apply well to the clinical setting. Because clinical nutrition managers are being asked to restructure their processes, they must be prepared with the tools to do this effectively so that the important tasks are not left by the wayside. Not only will they need to describe and prioritize tasks, but they will be expected to be able to establish the amount of time required to perform these tasks. To determine average time spent

Exhibit 4–2 Sample Policy and Procedures for Enteral Nutrition

---

Department: Dietetic Services   Date Issued: 2/92   Date Revised: 2/95
Subject: Enteral Tube Feedings   Approvals _____

Policy

It is the policy of the dietetic services at Forbes Nursing Center that enteral tube feedings shall be available to residents who cannot eat adequately, but shall not be forced on those persons or families whose advanced directives suggest otherwise.

Procedures

Responsible Person	Action
Director	1. Establish appropriate policies and procedures 2. Provide or ensure regular inservice training to include this topic 3. Monitor quality and outcomes 4. Provide available updates for enteral formulary, diet manual, and other product information as needed by the facility

Physician	1. The physician determines whether or not a tube feeding will be used because of:
	  a) inability to swallow without choking, aspiration, etc.
	  b) lack of alertness or coma
	  c) multifactorial malnutrition that is not corrected orally through liquid, pureed, or other consistency diets
	2. Orders may be written using the available tube feeding order form, which is developed with the assistance of the medical director.
	3. Discrepancies between resident-estimated needs and the tube feeding order are discussed with the physician. This may occur with the original order or with monthly or quarterly reviews.
	4. When an order does not meet the RDAs, a suggestion is made to order a multivitamin/mineral supplement.
	5. Water requirements are calculated as 30–35 mL/kg BW. Most products are 85% free water, although those which are more calorie dense (1.5 or 2 kcal/mL) are only 70%–75% free water. These latter products require additional flush to provide adequate free water.
	6. The following trends are monitored by the RD:
	  a) weight changes
	  b) lab changes (albumin, BUN, and glucose in particular)
	  c) hydration changes
	7. Residents who have acute or chronic problems are referred to the clinical coordinator for follow-up assessments.

Interdisciplinary Team	1. Tube feeding concerns are a part of the regular interdisciplinary team monitoring process involving nursing, dietetic services, and other disciplines.

Courtesy of Forbes Nursing Center, Pittsburgh, Pennsylvania.

Exhibit 4–3 Nutrition Care Tasks and Responsibilities for Long-Term Care: Framework and Guidelines for Practice

Tasks and Responsibilities	RD	Technician	Clerk
Menu Production			
1. Head and pull menus for patients			X
2. Ensure that all patients have a menu to select		X	X
3. Change menus when diet orders have changed; record changes			X
4. Check through all menus before service to ensure that a menu is present for all patients who are eating			X
5. Establish and maintain an inventory of menus and supplies		X	X
6. Transfer messages about "hold" or late trays and special items to the proper personnel in the kitchen			X
7. Calculate forecasting of food counts on all menus (e.g., the number of special items)		X	
8. Collect menus that patients have marked; review the menu with patients when there are questions		X	
9. Write special menus for patients unable to select	X	X	
10. Mark special, regular, or routine menus that patients cannot or do not want to choose themselves		X	
11. Calculate meal patterns for patients on highly specialized (e.g., renal) diets. Calculate needs for total and partial parenteral nutrition patients, with consult order	X	X with RD	
12. Calculate meal patterns for routine modified diets		X	
13. Plan nourishment requests for patients on routine diets		X	
14. Calculate tube feedings and commercial formulas for patients	X	X with RD	
15. Check nourishment requests by monitoring nourishment intake		X	
16. File special diet patterns and calculations from discharged patients		X	
Patient Visitation and Screening			
1. Complete a nutrition screening to determine the usual diet at home, history of weight changes, etc.	III	I–II	
2. Review screening to determine appropriateness of diet order according to patient tolerance of oral intake	X	X	
3. Assign care levels to the nutrition screening to prioritize patient care	X	X with RD	
4. Record pertinent findings from the screening onto appropriate care cards	X	X	
5. Determine which patients will be given a diet history	X		
6. Complete a diet history with patient interview	X	X	

continues

Exhibit 4–3 continued

Tasks and Responsibilities	RD	Technician	Clerk
7. Assess patients' ability to consume meals as ordered during stay (feeding problems, dentures, etc.); perform meal rounds	X	X	
8. Determine patients' ability to comprehend written and verbal instructions or information		X	X
9. Follow up on patient complaints regarding food service, basic care services, missing items, etc.	X	X	
10. Determine an appropriate time to meet with family or other members of the health care team regarding patient care (e.g., diet instructions)	X		
Use of Medical Records and Charting			
1. Review charts for disease or disorder, diet order, demographics of patients, height and weight status, laboratory values, and other data	X	X	
2. Review medication orders and determine possible food–drug interactions to be addressed	X		
3. Monitor measurable outcomes: changes in blood pressure, weights, laboratory values, etc. in medical record when available	X		
4. Record nutrition care plan and actions in appropriate section of the medical record	X		
5. Communicate with physicians regarding notes or nutrition plans and activities	X		
Nutrition Assessment			
1. Review data regarding weight status, laboratory values, intake history, body temperature, input and output, medications, mode of feeding, etc.; complete consultation records for chart	X		
2. Communicate with other health care team members regarding desired activities for patient care as an outcome of completing the assessment	X		
Nutrition Education			
1. Provide simple diet instructions to patients who are on modified or special diets		X	
2. Develop an educational plan for patients and their family members	X		
3. Implement educational activities:			
(1) patient or family diet counseling	X		
(2) provide structured diet and nutrition classes, and	X	X with RD	
(3) document educational care in the medical record	X		
4. Provide referral to outside agencies or ambulatory nutrition services for continued education	X		

continues

Exhibit 4–3 continued

Tasks and Responsibilities	RD	Technician	Clerk
5. Monitor ability of patient to select a menu in accordance with meal plan	X	X	
Implementation of Protocols/Care Maps or Clinical Pathways			
1. Provide patient care in accordance with preestablished criteria in the form of protocols or care maps	X		
2. Communicate to all personnel regarding necessary actions in accordance with protocols	X	X	X
Quality Assessment and Performance Improvement			
1. Determine appropriateness of diet order for patient condition (e.g., dysphagia)	X	X	
2. Verify diet orders with nursing or medical records		X	X
3. Assign nutrition care levels as a result of nutrition screening data	X		
4. Monitor effectiveness of dietary interventions; provide follow-up to services and care	X	X	
5. Verify that all non orally fed patients are tolerating their tube feedings or parenteral nutrition	X		
6. Document actual intake of meals, nourishments, or tube feedings on Kardex or patient chart	X–TF	X–meals	
7. Document patient satisfaction, problems, and complaints on Kardex or patient chart	X	X	
8. Document likely adherence to dietary instructions or counseling with the consultation	X		
9. Document performance of physician-requested services in the medical record	X		
10. Verify timeliness of nutrition services rendered to patients	X		
11. Verify proper performance of nutrition assessments	X		
12. Provide follow-up to patients who are taking nothing by mouth or who are on unsupplemented clear liquid diets	X	X	
13. Periodically assess nutritional adequacy of menus and patient selections	X		
14. Review patient readmission for same nutrition problems (e.g., uncontrolled diabetes mellitus)	X		
15. Reevaluate patient needs and educational requirements	X		
16. Write and update clinical pathways or care maps at least annually	X		
17. Document performance improvement goals for clinical team members	X		

Source: Adapted from S. Escott-Stump, Hospital Nutrition Services: Establishing Outcome Evaluations, *Topics in Clinical Nutrition*, Vol. 5, No. 1, pp. 31–39. © 1990, Aspen Publishers, Inc.

for each staff member, managers conduct job analyses or time and motion studies for a selected time period. Staff members record the number of direct and indirect services and the number of minutes spent for each. Laramee (1995) states "*direct* patient care activities involve specific services provided to individual patients whereas *indirect* activities include attendance at medical or discharge planning rounds where discussion of care plans for several patients may occur, reviewing of [Kardex] files, ordering of enteral formulas or nourishments, and other activities that are completed for a group of patients."

The following guide can be used to sort out the various tasks performed by the clinical staff; indirect activities are usually tracked by actual time and are recorded in the closest 15-minute interval:

- Direct patient care
  1. Nutrition screening
  2. Nutrition assessment and care planning
  3. Consultation with health team members
  4. Monitoring, follow-up, or written referrals to continuing care agency
  5. Patient/family nutrition education
- Indirect patient care
  1. Medical or discharge planning rounds
  2. Review and updating Kardex files
  3. Meal rounds
  4. Tray assessments
  5. Ordering nourishments and special feedings
  6. Reviewing patient rosters
- Nonpatient or administrative activities
  1. Planning, organizing, directing, and quality improvement
  2. Staff and student evaluation, meetings, and training
  3. Preparation of education materials, classes, and workshops

Figure 4–3 shows a system for tracking direct care activities that are performed each day. It is important to note that the system illustrated tracks the time allocated to each different patient care unit to which the dietitian is assigned. This is especially important since the concept of grouping patients by care centers (see Chapter 3) became popular. Costs for nutrition services to each care center can then be tied into the budgets for these newly established units as members of the clinical nutrition staff are dispatched to perform functions there. The conversion of time into standard units of measurement, such as relative value units, is discussed later in this chapter. If the department is en-

Dietitian or Intern Activities	Descriptive Comment or Notation	Unit_____		Unit_____		Unit_____		Unit_____	
		No.	Time	No.	Time	No.	Time	No.	Time
Patient-Related Activities									
1. Diet calculations: Simple diets									
Complex diets									
Tube feedings									
TPN solutions									
2. Chart review for meds, labs, Hx									
3. Patient interview (usual intake, etc.)									
4. Conferences—MD, RN, others/rounds									
5. Completing assessment & meal pattern									
6. Preparing care plans									
7. Patient education: Individual									
Family conference									
Group class(es)									
8. Counseling for outcomes— Meal planning									
Diet for home use									
9. Evaluation of patient outcomes									
10. Referral to outpatient									
11. Medical record charting: Initial entries									
Follow-up									
12. Meal rounds (number of patients)									
13. NPO follow-ups									
14. Nutrition intake analysis									
15. Care map design									

continues

Nonpatient-Related Activities	✓	Time	# Adm.___	# Adm.___	# Adm.___	# Adm.___
1. Continuing ed./conferences/ workshops			# Disc.___	# Disc.___	# Disc.___	# Disc.___
2. Clinical management: Supervision			Census___	Census___	Census___	Census___
Menu auditing			Date:			
Performance evaluation			Staff person:			
Checking nourishments						
Inventories			Comments:			
Pt. problems/complaints			Other activities			Time
Training student/intern			Nonproductive time: lunch, walking to units			
Inservice for technician						

Figure 4–3 Job analysis for clinical staff.

gaged in restructuring or reengineering, tasks may need to be reassigned to the new job categories that are established.

Staffing

One essential role for the clinical nutrition manager is recruitment and retention of sufficient, competent, and appropriate staff. How services are organized after task analysis and assignment will determine the number and type of staff members needed.

Although it would be easy to think that the percentage of patients on modified diets, the percentage on tube feedings or total parenteral nutrition (TPN), and the percentage on general diets could establish the proper ratio, this analysis generally specifies the work of dietetic technicians or clerks. The work of a clinical dietitian is more complex and is related more to nutritional risk factors, diagnoses, prognosis, planned surgical or medical interventions, medical history, and nutritional knowledge of the patient/client. With so many variables, it has been difficult within the profession to establish one set of rules based on patients fitting standards. Every patient is unique.

Table 4–1 provides a snapshot of common staffing patterns in the late 1980s at six hospitals. It can be seen that facilities larger than 300 beds varied significantly in their staffing. From the data shown, it would be difficult to conclude that one particular staffing pattern works for all facilities. More data about the facility would be essential, such as types of clinical units. One might ask whether there is a bone marrow transplant unit with fewer total patients but more extensive work for the dietitian or whether there are several cardiac reha-

Table 4–1 Staffing of Clinical Nutrition Services

Number of Beds	Occupancy	Number of Dietitians	Registered Dietitian: Patient Ratio	Number of Registered Dietetic Technicians	Percentage of Patients at Risk
300	75%	8.3	1:12	0	45%
480	80%	8.1	1:18	3.75	40%
625	75–80%	12.6	1:17	8.8	45%
663	50%	6.3	1:21	1	40%
710	89%	9.2	1:32	7.6	47%
1,008	85%	16.5	1:20	0	40%

Source: Staffing of Clinical Nutrition Services, Copyright The American Dietetic Association. Reprinted by permission from the *Clinical Nutrition Management Newsletter*, 1988; Vol. 6, No. 2, p. 3.

bilitation units where the dietetic technician provides basic services, including teaching a cardiac nutrition class.

Proposing a staffing *rule* could be detrimental for the patient population. The clinical nutrition manager must constantly reassess how the patient population is changing as related to standards of practice, typical lengths of stay, number of readmissions that require varying interventions, and/or educational contacts. In many cases, tracking the types of *work left undone* provides useful information for the manager. Another consideration for staffing is the need for weekend and vacation replacement. All key elements of the department must be considered.

Depending on the availability of dietetic technicians, such able assistants may relieve the clinical dietitian of more common, routine tasks. In a long-term care facility, the dietetic technician may complete slightly different tasks, as shown in Exhibit 4–3. Recently, some technicians have also taken on new patient-focused assignments, such as taking blood pressures and vital signs. In addition, the initial interviews and screening tasks are beginning to be coordinated centrally to avoid the cost of duplicating efforts in the facility. Computers also are able to assist with the screening task. At Rush Presbyterian–St. Luke's Medical Center in Chicago, the position of dietetic technician was recently eliminated after a major reengineering effort and conversion to patient-focused care (Sowa, 1995).

Integrated patient assessment affects the work done by employees from several departments. There are several steps involved in both a traditional system and a revised system. The traditional system was set up so that each discipline screened patients separately. It was found that patients were asked at least 10 of the same questions by different staff members. In that model, initial assessment notes were placed in different sections of the medical record.

At the 395-bed Jerry L. Pettis Veterans' Administration Medical Center in Loma Linda, California, a centralized system for initial patient assessment was tested to reduce duplication of effort. Zappia and Watrous (1995) note "In most medical centers, patients are interviewed and assessed by many people upon admission: admission clerks, physicians, nurses, dietitians, social workers, and so forth" (p. 13). Assessments are placed in different parts of the medical record, and the process is time consuming and somewhat repetitious. This results in a complex and fragmented initial assessment process. The interdisciplinary team developed a new method to minimize redundancy, make assessment information more easily accessible to all providers of care, and reduce paperwork. A pilot occurred in two units, medical and psychiatric, whereby screening was performed by the nursing staff and specialists followed up on cases requiring more comprehensive evaluation. This plan already appears to have the Joint Commission's endorsement.

Job descriptions for the clinical dietitian will vary by the complexity and setting within the institution. In facilities where there is only a small number of clinical dietitians, one general job description may suffice, whereas facilities that have complex staffing patterns may have a *clinical ladder*. For these larger facilities, the job descriptions and performance standards will describe higher expectations for positions such as clinical nutrition specialist or *nutrition support dietitian*. Some of the functions and responsibilities often assigned specifically to a nutrition support dietitian are listed below (Fish et al., 1993; Nelson & Steinborn, 1992; Schatz, 1993; Skipper & Winkler, 1992); the specialists in nutrition support roles normally have a higher educational and skill requirement within their job description:

- Identifies patients at risk and performs periodic assessments for patients on nutritional support (tube feedings, TPN).
- Serves as a patient advocate for nutritional issues.
- Designs, implements, monitors, and evaluates enteral and parenteral therapies in all settings, including the home.
- Designs effective transitional feedings between modalities (including oral nutrition).
- Writes an appropriate, complete nutritional care plan and documents all relevant findings.
- Communicates key elements of the care plan to the patient and significant others.
- Educates providers and insurers about the importance and cost effectiveness of medical nutritional therapy.

- Documents for proper coding for reimbursement by identifying malnutrition as a complication or comorbidity factor.
- Participates in research studies, practical or formal.

If there is a nutritional support team, the nutrition support dietitian may not report directly to the director of dietetic services. Generally, this position reports to the primary physician who operates the team. The team generally consists of the physician as team leader, a nurse clinician or specialist, a clinical pharmacist, and sometimes a designated social worker. If the team completes services for a large number of patients, the reimbursement rate generally covers the costs of operating such a highly complex service. When the team has few patients, the nutrition support dietitian is assigned other patients within the dietetics department and reports to the clinical nutrition manager. This staffing pattern also depends on the patient population, level of nutritional risk and complexity, and type of facility (e.g., tertiary versus community hospital).

INTEGRATING AND COORDINATING

The most significant trend in clinical nutrition is the shift toward increased interdisciplinary patient assessment. According to the Joint Commission (1996):

> Over time, patients may receive a range of care in multiple settings from multiple providers. For this reason it is important for a hospital to view the patient care it provides as a part of an integrated system of settings, services, health care practitioners, and care levels that make up a continuum of care. The goal of the continuity of care function is to define, shape, and sequence the following processes and activities to maximize coordination of care within this continuum. (p. 225)

The standards then proceed to list the important processes that occur before admission, during admission, in the hospital, before discharge, and at discharge. Chapter 1 fully describes the trend toward integrated care within individual health care facilities and in the community in general. Continuity of care is stressed in all the Joint Commission standards, including those for long-term care, ambulatory care, home care, and health care networks.

Standards for the patient assessment process have also become more stringent. For example, one of the Joint Commission's (1996) hospital standards states "The patient's history and physical examination, nursing assessment, and other screening assessments are completed within 24 hours of admission" (p. 103). With the length of stay for hospitalized patients averaging from 5 to 6 days, there is a need to identify high-risk cases quickly and to complete assessments in a timely manner so that intervention can occur at the point in time when patients really need care. The Joint Commission does not require assessment of all patients after screening but recommends that nutrition status be assessed when warranted by the patient's needs or condition. Exact protocols for the elements to be included in screening and assessment have not been identified by the Joint Commission, but guidelines for reassessment during the hospital stay and discharge planning standards have been identified. The OBRA regulations for long-term care include detailed criteria for nutrition assessment and monitoring of high-risk residents, as do the standards that govern ICF/MR facilities.

Another trend in the standards set by regulatory agencies is seen in the increased attention to patients' rights. Patients, residents, and their family members should be involved in the assessment and care planning processes, and their stated desires need to be reflected accordingly. This includes not only giving patients a choice in the foods they receive but providing treatment alternatives when extraordinary treatments, such as parenteral or enteral feedings, are indicated. Informed consent entails discussing all viable treatment options with patients and their surrogate decision makers so that they can make the best possible determinations. It includes the more serious, life-threatening issues as well as the somewhat routine issues, such as which diets patients can tolerate the best and which foods should be included in their meal plans.

Because of time constraints, health care professionals often focus on the life-threatening issues and overlook the simpler issues that contribute to how patients really perceive the hospital and how safe and secure they feel in their new environment. It is only when practitioners are able to address both types of issues successfully, that high-quality patient care can result.

An increased number of standards have also appeared for patient education, staffing, competency, and eating disorders, and continued emphasis is being placed on the topics of food–drug interactions and quality improvement, with special emphasis on the outcomes of care. As noted in earlier chapters, there is a need for professionals to develop standards of care that can be eventually adopted in these regulations. One important trend is the integrated approach to standardization of patient treatment through the use of clinical pathways or care maps.

The coordination of activities that clinical dietitians are most frequently involved in during the course of their work is discussed below, together with nutrition screening, assessment, care planning, and documentation. The trend toward increased computerization in the field is also addressed. Chapters 5 and 6 present more information about the legal aspects of nutrition care and patient education because these two issues require special consideration. Suggestions for optimizing reimbursement for nutrition care services are provided in Chapter 7.

Nutrition Screening

To determine which patients are at nutritional risk, a screening process is used. Depending on the complexity and specificity of the institution, this process may be simple, or it may be defined for age groups or diagnoses. Policies and procedures regarding the screening process should clearly define the responsibilities of everyone involved in the screening process. Policies vary from facility to facility, but in all cases they should be planned by an interdisciplinary team and approved by the medical staff or nutrition committee. The forms and guidelines that are used for screening also need to be clear and concise, leaving little room for error. An example of typical guidelines that can accompany a department's policies is shown in Exhibit 4–4.

Some practitioners have difficulty screening patients because data are not always available. For example, in the early 1990s when the American Dietetic Association first embarked on a 3-year project to develop clinical indicators for the Joint Commission, patient weight was naturally included as one assessment tool. It soon became apparent in the 14 hospitals used for field testing that weight could not be used because documentation in the medical record was not consistently available. According to Queen, Caldwell, and Balogun (1993), "The task forces all agreed, however, that even though the documentation on weight was not as it should be for some indicators, these indicators should be retained in order to drive practice and facilitate better documentation of this data element needed to evaluate key indicators" (p. 344).

As mentioned earlier, the research reported by Foltz et al. (1993) covered screening practices in 388 hospitals across the nation. These investigators found diagnosis, anthropometric measures, and albumin to be used most often, specifically weights (85.6%), heights (83.8%), diagnosis (83.5%), recent weight loss (83.0%), and albumin (79.6%). Less frequently used were food intolerance (58.8%), allergies (52.1%), functional status (45.9%), and food intake history (40.2%). Other parameters were used (cholesterol, hemoglobin/hematocrit, total lymphocyte count, medications, chewing/swallowing disorders, dietary order, and nausea), but they were all found in less than 5% of the hospitals.

Some clinical managers increase the number of parameters used for nutrition screening so that the process can be more accurate; others are experiencing staff reductions and are trying to simplify the process and decrease the number of parameters to one or two important factors. For example, Sowa (1995) reported that, at one institution before the clinical service underwent reengineering, several detailed items were included in the screening assessment. For the same population, when the screening results from that method were compared with those from a system that used patients' weight alone, significant differences were not found. It was therefore concluded that weight was a good predictor of

Exhibit 4–4 Nutrition Screening Guidelines

Height/Weight—Patient <85% of IBW						High-Risk Diagnoses
Height		Men Weight		Women Weight		abdominal surgery/resection
feet	cm	lb	kg	lb	kg	AIDS amputations
4'9"	145	—	—	101	45.9	anorexia nervosa/bulimia bowel obstruction
4'10"	147	—	—	104	47.3	burn cancer
4'11"	150	—	—	107	48.6	cardiac cachexia celiac disease
5'	152	—	—	110	50.0	chylous leak COPD
5'1"	155	128	58.2	113	51.4	cystic fibrosis pressure ulcer/nonhealing wound
5'2"	158	132	60.0	118	53.6	FTT
5'3"	160	134	60.9	120	54.5	GI fistula high-risk pregnancy
5'4"	163	138	62.7	125	56.8	inborn error of metabolism liver disease
5'5"	165	141	64.1	129	58.6	malabsorption multiple trauma
5'6"	168	146	66.4	133	60.5	pancreatitis prematurity of infants
5'7"	170	151	68.6	137	62.2	renal failure sepsis/prolonged infection
5'8"	173	155	70.5	141	64.1	others at RD discretion
5'9"	175	160	72.9	146	66.5	**Lab Data**
5'10"	178	163	74.1	149	67.7	Albumin < 3.5 mg/dL; Cholesterol < 150 mg/dL
5'11"	180	168	76.4	153	69.5	TLC < 900 cells/mm³
6'	183	173	78.6	—	—	TLC Mild depletion—1500–1800 Moderate depletion—900–1500
6'1"	185	178	80.9	—	—	TLC = % lymphs × WBC (in thousands—usually correlates with
6'2"	188	183	83.2	—	—	albumin levels) Not an absolute marker of nutritional
6'3"	191	187	85.0	—	—	status—decreased levels seen with infection, Ca, stress, steroids, &
		Large frame used		Small frame used		post-op

continues

Exhibit 4–4 continued

Levels of Risk

Low Nutrition Risk—I
0–1 risk criteria are present
Action:　Circle risk level in nursing data base
　　　　　Place sticker in progress note
　　　　　Rescreen in 7–10 days
Moderate Nutritional Risk—II
2 risk criteria are present
Action:　Visit on meal rounds and offer supplements and snacks prn
　　　　　Place sticker in progress note
　　　　　Request consult if appropriate
　　　　　Rescreen in 7–10 days
High Nutritional Risk—III
3 or more risk criteria present
Action:　Document risk in nursing database
　　　　　Place sticker in progress note
　　　　　Request consult if appropriate
　　　　　Rescreen in 3-4 days
Moderate or High Nutritional Risk but Palliative Care Only
Action:　Visit on meal rounds
　　　　　Offer supplements, snacks prn
　　　　　Document nutrition risk, understanding of no code status, and availability via consult
　　　　　on sticker

　Courtesy of Geisinger Medical Center, Danville, Pennsylvania.

---

the other factors in that facility, and the process was streamlined. In the future, this issue is expected to become a moot point when computerized medical records become more widespread. The computer will do all the work and be able to handle as many factors as one wishes. The following factors are recommended for nutrition screening:

- height and current weight
- recent weight changes (past month, past 6 months, past year)
- calculation of actual weight compared with desirable weight for height and age
- problems with nausea, vomiting, diarrhea, and/or anorexia lasting more than 1 week
- problems chewing or swallowing
- recent surgery or trauma
- serum albumin levels (especially levels below 3.5 mg/dL)

- other laboratory data of significance to the patient's diagnosis
- diagnosis that warrants significant nutritional intervention (e.g., newly diagnosed diabetes mellitus, gastrointestinal disorders such as inflammatory bowel disease, cancer with involvement of the gastrointestinal tract, renal failure with or without dialysis, pulmonary or congestive heart failure, eating disorders)
- signs of malnutrition after physical assessment (dry, pale skin; magenta or scarlet tongue; cheilosis, pressure sore; etc.)
- medication use with potential or concurrent nutrient and gastrointestinal interactions (such as use of thiazide diuretics, corticosteroids, drugs causing anorexia or diarrhea)
- inability to consume oral diet to meet estimated needs

In the acute care setting, screening data should be collected for elective admissions during the preadmission evaluation. A simple questionnaire can be used and administered by others so that time is not wasted during the first day of the hospital stay for locating high-risk cases. A questionnaire can elicit data on nutrition history as well as food preferences so that the first meals that patients receive conform to their desires. Test results, height and weight, and even the admitting diet order can be obtained at that time. For emergency admissions and those not covered in a preadmission program, the nursing staff or dietetic technician can obtain the preliminary screening data. The structure for hospitals using the patient-focused care model differs from traditional structures, and the care team normally consists of professional, technical, and service level members. In this case, the technical level is best suited to the task of screening. After data are collected, patient care is ranked into levels signifying basic risk, moderate risk, and high risk, as shown in Figure 4–4. This figure is actually a sticker that is added to the medical record after it is completed.

In most facilities, the clinical dietitians focus their energy on the high-risk and moderate-risk patients. They proceed to determine whether a nutrition assessment is needed and perform one if indicated. The dietetic technician works in tandem with the dietitian for those patients, and also the low-risk cases, by providing basic services such as menu planning, simple diet instructions for home, meal rounds, calorie count estimations, and other related services that do not require in-depth assessment by the dietitian (see Exhibit 4–3). To comply with standards for reassessment, dietitians should perform followup screening at set intervals, as illustrated in Exhibit 4–4. Service personnel such as dietary aides, patient care assistants, food service aides, or hosts usually pass nourishments, deliver or collect trays, record food intakes, deliver nourishments, deliver and collect menus, and assist or determine food production tal-

Risk Factors for Malnutrition:	Low Risk	High Risk	Not Available	Comments
1. Percentage of ideal body weight	≥85%	<85%		
2. Unintentional weight loss in past 6 months	≤10%	>10%		
3. Chewing/swallowing problems	No	Yes		
4. Intake: NPO, clear liquids since or PTA Mechanical inability to take po Inadequate po due to poor appetite	<5 days	≥5 days		
5. Laboratory data: Serum albumin	≥3.5 mg/dL	<3.5 mg/dL		
Total lymphocyte count	≥900	<900		
Serum cholesterol	≥150 mg/dL	<150 mg/dL		
6. Other (i.e., high-risk diagnosis that may add to nutrition risk)	No	Yes		
Number of risk factors identified:				

Assessed Nutritional Risk:
- ❏ Low (I)
- ❏ Moderate (II)
- ❏ High (III)
- ❏ Palliative care only

Plan:
- ❏ Visit on meal rounds
- ❏ Offer supplements or snacks
- ❏ Recommend change of diet to: _____
- ❏ Request nutrition consult
- ❏ Other _____

_____   _____
Signature/Title   Date

Figure 4–4 Nutrition screening sticker. Courtesy of Geisinger Medical Center, Danville, Pennsylvania.

lies for the next day. A person at the technical level may assist or oversee these processes.

Referrals are the most common source of patients in the ambulatory care setting. After patients are referred, they often complete a questionnaire that enables dietitians to collect pertinent information. Figure 4–5 shows a sample form that can be used for this purpose. It can also be modified to include food preferences for use in preadmission screening. Data from the medical record, when available, should also be used as a basis for the type of care that is given. As in other types of health care settings, it has become increasingly important in

BACKGROUND QUESTIONNAIRE

Name _____   Date_____

In preparation for your nutrition counseling session, please complete the following background questionnaire. Your dietitian will review this with you during your initial appointment.

1. Personal and family medical history

   Please check the box in Column A if you currently have or have had any of the following health problems. Please check the box in Column B if any members of your immediate family have or have had any of the following health problems (include parents, sisters, brothers, grandparents).

	A. Yourself	B. Family		A. Yourself	B. Family
Overweight	❑	❑	Angina	❑	❑
Diabetes	❑	❑	Cancer	❑	❑
High blood pressure	❑	❑	Kidney disease	❑	❑
High cholesterol	❑	❑	Orthopedic problem	❑	❑
Heart attack	❑	❑	Other problems:	_____	_____
Stroke	❑	❑	(please specify)	_____	_____
Bypass surgery	❑	❑		_____	_____

2. Do you take any medications? No ❑   Yes ❑   (list name and dosage).

   _____

3. Do you smoke?   No ❑   I quit in _____/_____ (month/year)

   Yes ❑   How many packs per day _____

4. Do you drink alcohol?   No ❑   Yes ❑

   If yes, circle type: beer   wine   liquor   mixed drinks

5. Are there any foods you avoid for religious, health, or philosophical reasons (including food allergies)?   No ❑   Yes ❑
   If yes, describe:

   _____

6. Do you have any difficulty chewing or swallowing foods?   No ❑   Yes ❑

7. Do you do any regular physical exercise?   No ❑   Yes ❑
   If yes, describe type and how often:

   _____

8. Do you take any vitamin, mineral, or other nutritional supplements?   No ❑   Yes ❑
   If yes, please list:

   _____

9. What is your occupation? _____

10. Who do you live with? Circle one or more:

    spouse   children   roommates   group home   parent   live alone   other_____

11. In your household, who does the majority of the cooking?_____

continues

12. In your household, who does the majority of grocery shopping?_____

13. If you eat meals outside of your home, describe location and how often.

_____

❑ Never eat out

14. If you eat "take out" food at home (e.g., pizza, subs, Chinese food), describe type of food and how often:

_____

❑ I never eat "take out" food at home

15. Height/weight history (adults only)   Height_____   Usual Weight_____

Lowest adult weight _____ (at age ____)   Highest adult weight _____ (at age ____)

16. What would you like to weigh? _____

17. Has your weight changed in the past year?   No ❑   Yes ❑
If yes, how many pounds were lost or gained?   Lost _____ lb   Gained _____ lb
If yes, describe the significant events in your life that may have influenced this weight change:

_____

18. Have you ever been on a weight loss diet before?   No ❑   Yes ❑

19. Have you had any previous nutrition counseling?   No ❑   Yes ❑
If yes, who provided the counseling (please circle one or more):

registered dietitian   physician   weight counselor   nurse   other_____

If yes, what was the reason for nutrition counseling? _____

20. Have you made any significant changes in your eating recently?   No ❑   Yes ❑
If yes, please describe:

_____

Questions to ask your dietitian:

_____

_____

_____

_____

_____

_____

PLEASE BRING COMPLETED QUESTIONNAIRE TO YOUR NUTRITION SESSION

Figure 4–5 Background questionnaire for the ambulatory care setting. Courtesy of Boston Regional Medical Center, Boston, Massachusetts.

ambulatory care to establish a paper trail, which starts with the initial assessment, continues through nutrition intervention activities, and ends in the final billing documents. Any outsider reviewing the medical record should be able to substantiate the need for nutrition care, the type and extent of the care that was provided, and measurable outcomes of the care. Proper coding is essential for this to occur. Some good basic guidelines for this process are provided by Fox (1991), and exact billing codes and current procedural terminology codes are provided by the American Medical Association (1996).

Nutrition screening in the long-term care setting is quite different, especially in facilities that are governed by OBRA regulations, which require the use of minimum data sets. All residents are fully assessed upon admission. Quarterly and annual assessments are completed after that point. When there is a significant change in the medical condition of the resident or his or her dietary tolerance, or if hospitalization occurs, reassessments are mandated. Screening in this setting requires the ongoing monitoring of residents' nutrition status to determine whether intervention is needed outside the normal assessment routine. A similar process is used for ICF/MR facilities, with special emphasis on the functional abilities of residents. In fact, the tools that have been used to assess functional status in long-term care for years are slowly creeping into the acute care setting, and all dietitians should probably consider screening on the basis of how much assistance is needed with the normal activities of daily living and instrumental activities of daily living.

For home health care, dietitians are not reimbursed on a fee-for-service basis, but home health care agencies may choose to hire a dietitian. According to Westbrook (Jackson, 1995b), the role of the dietitian is different in this setting. Nurses are the primary service providers in home health care, and dietitians will probably set protocols and train home health care nurses to screen and assess patients during their home visits, just as dietetic technicians are trained in the hospital setting. Westbrook refers to nurses as the fact-finders for all disciplines and states "if the system is set up properly, they can easily follow a decision tree to determine when intervention by a dietitian is needed. In this manner, the dietitian becomes more of a team consultant or resource person who performs direct care as indicated" (Jackson, 1995b, p. 7). In the home setting, home health aides often provide some types of basic care. A good source for establishing screening systems for home care and other community programs is the *Nutrition Screening Manual for Professionals Caring for Older Americans* (Nutrition Screening Initiative, 1991).

Nutrition Assessment and Care Planning

The more complete nutrition assessment is carried out by dietitians for patients at moderate or high risk for protein-calorie malnutrition and those requiring nutrition intervention for other reasons as indicated by the screening process or by referral from physicians or other members of the medical team. When physicians order nutrition intervention or consultation, it is more likely to be reimbursed. The exact format used for completing nutrition assessments varies from facility to facility. Some clinical nutrition managers work with staff members to design a special form for this purpose; others chart directly in the progress notes without the use of a special form. A separate form is helpful for several reasons. First, it provides a structure for individuals to collect and analyze data in an orderly fashion. As a result, forms are preferred when technicians fill in parts of them for dietitians or when the individual completing assessments is not quite sure about his or her ability to proceed in a logical, orderly fashion as patients are assessed. Second, when a form is used, one can demonstrate more easily that important factors were considered for each individual case. This is helpful when charts are reviewed internally by quality improvement teams or by external regulatory agencies or third party payers. Third, a separate form is a recognizable part of the medical record. When members of the health care team are looking for specific information, they know it will be in a certain part of the form, which they become accustomed to seeing.

Lathrop (1993) states that for every dollar spent on direct patient care, three to four extra dollars are spent in arranging for it, getting to the area where it is to be done, and documenting it. Excess paperwork can be cumbersome, especially if forms require a lot of time to complete. People tend to focus on the goal as being completing the form rather than what is really happening to the patient and what can be done to provide excellent care. Often, forms also force people to *fill in the blanks,* even when the data are not pertinent, just so it can be shown that the practitioner did, indeed, consider all the factors that he or she should have. In addition, forms sometimes force a structured approach in the treatment of patients, who undoubtedly need individualized attention. One must weigh the advantages and disadvantages of structured forms and decide what is best for one's facility. If the clinical staff are competent and disciplined enough to consider all relevant factors on their own, if they routinely follow acceptable and standardized protocols as they assess patients, and if regulatory agencies do not require or prefer a special format, perhaps the unnecessary paperwork can be avoided.

Regardless of the format used, the goal of nutrition intervention remains the same: to meet the clinical and personal needs of patients by improving their nutrition status. This entails a comprehensive nutrition assessment, where the dietitian explains the nutrition status of the patient and then provides an individualized care plan that identifies what will be done to improve it. The process involves three separate steps: data collection, nutrition assessment, and care planning.

Data Collection

Data collection involves identification of pertinent information from subjective and objective sources. Subjective data are gathered from the patient, family members, and/or caregivers regarding weight history, diet history, appetite, eating problems and disabilities, food allergies and intolerances, current intake, cultural and religious factors, physical and clinical complaints, past and present diet education, and the patient's current knowledge and application of the dietary principles that are important in treatment. The focus on subjective data is greater now than in the past because survey teams now challenge practitioners to show how patients' rights are being honored. The trend toward patient-focused care has also raised an awareness of this issue. The expressed desires of each patient need to be considered. These desires range from decisions about extraordinary care to decisions about the foods patients *want to eat* and *how they want to eat it*. If this information is not known by the providers of care, optimal satisfaction will not result. If patients (or their surrogate caregivers) are not involved in the entire process of assessment and care planning, the chances of missing the target are great.

Objective data that are needed to complete an assessment include anthropometrics (height, weight, elbow breadth, etc.), observed clinical and physical signs, diagnoses, medications, laboratory values and results of other diagnostic tests, vital signs, current diet prescription, and current nutrient intake and output. To avoid duplication of effort, data from previous providers of care should be reviewed whenever available. Successful practitioners also rely on the input from other providers of care. Patient assessment and treatment are team processes, and the data collected by others in their assessments of the patient are invaluable.

To support complete and appropriate orders for tube feeding or parenteral nutrition, standardized forms may be useful, especially in the case of complex orders. Generally, the nutrition committee develops and approves the use of an enteral nutrition order form. The pharmacy department works in conjunction with the nutrition services staff for development of a standardized TPN order form.

Nutrition Assessment

To assess a situation means to evaluate it. Nutrition assessments explain the current nutrition status of patients by appropriately combining pertinent subjective and objective data. Instead of spending time in writing lengthy dissertations and presenting complex calculations, dietitians can construct simple statements such as "Patient is clinically obese (25% > ideal body weight) but has lost 20 lb in the past 3 months, which she feels is related to her depression and emotional trauma since the death of her husband and the physical inability to care for herself in the home." Brief statements such as this one can be constructed, as indicated, for clear and concise assessments of factors that make the particular patient different from the norm. The process entails a search for the *issues*, or a search for an answer to the question: What is the nutrition status of the patient and exactly what caused this to happen? The dietitian seeks to identify a common thread in the data that are available. For example, a patient may complain of being tired all the time, laboratory tests show that he is anemic, and he tells the dietitian that he does not like to eat vegetables and stays away from red meats because they are high in cholesterol. When these data are grouped together, a logical assessment explaining the patient's medical condition (iron deficiency anemia) can be made. Clinical dietitians should consider assessing the following:

- anthropometrics (including weight)
- medical condition as it relates to diet or diet–drug interactions
- nutrient needs as related to the diet prescription and patient intake
- eating and swallowing ability
- knowledge and implementation of the diet by the patient/family member

One common concern is the weight of patients, and dietitians need to have sound methods to track weight status, goals, and changes over time. This, of course, is important information to include in the medical record. In some long-term care facilities and clinics, a weight and vital sign record has been developed for use in weekly or monthly tracking (see Figure 4–6). This is an interdisciplinary tool for use by nursing and nutrition services staff and may be one of several documentation forms in a separate nutrition and weight record section in the medical record.

Weight tables are often used to compare the patient's current or previous status with that of other persons of similar height and age. Tables for pediatric, adult, and geriatric populations are available. Such comparisons allow the practitioner to evaluate current weight, compare it with others, and identify recent changes. Usual body weight and the patient's expressed wishes need always to be kept in mind as well. For example, a patient who at age 70 has always been 5 ft 10 in and 170 lb has recently lost weight as a result of cancer therapies and is now 150 lb. This patient might do best with a goal of returning to the range of 170 lb plus or minus 5%.

Guides are available regarding the normal ranges for other anthropometric measurements, laboratory values, and other diagnostic tests. The ranges that are selected for use must correlate with the characteristic of the patient (i.e., sex

Admission Date/Year: _____

Admission Data: Height_____ Actual Weight:_____ Vital Signs: _____

Ideal/Desirable Body Weight: (Dietary only) _____ pounds (See chart on back)

Month	Day	Weight	Reweigh (if ± 5 lb)	Heart Rate	Temperature	Blood Pressure	Initial	Comment
January								
February								
March								
April								
May								
June								
July								
August								
September								
October								
November								
December								

FORBES NURSING CENTER
VITAL SIGN/HEIGHT–WEIGHT RECORD

Guide: Use same scale, same time of month, same clothing.
Use Comment section for unusual factors. Call
Dietary if, on reweigh, the resident is ± 5 pounds.

Figure 4–6 Vital sign and weight record. Courtesy of Forbes Nursing Center, Pittsburgh, Pennsylvania.

and age) with consideration of his or her diagnosis and normal values. Whenever possible, a baseline value for specific patients can be obtained for evaluative purposes, and deviations from this value over time can be monitored. For example, baseline values might be obtained from physician records for a newly admitted adult patient on a dialysis unit. Laboratory results can be monitored over time with respect to the baseline value and the norms for dialysis patients. While one is conducting assessments, it is helpful to utilize *practice guidelines*, either those established by the institution or those developed by national organizations.

Care Planning

The era of "doing things *to* patients" has passed. Instead, things are now "done *with* patients." If the personal desires of patients are not known or addressed, it is highly unlikely that an appropriate plan for treatment and education can be successfully identified and implemented. All too often, health care providers try to fit patients into their system instead of planning the system around patients. One common sign of this is the tendency for practitioners to label their patients as noncompliant. It is important to realize that many people become noncompliant when the treatment plan does not suit their personal needs. In reality, it may be the system that is not complying with the needs and expectations of its patients, instead of the reverse.

Clinical dietitians have the opportunity to practice informed consent every day. Suppose an obese patient has been placed on a 1,000-calorie diet by the physician, and the patient is found to be extremely unhappy with the diet, helps himself to foods in the vending machine, and stashes food from outside sources in the bedside table. The dietitian can discuss alternative options with this patient for 1,200 and 1,500 calories, explaining that slower weight loss will occur but that he might be happier in the long term. The patient would then express his choice, this would be documented as a more viable option, and the dietitian would make a recommendation to the physician for a change. A part of the discharge plan could then be an exercise plan that fit into the patient's life style and follow-up in the outpatient clinic to monitor progress and help the patient further.

It has been found that physicians are more likely to liberalize diets than restrict them for their hospitalized patients (Skipper, Young, Rotman, & Nagl, 1994). They want their customers to be happy while still being able to meet their clinical goals. While considering increased patient involvement, practitioners need to realize that they have the ethical obligation to present the facts accurately and to help patients make choices from among the therapeutic alternatives that are consistent with good medical practice. Informed consent entails a patient's right of self-determination, which can be exercised only if the patient possesses enough information to make intelligent decisions, and it applies to routine treatment issues as well as life-threatening issues.

A study by Skipper et al. (1994) involved a review of 865 dietary recommendations at 35 Pennsylvania hospitals. They found that 42% of the recommendations were actually implemented. Physicians were found to be more likely to take recommendations resulting from their own requests for dietary consultation (50%) or for cases discussed with them (65%) than to take unsolicited recommendations from dietitians. The types of recommendations that were most frequently implemented were for initiating enteral/parenteral feeding (49%), liberalizing the diet (other than increasing energy, 49%), changing energy intake levels (44%), and ordering caloric intake monitoring (42%). Those least likely to be implemented were changing enteral/parenteral feedings (40%), ordering weight measurement (38%), ordering laboratory tests (37%), and restricting the diet (other than decreasing energy, 24%). The investigators also found that significantly more recommendations were implemented in teaching than community hospitals, in independently managed than contract-managed departments, for dietitians with more experience on their jobs, and when narrative notes were used than when subjective/objective/assessment/plan (SOAP) notes were used. Factors that did not make a significant difference were the location of the dietitian's note; the type of recommendation; and the dietitian's age, degree, continuing education, route to registration, and overall experience in the field.

For the ambulatory care setting, Sowinski, Shepherd, Dowling, and Wagner (1994) state "What seems to work best are face-to-face meetings—tell the physician who you are and what services you provide" (p. 530). They surveyed physicians at one facility and noted "If physicians know you as a person and as a professional, you've broken down a very big barrier to having them refer patients to you" (p. 530). They asked physicians about what encouraged referrals to an outpatient nutrition clinic and found that *value-added services* increased referrals. The statements that were rated "strongly agree" or "agree" by the 139 responding physicians were as follows: help the patient receive reimbursement (92.1%), provide a free initial meeting with the patient (82.4%), teach group cooking classes (81.3%), charge on a sliding scale (80.5%), send frequent follow-up reports (79.9%), provide objective measurements (79.1%), and provide patient education materials (74.1%). Fewer physicians agreed with the following: offer evening and weekend hours (62.6%), offer counseling in the physician's office (61.9%), offer statistics on the efficacy of dietary counseling (54.7%), provide inservices for physicians on the role of nutrition counseling (52.5%), provide statements of patient satisfaction (50.4%), employ dietitians with a master's degree (41.7%), provide free consultation for the physician (38.1%), provide a videotape for the waiting room on the benefits of dietary changes (32.3%), and provide a list of physicians using the outpatient clinic who can provide recommendations (28.8%).

As previously stated, the assessment process will yield brief, concise statements explaining the current nutrition status of patients and probable reasons why the problems that are observed exist. Once the issues have been identified, the clinical dietitian sets a plan of care. Most care plans are written for the following purposes:

- additional data
- changes in the plan of care

- follow-up
- referral
- nutrition education

Additional data can be obtained by the dietary staff during follow-up interviews with patients or family members or by others, as in the case of intake documentation for calorie counts and laboratory or diagnostic testing. Changes in the care plan can be made by the dietary staff (such as foods offered or consistency modifications) or others, as in the case where the physician's diet prescription needs to be changed. Follow-up or monitoring at specific time intervals can be identified as a plan of care for dietary intake, the patient's medical condition, or the patient's acceptance of the treatment plan. Referrals are needed when assessments by other team members are required, as in the case where patients may be experiencing swallowing difficulties. Nutrition education can be planned for before or after discharge.

While one is writing care plans, it is important to build accountability into them. It is helpful to everyone involved to specify who will implement the plans and to describe briefly how and when they will be done. Consultation with other members of the health care team, along with a cooperative effort on everyone's part, is needed for this to occur. In the ambulatory care setting, it is also important to realize that patients often stay in the hospital for a short time. Short-term plans can be written for the predischarge period, and discharge plans can be written for other providers to consider.

Discharge Plans

Ideally, discharge planning occurs from the point of admission. Discharge plans can include the same types of activities, that is, data collection, future changes in the care plan, follow-up, referral, and nutrition education. Dietitians who work in institutions should be fully aware of the community services that are available to patients after discharge so that proper referrals can be made. These include programs for home delivered meals, congregate feeding, home health care, specialty clinics, and so forth. A written communication summarizing medical nutrition therapy should be sent to the next provider of nutrition care. A specific nutrition discharge plan form can be designed to include the following items:

- current diet prescription
- supplemental feedings
- details regarding tube feeding or TPN

- food allergies and intolerances
- problems such as swallowing, difficulty chewing, nausea, vomiting, diarrhea, pressure sores, and other nutritional needs or problems
- weight, height, ideal body weight, and usual body weight
- recent weight changes (past month, past 6 months)
- summary of nutrition interventions
- summary of nutrition education/counseling given to patient or caregiver
- name and telephone number of referring dietitian

When it is determined that a patient will be discharged from one facility to another or to the home environment, the team must ensure that *continuity of care* will occur between agencies and practitioners in the various settings. The patient must not suffer any negative setbacks because of faulty communications or planning between institutions. In all cases, the patient is the central focus of planning; his or her wishes should be ascertained, documented, and communicated along with those of the team.

Clinical Pathways

One role of the clinical nutrition manager is to ensure that nutrition care is coordinated with other disciplines. Today, this is achieved in several ways. Clinical dietitians, technicians, clerks, or *patient-focused teams* participate appropriately in *collaborative practice teams*. A case manager may be assigned to each patient's care from admission to discharge, ensuring that costs are contained while maintaining a high quality of services. In many facilities, dietitians have been invited to serve as case managers. Often, these efforts involve the use of a *clinical pathway* or *care map*, where specific services, discipline specific and correlated with the typical length of stay, are planned and implemented. Figure 4–7 shows a clinical pathway for an uncomplicated open heart case.

When clinical pathways are used for disease states that require nutrition intervention, input from the clinical dietitian for both the development of the pathways and patient monitoring is important. The example shown in Figure 4–7 shows not only the pre- and postoperative diet that was decided by the care team but also nutrition counseling on the fourth day after surgery. Follow-up counseling is also provided after admission. If and when patients come off the care map, variations are noted on a separate form, which includes the date, patient unit, critical path day, nature of the variance, cause of the variance, and action taken. This form is used to substantiate any extensions in the patient's length of stay.

Pt. Origin:

Mount Clemens General Hospital Critical Path: Uncomplicated Coronary Artery Bypass	Admit Date: / /

	P.A.T. Date: Day:	O.P.S./D.O.S. Date: Day:	O.R./D.O.S. Date: Day:	L.C.U./D.O.S. Date: Day:	PO Day 1 Date: Day:
Assessments Evaluations	Nursing Assessment ___ Anesthesia Assessment ___ Intern H&P or letter ___ Chart requirements met ___ Consent ___ Admission Note ___	Nursing Assessment ___ SDA/OPS 0530-0600 ___ Anesthesia Assessment ___ Chart requirements met ___	Neg. Assessment ___ Chart requirements met ___ Anesthesia Assessment ongoing ___	Neg. Assessment ___ 7–3 ___ 3–11 ___ 11–7 ___ RT Assessment ___ Post-op VS till stable ___ VS protocol ___	Neg. Assessment ___ 7–3 ___ 3–11 ___ 11–7 ___ RT Assessment ___ Nutritional screen ___ VS protocol ___
Tests	Routine UA ___ EKG ___ Chest x-ray (PA&LAT) ___ Chem 20, CBC, PTT, Plt. ___ Type & cross ___ 4 units/6 units ___ Pregnancy test if ind. ___	EKG ___	ABG's ongoing ___ Heart profile: RBS, LYTES, Ca, Hgb, Hct ___ Co-Oximetry ___	Chest x-ray ___ EKG ___ ABG, CBC, BUN, Cr, PT, PTT, CBK, LDH, Isos ___	Pre/Post Extubation ABG's ___ CBC, BUN, Cr, LYTES, CPK, LDH, SGOT, PT, PTT, Plt count ___ EKG ___ Chest X-ray ___
Consults	Confirm medical eval complete ___ Catch report to chart ___			Pulmonary, Cardiology Co-manage ___ Cardiac Rehab. ___	
Treatments		Accurate height/weight ___ Shave/prep ___ Nasal O^2 ___	Insert PA catheter ___ Insert A-line ___ Apply cardiac monitor ___ Pulse oximetry ___ LABP standby ___ Intubate/ventilator ___ Prep ___ Drape ___ Surgery/bypass ___ Autotransfuser ___ Chest tubes ___ Pacer wires ___ Warning blanket ___ Dressings ___	Bed weight ___ Dressing assessed ___ Ventilator ___ RT treatments ___ Autotransfusion ___ Pulse oximetry ___ Hemodynamic monitoring ___ Chest tubes ___ Pacer standby ___ Warning blanket ___ Cardiac monitoring ___	Wean/extubate within 12 hours ___ Weight 06:00 ___ O^2 therapy per RT protocol ___ Dressing changes ___ Cardiac monitoring ___ RT treatments ___ Nurse C & DB ___
Medications	Confirm availability of autologous blood if ordered ___	Start 2 IV peripheral lines ___ Prophylactic antibiotic pre-op ___	Anesthesia sedation ___ Blood therapy ___	IV ___ IV meds ___ Post-op sedation ___	IV ___ IV pain meds ___ Post-op sedation ___
Activity		ABR ___	ABR ___	ABR ___ Cardiac Rehab ___	Up in chair ___ Cardiac Rehab ___ ROM ___
Diet	AHA ___	NPO ___	NPO ___	NPO ___	Cl. Liq. p Extubation prog. ___ to AHA low cholesterol
Elimination		Empty bladder ___ I & O ___	Insert foley cath ___ Insert NGT ___ I & O ___	Foley ___ NGT ___ I & O ___	DC foley ___ DC NGT ___ I & O ___
Education	Resp. therapy teaching ___ Pre-op teaching by P.A.T. staff ___ Tour of OR/ICU/TCU ___ Education Folder ___ Cardiac Rehab-Pre op teaching ___	Family visit ___ ID significant other ___	Family communication ongoing ___	Family Visits ___ Initiate discharge teaching protocol ___ Re-orient family to ICU ___ PM call to family ___ Cardiac Rehab visit family ___	Ongoing patient & family support ___ Cardiac Rehab visit ___ Incentive spirometry teaching reinforced ___ Reinforce C&DB ___
Discharge Planning	Utilization Review/ Discharge ___ Planning requirements met ___	Transfer to OR #2 at 07:00 ___	Transfer to ICU on weight bed & eggcrate mattress ___	ID significant other ___ Begin discharge planning ___ Social worker ___	Clinical Social Work ___ Diet ordered ___

SIGNATURE CODES	SIGNATURE _____	INITIALS _____	SIGNATURE _____	INITIALS _____

INSTRUCTIONS:
1. Fill in dates and days of week for entire path on top of each column.
2. Fill in initials and signature at bottom of page.
3. When you have verified that the stated event has occurred, initial the corresponding box for that day. If the stated event has *not* occurred, you must do the following:
   a. evaluate why,
   b. take corrective action to ensure it does occur before the end of the day.
4. If the stated event cannot occur within prescribed date, document fully on the variance report.

Discharge Date: / /	Expected L.O.S. / /	Actual L.O.S. / /	DRG # 107		

PO Day 2 Date: Day:	PO Day 3 Date: Day:	PO Day 4 Date: Day:	PO Day 5 Date: Day:	PO Day 6 Date: Day:	PO Day 7 Date: Day:
Neg. Assessment 7–3 ___ 3–11 ___ 11–7 ___ VS protocol ___	Neg. Assessment 7–3 ___ 3–11 ___ 11–7 ___ VS protocol ___	Neg. Assessment 7–3 ___ 3–11 ___ 11–7 ___ VS protocol ___	Neg. Assessment 7–3 ___ 3–11 ___ 11–7 ___ VS protocol ___	Neg. Assessment 7–3 ___ 3–11 ___ 11–7 ___ VS protocol ___	Neg. Assessment 7–3 ___ 3–11 ___ 11–7 ___ VS protocol ___
EKG CBC, BUN, Cr, LYTES, CPK, LDH, SGOT, PT, PTT, Platelet count Chest X-ray	EKG ___ CBC, LYTES, CR, BUN ___ Chest X-ray ___				
Pulmonary Rehab teaching	Pulmonary Rehab teaching ___				
Weight 06:00 Incision checks ___ Incision care ___ DC dsg prior to transfer ___ RT treatment ___ Assess for DC chest tubes, pacer lines ___ Cardiac Monitor O² therapy per RT protocol ___ Incentive Spiro ___ C & DB ___	Weight 06:00 Incision checks ___ Incision care ___ Cardiac monitoring ___ O² therapy per RT protocol ___ Incentive Spiro ___ C & DB ___ Pulse Ox with amb per RT protocol ___	Weight 06:00 Incision checks ___ Incision care ___ Cardiac monitoring ___	Weight 06:00 Incision checks ___ Incision care ___ Cardiac monitoring ___	Weight 06:00 Incision checks ___ Incision care ___ Cardiac monitoring ___	Weight 06:00 Incision checks ___ Incision care ___ DC staples ___ DC cardiac monitor ___
IM to PO pain Rx DC IV lines main. ___ Routine meds ___ 1 IV ___	Routine meds ___ Changes to heplock ___ PO meds ___	Routine meds ___ DC heplock ___ PO meds ___	Routine meds ___ PO meds ___	Routine meds ___ PO meds ___	Routine meds ___ PO meds ___
Amb in room with assistance Cardiac Rehab ___	Amb in hall ___ Cardiac Rehab ___ Shower ___	Amb in hall ___ Cardiac Rehab ___ Shower ___	Amb in hall ___ Shower ___ Cardiac Rehab ___	Amb in hall ___ Shower ___ Cardiac Rehab ___	Amb in hall ___ Cardiac Rehab ___
As tolerated ___	As tolerated ___	As tolerated ___	As tolerated ___	As tolerated ___	As tolerated ___
I & O ___	I & O ___	I & O ___	I & O ___	I & O ___	I & O ___
Incentive spiro Post-op reinforce C&DB, splinting ___ Ongoing pt & family support ___ Cardiac Rehab X2 ___	Ongoing pt & family support ___ Cardiac Rehab X2 ___	Ongoing pt & family support ___ Cardiac Rehab X2 ___ Nutritional Counseling ___	Ongoing pt & family support ___ Cardiac Rehab X2 ___	Ongoing pt & family support ___ Review of discharge activity instructions by Cardiac Rehab. ___	Review meds & follow-up appts. c. pt. or S/O ___
Transfer to TCU ___ Home care planning ___ Home care referral ___	ID placement & support ___	Confirm discharge date with surgeon ___	Notify family of discharge date ___	Order Cardiac Rehab OP program 7–10 days after DSCH ___	DC orders written ___ Rx written ___ DC before 1100 ___
SIGNATURE _____	INITIALS _____	SIGNATURE _____		INITIALS _____	

Figure 4–7 Critical pathway for uncomplicated open heart patients. Courtesy of Mount Clemens General Hospital, Mount Clemens, Michigan.

Documentation of Services

Documentation of medical nutrition therapy, recommendations, and services is essential. Charting in the medical record must include all relevant facts without repetition of information found elsewhere in the chart. The professional dietitian and dietetic technician are generally the only dietetic staff members who document in the medical record. Approval of where and how often documentation occurs, who documents, and what is documented is within the jurisdiction of the institution's medical record committee. Support of the desired location for these entries is needed from the medical director or other key physicians serving on this committee.

Style and Location of Notes and Recommendations

The style of charting may vary from one institution to the next. There is no one perfect charting method. One style, known as SOAP charting, has been common in hospitals for a number of years. Other styles, such as problem/intervention/evaluation charting and focused charting (with data/action/response), have become popular in recent years. There also has been a movement toward diagnostic charting using nutritional diagnoses, much like those introduced by nursing in the past. Some practitioners use a general narrative format; in an effort to minimize paperwork, others now use what is called charting by exception, although this method has not yet been standardized. There is no consensus about which style is best, so that staff must work with other disciplines to ensure that communication is effective for all. When Skipper et al. (1994) reviewed physicians' responses to different formats, they found that dietitians' recommendations were more likely to be implemented when narrative, rather than SOAP, formats were used.

When preestablished charting forms are used, they are usually placed in a separate nutrition or consultation section of the record. Ideally, an assessment form is placed in the designated section, with progress notes on follow-up care being charted with the integrated progress notes of the record. Where this integration is not permitted or feasible (because of lack of access to the individual patient record, as in outpatient or home care), a separate nutrition progress note form is suggested to standardize and simplify the follow-up process. It is recommended that forms that are developed for any site be planned in conjunction with the appropriate team members who will use the information for their decision making. Often in settings where the referring physician is not readily available, communication will be dependent upon the transmittal of records to and from the physician's office and possibly delayed.

Lengthy chart notes are generally kept to a minimum. PiSunyer (Jackson, 1995a) encourages dietitians to sharpen their writing skills and communicate in well organized, brief, and concise notes: "Don't make notes too lengthy. Long notes lose their bite and physicians may not have time to read them all" (p. 3). Regarding dietary recommendations, PiSunyer states "The most important thing is for dietitians to be knowledgeable in the rationale behind the changing of an order. This makes them more self confident and articulate in presenting reasons for a change. Then the physician will be more likely to follow their recommendation" (p. 4). PiSunyer notes that, when dietitians are well informed, they can be more effective in changing a physician's mind. Even though dietitians are busy with high caseloads, it is best to contact a physician personally with a short telephone call: "Briefly say that you put a note in the chart, why your recommendation was made, and how the patient will benefit" (p. 7). In addition, PiSunyer recommends that nurses not be used as mediums of communication from the dietitian to the physician because they are also busy and have a different point of view. Dietitians should approach physicians directly because they know the changes they would like to see and the rationale behind their recommendations and can answer any questions that the physician may have.

According to PiSunyer, "It is always helpful when the dietitian makes rounds with the team. This promotes rapport and allows dietitians to make themselves heard while presenting the rationale for their recommendations" (Jackson, 1995b, p. 7). To support a recommendation, it is acceptable to provide the physician with a scientific research article, but one should be cautious about using materials from companies or manufacturers that promote certain nutrition products. As dietitians try to improve the effectiveness of their dietary recommendations, continuing education is of the utmost importance. The *Journal of the American Dietetic Association*, the *American Journal of Clinical Nutrition*, the *Journal of Nutrition*, and the *British Journal of Nutrition* are the primary professional journals for the field. To locate other sources of important nutrition information, dietitians can consult the *Index Medicus*.

For simplified documentation of nutritional care, the dietitian and physician will find it useful to have a note or sticker that summarizes findings and key recommendations. A sticker may provide standard information as obtained from a nutritional screening, a request for further intervention, a summary of recommendations, or documentation of patient education that has been provided. Stickers are also easily carried in the pocket or a folder, making them transportable to any location where services are rendered. They also allow dietitians to make more efficient use of their time by preparing chart entries at times when the medical record may not be available. The sticker shown in Figure 4–4 summarizes nutritional screening data. A chart sticker may also provide a succinct format to summarize recommendations, giving clear suggestions to the physician as an action plan. Figure 4–8 shows an example of one that can be used for this purpose. One must first check the legalities of using certain stickers as a permanent part of the medical record.

Legal Considerations

Regardless of the type of documentation or the specific format used for documentation, the chart note author must consider a few key facts. One is that chart notes are part of a legal document. Another is that this document serves as a communication tool. Biesemeier states that dietitians will benefit from the more global view of those who actually use the medical record (Jackson, 1996). Besides the clinical care team, one should consider the following individuals and institutions involved in reading chart entries:

- patients and families
- accountants
- administrators
- quality improvement personnel
- medical record staff
- risk managers

Nutrition Findings and Recommendations

❑ As a result of nutrition consult, it is recommended that the current diet/TF/TPN order be continued.

❑ As a result of nutrition consult, it is recommended that the current diet/TF/TPN order be changed to:

_____

❑ Further intervention needed. Recommendation:

_____

Dietitian's signature _____ Date/time_____

Figure 4–8 Chart sticker for recommendations.

- alliances and systems of care
- outpatient surgery centers
- donor organ banks
- health maintenance organizations
- other facilities (hospitals, nursing homes, rehabilitation centers, etc.)
- hospices
- home care agencies
- staff from physician offices
- peer review organizations
- quality assurance and risk management companies
- government agencies
- review agencies
- disease registries

As a result of shortened lengths of stay, increased consumer awareness, and shrinking budgets, dietitians are being pressured to improve productivity while attempting to meet the needs of their patients. This directs the focus toward high-risk issues, those that can potentially result in major losses to hospitals and the professionals they employ. The concept of informed consent has already been discussed. Health care professionals have the ethical obligation to present the facts accurately and to help patients (or their designees) make choices from among the therapeutic alternatives that are consistent with good medical practice. Patients have a right to request and read their medical records and to be involved in determining the plan of care.

Conformance to patients' living wills and advance directives is also a common legal issue. While assessing patients, one should review the documents that portray their personal desires and honor them in nutrition care plans. The American Medical Association and the U.S. Supreme Court have both concluded that artificial feeding by means of an alimentary tube or intravenous infusion is the same as other life-prolonging medical treatments. Hospital policies and signature forms need to ensure full understanding that advance directives to forego or withdraw life-sustaining treatment include technologically supplied food and fluids. According to King (1991), "Health professionals tend to be the most avid death-denying segment of our society. Death is perceived as a failure of medicine and therefore their failure. Withholding or discontinuing nutrition support may sound like professional heresy to the nutritionist" (p. 1). Nevertheless, the professional's values cannot supersede those of the patient; the professional's role is best practiced as the provider of information about alternative feeding modalities and continued moral support of patients and family members regardless of the choice that is made. For terminally ill patients, the American Dietetic Association (1992) has provided specific guidelines for practitioners.

Failure to follow existing hospital policies or professional standards regarding assessment and treatment of patients is a frequent basis for legal action. Often, the medical record contains definite clues that are not considered during the assessment process, and legal hassles result. One case in point involved an elderly diabetic patient with severely infected pressure ulcers and other complications (Jackson, 1995a). The patient was on a 1,800-calorie diet and had nursing documentation showing poor intake. Frequent entries were made in the medical record by the dietitian and diet technician, such as "1,800-calorie diet was being provided as ordered . . . the diet met the recommended dietary allowances . . . the patient was feeding herself." No one dealt with the issue of poor intake, however, and the fact that the patient was not getting sufficient nutrients for healing. In a lawsuit that was ultimately filed by family members, the staff were cited for inappropriate nutritional care of this patient.

Legal action may involve foods that cause illness or complications in a patient's medical condition. Such may be the case when food allergies are not honored or when sufficient instruction and precautions for potential food–medication interactions are not observed. Foodborne illnesses affect more than 15,000 individuals in the United States each year and are frequently followed by lawsuits on behalf of persons who are severely affected. According to Cody (1991), the most susceptible are the elderly, children, immune-suppressed individuals, and those recovering from illnesses. Aspiration due to choking on food is another common ground for legal action. In one legal case, an inappropriate diet was served to a patient with a history of stroke who was characterized as being a fast eater. After two episodes of choking on regular foods, the physician changed the diet to mechanical soft foods, and dysphagia was added to the problem list. Even though the facility's diet manual stated that chopped meats were to be used for this diet, a mixed dish with chicken pieces was served because the dietary staff believed that the meat in this entree was soft enough for patients on this diet. After the patient failed to chew the meat properly, he aspirated and expired. The family's case was supported by autopsy results, and liability rested with the provider of care.

Not only do suspected cases of abuse have to be reported, but the institution is frequently held accountable for abusive behavior on the part of its employees. Inservice training and supervision serve to promote proper conduct on the job, and even subtle incidents of abuse should result in counseling or disciplinary action for employees who display such tendencies so that their improper behavior can be effectively curtailed. If an employee feels that involvement in a patient's care conflicts with his or her personal values or religious beliefs, he or she can request not to participate in care. The Joint Commission standards address this issue to ensure that patients' care is not negatively affected.

According to the Joint Commission, an initial assessment of each patient's physical, psychological, and social status determines the need for care, the type of care to be provided, and the need for any further assessment. Although each hospital has liberty to determine the exact screening criteria, patients who are found to be malnourished or those at moderate or high risk of malnourishment must receive further assessment, and their therapeutic responses should be monitored and documented. Unfortunately, screening according to acceptable protocols does not occur for all patients, as described at the beginning of this chapter.

To avoid potential risks, immediate attention can be given to identifying and treating high-risk cases properly. The clinical nutrition manager can work with the clinical staff to learn exactly how many patients are being overlooked and why. The staff can be supported in efforts to provide timely and high-quality care, and managers can assist them in restructuring their jobs so that this can be done. Assistance can also be obtained from other members of the health care team who are involved with quality improvement, patient advocacy, risk management, ethical practice, and management information. The clinical nutrition manager has the responsibility of communicating any potential problems that could result in poor care and possible legal disputes and of assisting in resolving these issues.

Readers are referred to Chapter 6 to learn about current issues of patients' rights that need to be considered. A case study is presented in that chapter that illustrates how these concepts can be integrated into the plan of care.

Standard Operating Procedures

A clearly defined scope of practice for the profession, whether part of state licensure or an accepted national norm, serves to represent current standards (i.e., what would any other *reasonable dietitian* have done in a similar case?). This thought must always be in the mind of the person who is documenting care: "Have I done all that is reasonable and expected in a case of this nature?" Malpractice suits, although not common against dietitians as isolated practitioners, sometimes affect this area of practice because they implicate all disciplines.

The clinical nutrition manager can establish standards at two levels. The first level is *standard operating procedures* that govern processes such as communications and methods that are used by team members to do their work. The second level entails what are commonly called *standards of practice*, the exact protocols that guide clinical assessment and treatment of patients and other customers. They are covered below.

An integrated approach can be taken to the establishment of standardized operating procedures. In the beginning of this chapter, the topic of planning was covered, and this applies to the development of departmental standards. Internally, the nutrition services staff members can work together to develop the procedures, methods, and forms needed for ensuring effective and efficient care, such as the dietary Kardex, calorie count forms, supplement records, nothing by mouth/clear liquid tracking forms, and others. These tools are useful to reduce rework and to communicate accurately the information used during case management of patient and clients. There should be a paper trail that leads from one stage to another. For example, if the dietitian requires additional data regarding the actual intake of a patient, the nutrition care plan includes these data, and in many instances a recommendation is made to the physician to order a 3-day calorie count. A form can be developed for data collection so that this can be done with accuracy. This form is used by nursing to document actual intake, and the nutrition care staff estimate the nutrient value of the foods they list. If patients have increased needs for specific nutrients other than protein, carbohydrates, and fats, they can be included in the analysis. Figure 4–9 shows an example of a form that can be used for data collection and analysis.

A note can be then entered in the medical record that shows patients' nutritional needs, the nutrients that are provided with the current physician's order, and results of the analysis. A chart sticker for this note is shown in Figure 4–10. To guide physicians properly to the best possible diet prescription, the nutritionist must convey the nutrient composition of the current diet and foods.

This leads to a discussion of nutrient analysis of menus. According to health codes, menus used for patient service must be nutritionally balanced and meet all requirements for the population served. It is common for surveyors to ask about the nutrient composition of menus to determine whether foods that are served actually meet the stipulations cited in the facility's diet manual. If a certain diet has unusually low nutrient profiles, this should be stated in the manual so that physicians know they are ordering an inadequate diet.

It should be understood that nutrient analysis of menus only yields *estimated* amounts of nutrients, for several reasons. First, nutrient databases reflect data taken from manufacturers, which use modeling techniques rather than direct analysis of their foods. Second, it cannot be denied that foods have inherent variability; they differ in genetic make-up, in environmental conditions, and as a result of food processing, storage, and preparation methods. Third, and perhaps most important, the biggest discrepancy exists when one considers the fact that recipes and food service handling practices vary from facility to facility and from day to day. Nutrient losses often occur during storage and prolonged holding of foods after preparation. Databases are primarily based upon food

Directions: Nursing records all foods, fluids (except water), tube feedings, IVs, and between-meal snacks for each patient for the total 24-hour period. The nutrition care staff calculate estimated nutrient content for each item and day.

Meal	Food, Beverage, Snack, or Supplement	Quantity (%)	Comment	Initials	CHO (g)	Protein (g)	Fat (g)	Kcal	Other Nutrients __ __ __		
Breakfast											
Lunch											
Dinner											
Snacks											
Total											

Patient_____ Room_____

Signature_____

Date_____

	Oral						
	Tube						
	IV						
	Total						

Figure 4–9 Calorie count record.

Calorie Count Findings and Recommendations

Estimated Nutrient Needs	Provision with Current Diet Prescription	Actual Intake (Average for ____ days)
Calorie _____	_____	_____
Protein _____	_____	_____
Carbohydrate _____	_____	_____
Fat _____	_____	_____

Other pertinent nutrients:

_____   _____   _____

_____   _____   _____

_____   _____   _____

❏ As a result of this calorie count, it is recommended that the current diet/TF/ TPN order by continued.

❏ As a result of this calorie count, it is recommended that the current diet/TF/ TPN order be changed to:

_____

❏ Further intervention needed. Recommendation:

_____

Dates of calorie count _____

Dietitian's signature _____ Date/time _____

Figure 4–10 Chart sticker for calorie count.

samples that are handled under controlled conditions without long-term holding before consumption.

For a complete and accurate paper trail to exist, dietitians must be sure that their diet manuals reflect the nutrient composition of the diets, tube feedings, and parenteral formulas they offer. They also need to decide the most appropriate group for which adequacy is to be evaluated. The dietitians at Yale–New Haven Hospital, for example, present data in their diet manual for both reference adult males and females and for other groups, such as pregnant mothers and pediatric patients (Ford, 1990). Their diet manual states "the key to using any nutrient analysis data for determining the nutritional adequacy of a diet is to remember that the word RECOMMENDED should not be interpreted as a fixed immutable FACT" (p. 1). A computer system, along with the standards for nutritional adequacy listed below, is used for nutrient analysis; other nutrients are included when indicated by certain types of diets:

- recommended dietary allowances for calories, protein, vitamin A, thiamin, riboflavin, niacin, vitamin B6, vitamin B12, folacin, vitamin C, vitamin E, calcium, iron, magnesium, phosphorus, selenium, and zinc (National Research Council, 1990)
- estimated safe and adequate daily dietary intakes for pantothenic acid and copper (National Research Council, 1990)
- estimated minimum requirements for potassium and sodium (National Research Council, 1990)
- dietary goals for the United States for cholesterol and percentages of calories from carbohydrate, protein, and fat (U.S. Select Committee on Nutrition and Human Needs, 1977)
- the American Dietetic Association's and Food and Drug Administration's recommendations for dietary fiber (American Dietetic Association, 1988)

Standard operating procedures can be set for establishing policies, procedures, and methods for formularies, writing diet orders, and many other processes that occur routinely.

Standards of Practice

According to Biesemeier

Unlike the nursing profession which already has minimum data sets and defined nursing care process, dietitians do not have a nutrition care process and . . . this is a great deficit. Many dietitians use a standard assessment process but do not see themselves to have the role of identifying nutrition problems. Rather, they perceive their role as providing interventions for problems that other caregivers define. (Jackson, 1996, p. 6)

Clinical nutrition managers can empower dietitians to work at higher levels and for role definition in the field.

The American Dietetic Association does not mandate guidelines, but it supports those from the American Hospital Association for patient assessment, which were first issued in 1980 and reaffirmed in 1990. There is no specific format recommended in these guidelines. Two models for the nutrition care process have been presented in the literature (Gates, 1992; Kight, 1985). Both these models, according to Biesemeier, are very promising. Gates (1992) presents a circular model, whereby dietitians collect data, identify and prioritize problems, analyze alternatives, set goals, plan and implement interventions, and evaluate the effectiveness of the plan. Kight's (1985) model is similar but much more specific with regard to standardizing names for problems, definitions, codes, etiologies, interventions, and outcomes. "This system has been validated, and it reflects evidence based practice" (Jackson, 1996, p. 7).

Prudent practices and comprehensive documentation according to facility standards are two ways to protect against malpractice. Dietitians can work with members of the health care team to develop integrated standards for the assessment and treatment of patients. These can be expressed as clinical pathways or care maps focused on specific diagnoses, as described earlier in this chapter, or standard practice guidelines for the nutrition component alone can be developed. A good reference for standard protocols is now available from the American Dietetic Association (1996). Exhibit 4–5 shows a standard guideline for a specific diagnosis (human immunodeficiency virus infection/acquired immunodeficiency syndrome).

Nutrition Education

One intervention that cannot be underestimated in its potential to reduce costs associated with nutrition excesses or deficits is patient education. As a result of recent emphasis in the industry on patient and community education, Chapter 5 is dedicated to this topic. Clinical nutrition managers can help their patients best if they focus on education and emphasize the need for a practical approach. For example, the patient with newly diagnosed diabetes mellitus would receive in-depth instructions on self-management techniques (i.e., how to match diet to administration of drug therapy, how much and when to eat, how to avoid problems when traveling, how to manage illness and eating in restaurants, and how to detect and treat symptoms of hypo- and hyperglycemia). The role of the dietitian cannot be overlooked among those of the other team members who can reduce the need for hospitalizations, excess medication costs, and lost job productivity.

In addition to the provision of information and instructions, counseling over time is recommended as the patient progresses in self-management. Once home, patients encounter challenges in their environments and daily lives that may preclude their following the dietitian's instructions. With follow-up counseling, the dietitian is able to provide additional insights, suggestions, and encouragement to the patient. This step is of the utmost importance in allowing the patient to gain independence and self-confidence, both of which are goals of the dietitian as patient educator and counselor. In addition to instructions rendered (the practitioner's process), the results (the patient's outcome) must be recorded. After education has occurred, it is best if the dietitian notes how the

Exhibit 4-5 Sample Patient Care Guidelines: Nutrition and Human Immunodeficiency Virus Infection/Acquired Immunodeficiency Syndrome

HIV Protein: Follow usual guidelines for protein repletion
 Energy: Stress factor is 1.1 for asymptomatic or symptomatic HIV. Add 500 kcal for weight gain.
AIDS Protein: 1–2.5 g/kg
 Energy: 35–40 kcal/kg or Harris-Benedict equation × activity factor × stress factor. Stress factor is 1.25 for H/O AIDS; 1.3 for H/O AIDS with secondary infections.
 Fluids: Per general recommendations: 100 ml for each of the first 10 kg
 50 ml for each of the second 10 kg
 10–20 ml for each kg over 20 kg
 or
 35 ml/kg—average adult (25–50 yrs)
 40 ml/kg—young active adult (16–30 yrs)
 30 ml/kg—older person (55–65 yrs)
 25 ml/kg—elderly persons (> 65 yrs)

Interim Dietary Recommendations for Early Stage HIV-Infected Persons

Nutrient	Multiples of RDAs	Daily Amount
Riboflavin	6	9 mg
Vitamin B_6 (pyridoxine)	>10 mg	>20 mg
Vitamin B_{12} (cyanocobalamine)	25 µg	50 µg
Vitamin A	10	10,000 µg RE[1]
Vitamin C	10	360 mg
Vitamin E	6	60 mg
Zinc	5	75 mg

[1]RE = retinol equivalents. 1 RE = 1 µg retinol or 6 µg β-carotene. Vitamin A sources vary in vitamin activity.
Note: Recommendations are referenced as multiples of the recommended dietary allowances (RDAs) from the National Research Council. (*Source:* Baum, M.K., et al. Interim dietary recommendations to maintain adequate blood nutrient levels in early HIV-1 infection. Biopsychosocial Center for AIDS, University of Miami School of Medicine, Miami, FL. Poster #POB3675—International Conference on AIDS, Amsterdam, 1992).

Other Vitamin/Micronutrient Information: Selenium and folate supplementation is currently being researched. Regarding zinc, supplementation > 25 mg may cause gastrointestinal distress.

Other Nutritional Considerations: With a normally functioning gastrointestinal tract, a high-calorie, high-protein diet with oral supplements should meet patients' needs.

continues

Exhibit 4–5 continued

Consider a lactose-free or low-fat diet with gastrointestinal malabsorption. If enteral nutrition is indicated, an elemental formula with MCT and low osmolality may need to be considered.

HIV-Infected Child   Energy: Use RDAs unless catch-up growth is required
Protein: 1.5–2 × RDAs
Supplementation of vitamins and minerals at levels not to exceed one to two times the RDA may be recommended for these children.

Formulas estimating requirements during catch-up growth:
Kcal/kg = RDA calories for weight and age × ideal weight for height/actual weight
Grams protein/kg = RDA calories for weight and age × ideal weight for height/actual weight

Source: Data from C. Grunfeld, et al., Resting Energy Expenditure, Caloric Intake, and Short Term Weight Change in Human Immunodeficiency Virus Infection and the Acquired Immunodeficiency Syndrome, *American Journal of Clinical Nutrition,* Vol. 55, pp. 455–460, © 1992, American Society for Clinical Nutrition; D.P. Kitler, Enteral Alimentation and Repletion of Body Cell Mass in Malnourished Patients with Acquired Immunodeficiency Syndrome, *American Journal of Clinical Nutrition,* Vol. 55, pp. 449–454, © 1991, American Society for Clinical Nutrition; and K.E. Peterson, J. Washington, and S.M. Rathbun, Team Management of Failure to Thrive, *Journal of the American Dietetic Association,* Vol. 84, pp. 810–814, © 1994, American Dietetic Association.

information was received. When possible, a written or oral quiz should be given to determine retention of information. In some cases, such as after menu planning, a return demonstration by the patient is suggested to evaluate the depth of understanding of the principles that were taught. In the institutional setting, evaluation can include a review of the patient's menu selections to determine whether principles were successfully applied. Figure 4–11 is a sample chart sticker for documenting educational actions and dietitians' recommendations for further inpatient or outpatient education.

PERFORMANCE APPRAISAL

Productivity factors must be tied to performance evaluation of staff members. Generally, performance appraisal tools are most effective if 8 to 10 standards are set and if no more than three evaluative measures are used (i.e., "meets standard," "does not meet standard," and "exceeds standard"). When expectations are written clearly and determined fairly, staff members are more likely to be able to meet or exceed the standards.

Nutrition Education and Recommendations

Patient has received nutrition information on:

❑ Cardiac nutrition   ❑ Diabetes self-management
❑ Prenatal nutrition   ❑ Weight loss
❑ Breastfeeding guidelines   ❑ Eating disorders
❑ Age-specific nutritional guidelines for life cycle stage:
      infant   adolescent   geriatric
      child   adult male/female
❑ Potential drug–nutrient interactions for _____
❑ Other _____

Method: ❑ Individual counseling with: ❑ patient ❑ family or caregiver
          ❑ Group counseling including: ❑ patient ❑ family or caregiver

❑ As a result of this education, it is recommended that:

_____

_____

Date of education _____

Dietitian's signature _____ Date/time _____

Figure 4–11 Chart sticker for nutrition education.

In many institutions now, benchmark standards have been established for certain job descriptions. These benchmarks should be available in any job with the same title anywhere in the country. For example, a dietetic technician should be expected to modify menus accurately according to physician orders within a given time frame. A clinical dietitian should be expected to conduct a thorough nutritional assessment, including all key parameters of nutritional status, from a medical record in any area of the nation. Chapter 14 contains more detail on benchmarking.

Individual standards are then established for the specific job. In home care, the dietitian may have a standard stating "nutritional consultations are completed within 24 hours, with a documented report sent to the physician within 48 hours." In long-term care, the consulting dietitian may report all findings of

Competency Statement for Enteral Assessment and Monitoring

Demonstrates the ability to assess appropriately the nutrition needs, develop tube feeding care plan, and monitor tolerance and changing needs of the patient receiving tube feeding.

Validator's Initials and Dates	Critical Behaviors
	1. Demonstrates knowledge of indications/contraindications of the use of tube feeding in the hospitalized patient.
	2. Demonstrates ability to assess a patient's nutritional needs based on metabolic aberrations necessitating tube feeding support.
	3. Demonstrates knowledge of the classification and composition of feeding formulas.
	4. Demonstrates knowledge of enteral access routes and their impact on tube feeding formulation and delivery.
	5. Demonstrates knowledge of the different enteral administration methods.
	6. Demonstrates ability to determine appropriate initiation and progression of tube feeding schedule.
	7. Demonstrates ability to recommend appropriate monitoring of tube feeding support.
	8. Demonstrates ability to interpret tube feeding monitoring data and recommend appropriate changes.
	9. Demonstrates knowledge of potential drug–nutrient interactions related to tube feeding.
	10. Demonstrates ability to communicate nutritional needs and tube feeding recommendations to hospital staff verbally and in written form.
	11. Demonstrates knowledge of postdischarge tube feeding needs.
	12. Demonstrates ability to instruct caregiver(s) on postdischarge tube feeding regimen as appropriate.

Learning Activities
1. Read CMHA Clinical Nutrition Manual, Enteral Nutrition Chapter.
2. Complete ASPEN Enteral Nutrition Self-Assessment Program.
3. Demonstrate management of the provision of the tube feeding care process under the supervision of the Clinical Specialist/Supervisor.

continues

Competency Questions/Demonstration Activities
1. T or F—Nutrients are metabolized and utilized more effectively via the enteral than the parenteral route.
2. Identify two situations in which a fiber formula would be beneficial.
3. Describe the symptoms of a patient's intolerance to a formula with high osmolality.
4. Describe the difference between continuous feeding, intermittent feeding, and bolus feeding. What are the advantages of each?
5. What precautions can be taken to avoid aspiration pneumonia in tube-fed patients?
6. List the modular products available at CMC.
7. What is the difference between a polymeric and partially hydrolyzed tube feeding formula?
                              Score_____

Evaluation	The policy and procedure will be followed upon completion of this clinical validation of the competency.	
	Date	**Validator's Signature**
Attempted	_____	_____
Validated	_____	_____
	_____	_____

Figure 4–12 Clinical nutrition competencies for enteral assessment and monitoring. *Source:* © 1995: The Charlotte-Mecklenburg Hospital Authority. Department of Dietetic Services, P.O. Box 32861, Charlotte, NC 28232.

violations in diet order management to the director of nursing within 24 hours of completion of the facility visit.

Standards should be written to include consideration of patient population characteristics (pediatric, adult, and geriatric), scope of nutritional therapy, knowledge and skills required, and level of supervision or management expected from the position. Complexity of patient cases may be included, such as extensive involvement with enteral and parenteral nutrition therapies, support team services, and reimbursement documentation.

STAFF DEVELOPMENT

Competency documentation is also required by the Joint Commission. In addition to background checks, interviews, and verification of credentialing at the time of hire, critical behaviors related to competency must be reviewed and summarized at least annually. These competency assessment tools become an important part of the appraisal process and set the stage for staff development plans. Figure 4–12 is a sample competency documentation checklist.

Effective staff development begins at the time of hire. Orientation should be of sufficient duration to establish a baseline for an individualized plan. Each staff member's personnel file should contain a record that includes an outservice and in-house educational log of meetings and workshops that have been attended. After new hires are sufficiently oriented and trained in their assignments and standards, an annual educational needs assessment is suggested. Staff members should be able to select those areas of further growth and development that meet their professional goals. In addition, the clinical nutrition manager will want to include areas where the performance appraisal document, productivity studies, and quality improvement studies have shown weaknesses. A sample form is shown in Figure 4–13.

Finally, staff development considerations must include the goal of promotion and retention of staff. Clinical ladders, mentioned earlier in this chapter, should be considered one method for offering growth in the clinical specialty areas. Advancement to clinical specialist positions should allow the seasoned practitioner to demonstrate expertise and valuable skills while maintaining a commitment to direct patient care.

To meet your needs and interests, please indicate your level of agreement with the following topics planned for 1997:

1. Quality Indicators   ❑ Agree   ❑ Uncertain   ❑ Disagree
2. Stress Management   ❑ Agree   ❑ Uncertain   ❑ Disagree
3. Dysphagia Management   ❑ Agree   ❑ Uncertain   ❑ Disagree
4. Nutrition and Pressure Sores ❑ Agree   ❑ Uncertain   ❑ Disagree
5. Nutritional Pharmacology   ❑ Agree   ❑ Uncertain   ❑ Disagree
6. Cancer Therapy Updates   ❑ Agree   ❑ Uncertain   ❑ Disagree
7. Tube Feeding versus TPN Today ❑ Agree   ❑ Uncertain   ❑ Disagree

Check two preferred methods of presentation that you consider most helpful to you:

❑ Lecture/discussion   ❑ Self-learning packets   ❑ Interdisciplinary rounds
❑ Demonstration/practice   ❑ Patient case studies   ❑ Handouts
❑ Journal club   ❑ Audiovisuals (slides, videos)

How often do you want an inservice?

❑ Weekly   ❑ Twice a month   ❑ Monthly   ❑ Every other month

What are the best times for you to attend an inservice?

❑ Before a shift   ❑ After a shift   ❑ During a shift
❑ On a day off   ❑ Full-day workshop   ❑ Weekend retreat

How long should the program last?   ❑ 30 minutes   ❑ One hour   ❑ Over 1 hour

Figure 4–13 Annual clinical needs assessment survey.

QUALITY MANAGEMENT IN NUTRITION SERVICES

After the groundwork has been laid for the department's success (with proper mission, goals, design, and staffing), the last but most important step is the management of continuous quality improvement. It is not only the manager's role, but everyone's role, to review continuously what is being done, the impact of those actions, and how to improve services to meet the needs of the customer. Chapter 14 deals with the topics of quality improvement and benchmarking for clinical nutrition and food service functions.

CONCLUSION

The goals of a superior nutritional program are to meet or exceed customer expectations, to contain costs, to empower staff members, and to achieve excellence. *Employee commitment, teamwork,* and *proactivity* are effective buzzwords for this decade and for the 21st century. Survival of the fittest, and the finest, requires leadership and the astute management of resources. In the nutritional services arena, these resources focus on cost effectiveness (i.e., costs in dollars divided by outcomes in units) and outcomes management. Early prediction of length of stay in acute care settings, decreasing use of intensive care units, and improvements in multidisciplinary collaborative care across the health care continuum will be the norms of the future.

In the current environment of health maintenance organizations and managed care organizations, those services that save or reduce costs will become more visible and more valuable. Benchmarking, or comparing costs and standards of care among institutions, will become commonplace when consumers dictate where they will seek health care. Decreasing the costs related to malnutrition in any setting is not only possible but essential. With an organized nutritional services program, dietitians can provide individualized screening, assessments, medical nutrition therapies, and counseling. These interventions can lead to changes in food habits, decreased risk factors, improved health outcomes, decreased hospital stay, and economic benefits. In this era, no health care system can afford to provide less.

REFERENCES

American Dietetic Association. (1988). Position of the American Dietetic Association: Health implications of dietary fiber. *Journal of the American Dietetic Association, 88,* 216.

American Dietetic Association. (1992). Position of the American Dietetic Association: Issues in feeding the terminally ill adult. *Journal of the American Dietetic Association, 92,* 996–1002.

American Dietetic Association. (1996). *Medical Nutrition Therapy Across the Continuum of Care.* K.G. Smith & E.Q. Johnson (Eds.). Chicago: American Dietetic Association.

American Medical Association. (1996). *Physicians' current procedural terminology.* Milwaukee: Author.

Cody, M.M. (1991). *Food Safety for Professionals.* Chicago: American Dietetic Association.

Fish, J., Hunter, A., Chernoff, R., et al. (1993). Evolution of the nutrition support team. In M. Gottschlich, et al. (Eds.), *Nutrition support dietetics core curriculum* (pp. 1–14). Silver Spring, MD: ASPEN.

Foltz, M.B., Schiller, M.R., & Ryan, A.S. (1993). Nutrition screening and assessment: Current practices and dietitians' leadership roles. *Journal of the American Dietetic Association, 93*(12), 1388–1395.

Ford, D.A. (1990). Interpreting the nutrient analysis data. In *Manual of Clinical Dietetics* (pp. 1–7). New Haven: Yale–New Haven Hospital.

Fox, M.K. (Ed.). (1991). *Reimbursement and insurance coverage for nutrition services.* Chicago: American Dietetic Association.

Gates, G. (1992). Clinical reasoning: An essential component of dietetic practice. *Topics in Clinical Nutrition, 7,* 74–80.

Jackson, R. (1995a). Avoiding legal disputes. *Hospital Food & Nutrition Focus, 11*(5), 3, 4, 7.

Jackson, R. (1995b). Making effective dietary recommendations. *Hospital Food & Nutrition Focus, 11*(10), 7–8.

Jackson, R. (1995c). Medicare/Medicaid reimbursement for home care. *Hospital Food & Nutrition Focus, 11*(9), 6–7.

Jackson, R. (1996). Computerized medical records. *Hospital Food & Nutrition Focus, 12*(6), 6–8.

Joint Commission on Accreditation of Healthcare Organizations. (1996). *1996 Accreditation manual for hospitals.* Oakbrook Terrace, IL: Author.

Kight, M.A. (1985). Working with diagnosis related groups (DRGs): Diagnosis in the practice of selected health-medical team members. *Nutrition Support Services, 5,* 39–46.

King, D.G. (1991). Nutrition support: Quandaries of morality and mortality. *Wyeth-Ayerst International, 4,* 1–3.

Laramee, S. (1995). Monitoring productivity of the clinical staff. *Hospital Food & Nutrition Focus, 11*(10), 4–5.

Lathrop, J.P. (1993). *Restructuring health care. The patient focused paradigm.* San Francisco: Jossey-Bass.

National Research Council. (1990). *Recommended Dietary Allowances* (10th ed.). Washington, DC: National Academy Press.

Nelson, J., & Steinborn, P. (1992). Who are we, where are we, where are we going? *Nutrition in Clinical Practice, 7,* S18–S21.

Nutrition Screening Initiative. (1991). *Nutrition screening manual for professionals caring for older Americans.* Washington, DC: Author.

O'Rourke, L.M., & Bader, B.S. (1993, March). A process for developing a board quality and performance report. *Quality Letter,* p. 9.

Queen, P.M., Caldwell, M., & Balogun, L. (1993). Clinical indicators for oncology, cardiovascular, and surgical patients: Report of the ADA Council on Practice Quality Assurance Committee. *Journal of the American Dietetic Association, 93,* 338–344.

Schatz, G. (1993). Coding for nutrition services: Challenges, opportunities and guidelines. *Journal of the American Dietetic Association, 93*, 471.

Skipper, A., & Winkler, M. (1992). The changing role of the dietitian in clinical practice. *Nutrition in Clinical Practice*, S5–S8.

Skipper, A., Young, M., Rotman, N., & Nagl, H. (1994). Physicians' implementation of dietitians' recommendations: A study of the effectiveness of dietitians. *Journal of the American Dietetic Association, 94*(1), 45–49.

Sowa, D.C. (1995). *Launching a clinical nutrition practice model for the 21st century.* Presented at the annual meeting of the American Dietetic Association, Chicago, IL.

Sowinski, S.A., Shepherd, S.K., Dowling, R.A., & Wagner, M.H. (1994). Value-added services that increase physicians' intent to refer patients to an outpatient clinic. *Journal of the American Dietetic Association, 94*(5), 529–532.

U.S. Department of Health and Human Services. (1990). *Healthy people 2000: National health promotion and disease prevention objectives.*Washington, DC: Public Health Service.

U.S. Select Committee on Nutrition and Human Needs. (1977). *Dietary goals for the United States* (2nd ed.). Washington, DC: Government Printing Office.

Zappia, P., & Watrous, J. (1995). Designing an integrated, initial patient assessment. *Joint Commission Perspectives, 15*(1), 13–15.

Outcome-Based Nutrition Education

Laura K. Guyer

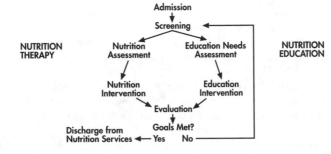

Patient education is an essential component of comprehensive health care, and dietitians have long recognized the role of nutrition education in recovery from illness, shortened length of hospital stay, and return to activities of daily living (American Dietetic Association, 1995). Nutrition education and counseling are the tools used by dietitians to transmit information to individuals about the relationships among food, behavior, and health. As preventive health care becomes increasingly important, there has been more emphasis in recent years on education in the field. The Joint Commission on Accreditation of Healthcare Organizations (Joint Commission) has even included a separate section in its standards for this topic. The following is from the preamble of this section of the *1996 Accreditation Manual for Hospitals* (Joint Commission, 1995, p. 125):

> Education promotes healthy behaviors, supports recovery and a speedy return to function, and enables patients to be involved in the decisions about their own care. The goal of the patient and family education function is to improve patient health outcomes by promoting healthy behavior and involving the patient in care and care decisions.

Nutrition education and counseling are two interdependent activities. Education provides information that empowers individuals to make informed decisions about food, and counseling enables a change of inappropriate attitudes and eating behaviors. The goal of each is to improve nutritional well-being.

THE TRADITIONAL HEALTH CARE MODEL

Since the 1970s the role of the dietitian has changed, and through nutrition assessment and intervention practitioners have moved from provision of passive support to active care. Recently, dietetic practice has expanded and advanced through scientific discoveries, and new responsibilities have emerged for the dietitian in both traditional and nontraditional settings. In spite of progress in many areas, nutrition education and counseling, as components of practice, have changed little.

Comprehensive nutrition assessment and intervention include patient education. As a component of the nutrition program, however, the delivery, outcomes, and rewards of nutrition education are often less than ideal for practitioners and patients alike. This is why education is being stressed more. Its role as a preventive measure is being realized more now than in the past.

Many reasons have been offered to explain why the nutrition education and counseling exchange has not been satisfactory. First, the delivery of quality instruction is time consuming. Second, barriers to success include a lack of coordination among health care providers, limited preparation of the health care professional for the teaching role, and assignment of low priority by administration to patient education (Webber, 1990). Third, the lack of tangible reward or recognition for the effort spent in education leads many practitioners to allocate time to the more recognized, and thus more satisfying, aspects of care. Fourth, the discharge instruction given at the bedside does not enable the development of a relationship between dietitian and patient. This results in a less effective, and therefore less satisfying, education exchange. Effective instruction requires time to identify patient needs and build a relationship of trust and support.

Integrating Nutrition Education

It is time for dietitians to think about nutrition therapy and education as dependent yet distinct programs, as illustrated in Figure 5–1. It can be seen in this model that patients are not discharged from nutrition therapy until their goals are met. Even if they are discharged from the facility, they can continue to receive nutrition therapy and/or nutrition education on an outpatient basis. The concept of integrated health care delivery therefore can be practiced as patients and other customers travel through the continuum of care. As defined, medical nutrition therapy is an assessment of nutrition status to identify risk factors. After assessment, patient management requires provision of specialized

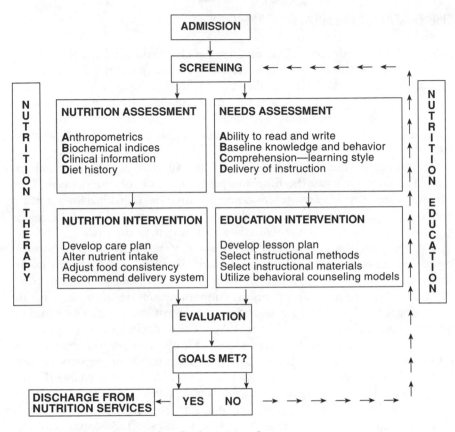

Figure 5-1 Components of medical nutrition therapy.

nutrition therapies such as diet modification, medical foods, parenteral nutrition, and/or counseling (American Dietetic Association, 1995).

In dietetic practice, education assessment and intervention are less well defined and developed than nutrition assessment and intervention. To move forward, dietitians must discontinue the routine practice of providing patient instruction at the time of discharge and assume a leadership role in planning and directing the process of nutrition education and counseling. Directors of nutrition services are encouraged to support them in this effort.

The knowledge and skills possessed by dietitians through education and training are often underutilized. Dietetic education provides broad and comprehensive training for registered dietitians, according to the American Dietetic Association's *Standards of Education* (1994). The 24 knowledge and 18 performance requirements shown in Exhibit 5-1 guide the design of under-

Exhibit 5–1 Standards of Education Knowledge and Performance Requirements

Knowledge Requirements for Entry Level Dietitians

1. Knows principles of effective oral and written communication and documentation.
2. Knows fundamentals of human relations and group dynamics.
3. Knows techniques of interviewing and counseling.
4. Knows principles of education and effective methods of teaching.
5. Knows use of computers for data processing and information management in dietetics.
6. Knows basic concepts of research methodology and statistical analysis.
7. Knows fundamentals of quality assurance.
8. Knows laws, regulations, and standards affecting dietetic practice.
9. Knows principles of human anatomy and physiology, microbiology, organic chemistry, and biochemistry.
10. Knows principles of behavioral and social sciences.
11. Knows the physiological, biochemical, and behavioral bases for nutrition intervention in health and disease.
12. Knows the influence of socioeconomic, cultural, and psychological factors on food and nutrition behavior.
13. Knows energy and nutrient needs for various stages of the life cycle.
14. Knows principles of food science and techniques of food preparation.
15. Knows nutrient composition of food and appropriate sources of data.
16. Knows principles of menu planning for optimal nutrition of individuals and groups in health and disease.
17. Knows principles of nutrition screening, assessment, planning, intervention, evaluation, and documentation.
18. Knows resources for delivery of nutrition care in community programs.
19. Knows principles of procurement, food production, distribution, and service.
20. Knows fundamentals and techniques of financial management.
21. Knows principles of organization and management.
22. Knows principles and techniques of human resource management.
23. Knows fundamentals of marketing food and nutrition services.
24. Knows fundamentals of the political and legislative process.

Performance Requirements for Entry Level Dietitians

1. Utilizes effective oral and written communication skills in the practice of dietetics.
2. Promotes effective professional relationships in the practice of dietetics.
3. Provides education to consumers, clients, other professionals, and support personnel.
4. Utilizes computer and other technologies in the practice of dietetics.
5. Applies current research information in the practice of dietetics.
6. Participates in quality assurance programs.
7. Utilizes knowledge of political, legislative, and economic factors that affect dietetic practice.
8. Complies with the Code of Ethics and Standards of Practice for the Profession of Dietetics.
9. Provides nutrition care for individuals and groups through systematic screening, assessment, planning, intervention, evaluation, and documentation.

continues

Exhibit 5–1 continued

10. Provides nutrition counseling and education to individuals and groups for health promotion, maintenance, treatment, and rehabilitation.
11. Participates in the management of cost-effective nutrition care systems.
12. Utilizes food, nutrition, and social service resources in community programs.
13. Ensures that food service operations meet the food and nutrition needs of target markets.
14. Utilizes menus as focal points for control of the food service system.
15. Participates in the management of food service systems, including procurement, food production, distribution, and service.
16. Participates in the management of human, financial, material, physical, and operational resources.
17. Integrates food and nutrition services with other services in the practice setting.
18. Participates in activities that promote improved nutrition status of consumers and market the profession of dietetics.

Courtesy of Standards of Education. Chicago: The American Dietetic Association, 1994, Chicago, Illinois (with permission).

---

graduate curricula and have their foundations in basic and applied sciences; they include supporting courses from the social and behavioral sciences to prepare students for entry level practice.

As health care providers, dietitians are well prepared by their education and experience for competition in a dynamic and changing environment. Today's dietitians must recognize that the uncertainty created by change provides new opportunity, and those with vision, confidence, and plans of action will change dietetic practice and the direction of our profession as we move into the 21st century. The climate today is as ripe for change as it was in the 1970s, when "The Skeleton in the Hospital Closet" (Butterworth, 1974) moved the dietitian to active membership on the health care team.

Health care is changing rapidly, and providers are facing many new challenges: increased work load, decreased average length of patient stay, increased number of patients with acute illness upon admission, and increased number of patients discharged with the responsibility to manage their own care (Nielsen & Sheppard, 1988). Today's health care organizations are using new strategies to meet society's mandate for quality care. Dietitians will either follow the leadership provided by others or identify areas where they choose to lead.

The Joint Commission Standards: Opportunity for Change

Recent Joint Commission standards offer hope and opportunity for those whose practice includes nutrition education and counseling. The new standards prescribe an interdisciplinary, performance-based model of health care that focuses on the outcomes of care. They require assessment of patient learning needs, readiness to learn, and learning ability (Dougherty, Bankhead, Kushner, Mirtallo, & Winkler, 1995; Krasker & Balogun, 1995). This provides an opportunity for dietitians to require and provide nutrition education and counseling as components of comprehensive care. Maximum benefit will be achieved if dietitians design education systems that encourage the identification and documentation of the outcomes of successful education intervention.

The goals of the Joint Commission's standards are to empower patients and ensure that their rights are protected. To accomplish these goals, patients must become involved with health management before discharge. The hospital of the future will be a learning laboratory. With this in mind, dietitians must discontinue the ineffective practice of instructor-controlled didactic instruction and expect that patient knowledge, attitudes, and behaviors will change. The goals of education will be accomplished as dietitians identify the barriers to learning in their institutions, in their patients, and in themselves and forge effective interdisciplinary relationships with other health care providers.

Since the 1980s, dietitians have been encouraged by the American Dietetic Association to document the outcomes of nutrition care to establish a research database (Guyer, Roht, Probart, & Bobroff, 1993) and support third party reimbursement efforts. Outcomes research showing impact on quality of life, cost savings, and efficacy is needed to move our profession forward (Derelian, Gallagher, & Snetslaar, 1995). Documentation used to focus on the process of care. Today's competitive market requires documentation of outcomes. Enterprising practitioners will use the 1995 Joint Commission standards to continue quality improvement efforts, and they will document the outcomes of nutrition education intervention to expand and/or maintain their practices.

THE PROCESS OF EDUCATION: IDENTIFYING INDIVIDUAL NEEDS

To implement an effective nutrition education program, it is important to understand the learning process. Each patient presents with a different set of learning skills and motivational behaviors. These things, among others, make a difference in the way patients learn.

How Adults Learn

Adults are capable of learning and changing their behavior throughout the life span. They are self-directed, motivated, and independent learners with more experiences than the young. In addition, they have more well-defined learning styles, personalities, interests, and needs. The adult possesses memory of what was learned in the past, awareness of the present, and expectations for the future based on past experiences. In some instances, adults have "learned disabilities" that must be restructured because they hinder new learning (Even, 1987).

The adult is interested in applying what is learned to current problems and situations (Knowles, 1970); consequently, learning activities should utilize a problem-solving approach. Mentally, the adult interacts with new ideas while deciding whether to enter them into memory (Holli & Calabrese, 1991).

According to Knowles (1970), adult learning is enhanced when the learner is actively involved in the learning process and has freedom to express individual opinions and concerns. Individual differences must be treated with respect. Instruction should build on the experiences of the learner and include activities organized around life problems rather than subject topics.

Because the experiences and personalities of adult learners vary greatly, instructors should not assume that all adults learn equally when given the same instruction. Rather, a variety of instructional strategies, materials, examples, and activities will allow each learner to identify and integrate important information. Variety is the key to success when working with adults (Even, 1987).

For maximum effectiveness, nutrition education should progress systematically through the following steps. First, assess cognitive (knowledge), psychological (emotional), and psychomotor (skill) needs because learning will be affected by deficits in these three areas. Second, include each learner in the development of measurable, realistic learning objectives. Third, determine the content of instruction based on results of the assessment and objectives. Fourth, use appropriate instructional methods and materials. Fifth, provide guided practice opportunities that are practical and relate, as much as possible, to the learner's previous experiences. Sixth, provide feedback about performance at regular intervals. Seventh, document the outcomes of instruction, discharge plans, and plans for referral or follow-up (Holli & Calabrese, 1991), and involve the learner in each stage of documentation.

Figure 5–2 shows an example of how one hospital conducts a formal assessment of barriers to learning, readiness to learn, and outcome of patient education. It is an interdisciplinary flow sheet that demonstrates involvement of patients and/or family members in the process and includes a definition of the content and methods used.

Learning Style

Each individual possesses a learning style, a preferred way to learn, that is uniquely determined and influenced by environmental factors. It is important for instructors to understand the effect of learning style on successful learning. It is equally important to understand that learning style has a powerful influ-

INTERDISCIPLINARY FLOW SHEET

CLINICAL RECORD	PATIENT & FAMILY HEALTH EDUCATION INTERDISCIPLINARY FLOW SHEET	
Barriers to Learning Circle the appropriate code(s) **L** = Language barrier **E** = Emotional barrier **A** = Activity limitation **R** = Religious practice **N** = No desire or motivation **S** = Sensory N/A = Not applicable	**Assessment—** **Readiness To Learn** Circle the appropriate code(s) **A** = Asking questions **D** = Demonstrates interest **U/D** = Unable to determine	**Outcome Code of Patient's** **Learning** Circle the appropriate code(s) **V** = Verbalizes content adequately **D** = Demonstrates procedure safely **R** = Reinforcement of content procedure needed **N/R** = Not receptive to learning at this time **U/E** = Unable to evaluate

Date	Barrier to Learn	Problem/Knowledge Needs	Assess Readiness To Learn	Content and Method	Outcome	Signature & Title
	L E A R N N/A	**Advance Directives** Have advance directives ___ Yes ___ No Adv. direct. booklet given? ___ Yes ___ No	A D U/D	1. Adv. direct. discussed? ___ Yes ___ No 2. Adv. direct. given? ___ Yes ___ No 3. Adv. direct. completed? ___ Yes ___ No	V D R N/R U/E	

Patient or Family Member Signature _____

Date	Barrier to Learn	Problem/Knowledge Needs	Assess Readiness To Learn	Content and Method	Outcome	Signature & Title
	L E A R N N/A	**Unit Orientation**	A D U/D	___1. Call bell system ___2. Environment ___3. Interdisciplinary team ___4. Patient handbook ___5. Dr. rounds ___6. Bed operation ___7. Bathroom ___8. Visiting hours ___9. Meal times	V D R N/R U/E	

Patient or Family Member Signature _____

continues

continued

Date	Barrier to Learn	Problem/Knowledge Needs	Assess Readiness To Learn	Content and Method	Outcome	Signature & Title
	L E A R N N/A	Orientation to Safety	A D U/D	___Nurse call bell demo ___Safe footwear ___Obey hospital signs ___Side rail usage ___Bed—low position ___W/C—wheels locked	V D R N/R U/E	

Patient or Family Member Signature _____

Date	Barrier to Learn	Problem/Knowledge Needs	Assess Readiness To Learn	Content and Method	Outcome	Signature & Title
	L E A R N N/A	Hazards of Smoking	A D U/D	___1. Physiological side effects of smoking ___2. 3 Ways of being hooked on smoking ___3. Benefits of quitting smoking ___4. Approaches to stopping smoking	V D R N/R U/E	

Patient or Family Member Signature _____

Date	Barrier to Learn	Problem/Knowledge Needs	Assess Readiness To Learn	Content and Method	Outcome	Signature & Title
	L E A R N N/A	Diet:_____ Increased knowledge and understanding of pre-scribed diet.	A D U/D	___1. Diet handbook ___2. Individual instruction regarding prescribed diet	V D R N/R U/E	

Patient or Family Member Signature _____

Date	Barrier to Learn	Problem/Knowledge Needs	Assess Readiness To Learn	Content and Method	Outcome	Signature & Title
	L E A R N N/A	Disease Process Increased knowledge and understanding of disease process.	A D U/D	___1. Individual instruction regarding disease process.	V D R N/R U/E	

Patient or Family Member Signature _____

continues

continued

Date	Barrier to Learn	Problem/Knowledge Needs	Assess Readiness To Learn	Content and Method	Outcome	Signature & Title
	L E A R N N/A	Oxygen Use Safety	A D U/D	___Unit instruction ___No smoking ___Nurse adjust flow rate ___Engineering check electrical appliances ___No flammables near O2	V D R N/R U/E	

Patient or Family Member Signature _____

Date	Barrier to Learn	Problem/Knowledge Needs	Assess Readiness To Learn	Content and Method	Outcome	Signature & Title

	L
	E
	A
	R
	N
	N/A
		Use of Inhalation in Asthma and COPD	A
			D
			U/D
				___1. Technique
				  • Shake well
				  • Puffer up to mouth
				  • One puff while
				    inhaling
				  • Wait 1 minute
				  • Repeat process 1×
				  • Rinse mouth with
				    water
				___2. Frequency of Tx
				___3. Untoward signs/
				    symptoms
					V
					D
					R
					N/R
					U/E	

Patient or Family Member Signature _____

Figure 5–2 Patient and family health education: interdisciplinary flow sheet. Courtesy of Department of Veterans Affairs Medical Center, Lake City, Florida.

ence on learner motivation and interest (Merriam, 1988). Some of the learning style patterns that may be encountered include the following: generalists who need to understand the big picture before seeing the details, explorers who learn by actively manipulating objects, social learners whose learning is enhanced by communication with others, verbal learners who learn by repeating what is said in their own words, and structured learners who need logic and systematic presentation of new information (Guild, 1989).

In addition, learners differ in their sensory preferences. Some are tactile (hands-on), and others are kinesthetic (involving the whole body), auditory, or visual. Learning styles cause some instructional methods to be more effective than others for each person, and it has been shown that learning is enhanced when the preferred learning style is used. Most instructors teach by using the instructional methods of their instructors and their own learning style preferences (Dunn, Beaudry, & Klavas, 1989). It is interesting to watch new graduate students teach medical nutrition therapy to patients. These students lecture to patients because this is the most common method of instruction used in universities. The lecture method of instruction, however, is among the least effective ways to teach new skills to an adult in a one-on-one session.

Because it is not possible to know the learning style of each patient, it is best to use a variety of instructional methods and materials. Consider these examples. Use food models that can be visualized and manipulated, and provide tactile experiences while simulating meal planning. Follow discussion of the fat content of foods in the American diet (big picture) by reading (visual style) food labels aloud (auditory style) to show the applied details. After reviewing *Guidelines for Meal Planning* (American Diabetes Association & American Dietetic Association, 1986) with a diabetic patient, ask him or her to restate (verbal style) the medical nutrition therapy and meal planning using his or her own words.

Motivation and Interest

Motivation is an internal characteristic that gives intensity and direction to life pursuits. It is measured by observed behavior. Motivation is affected by both internal and external factors and is a function of characteristics of the learner, interest in the topic being taught, the learning materials, the instructional methods used, and characteristics of the instructor. In a nutrition counseling session, only some of these factors are under the instructor's control. Therefore, the effective instructor is one who learns to make the learning situation more ideal (Frymire, 1985).

The process of motivation requires identification of the internal and external factors that are important to each person. For example, some will be motivated to change their eating behaviors because of an internalized value for health or a belief that health will improve when food habits change. Others will be motivated to change because of external motivators such as praise, reward, or punishment.

The goal of nutrition education intervention is to increase knowledge and change behavior. As a powerful influence on behavior, motivation is affected by change in knowledge, which in turn affects awareness, internal and external factors, the process of setting and reaching short- and long-term goals, emotions, and beliefs (Holli & Calabrese, 1991). Because so many variables are related to motivation, dietitians must build relationships with those whom they teach and counsel. Intervention is successful only when there is an honest, mutual exchange of information followed by the support needed for skill development.

Interest is strongly related to motivation, and no discussion of motivation would be complete without an investigation of the factors affecting its development.

Seven factors are salient in this regard: previous experience; degree of compulsion; meaningfulness of the subject; sequencing, pacing, spacing, and repetition of instruction; complexity of the subject; personal values; and self-concept. Effective instructors are those who identify the interests of each person and use them to heighten their interest in the topic. Interest is related to previous experience, and positive experiences usually result in increased interest. When interest increases, the learner usually seeks more experiences in that area.

Compulsion to become involved with an experience because of external forces is an interesting factor. The key is for dietitians to identify the feeling of compulsion that may be present in some individuals. For example, two individuals may follow a Step 1 diet but express different feelings about the experience. One may feel compelled to follow the regimen because of family pressure and physician expectations, and the other may follow it willingly because of interest in improving health and preventing disease.

Interest is related to the meaningfulness of the subject and is tied to the perceived usefulness of information. Dietitians assume that all people perceive food as important for life. The meaningfulness (usefulness) of knowing the best food sources of calcium may be low, however, until those susceptible to osteoporosis learn to relate the information to their diets to prevent disease onset.

Once interest in a topic is stimulated, instructors should move from the manager to the facilitator role to teach the learner to sequence, pace, space, and repeat instruction. One important goal of teaching is to involve the learner actively so that he or she will take control of the learning situation. To accomplish this goal, dietitians should provide a variety of instructional materials for patients to use independently and at their own learning pace.

Interest is stimulated when new information is taught systematically and tied to previous learning. Although complex subject matter is more interesting than simple, all subjects should be taught so that the content of instruction moves from basic to more complex. It is important to provide flexibility in the learning environment because some learners prefer more structure and less autonomy and others prefer less structure and more independence.

Finally, personal values affect interest in the topic to be learned, and people are drawn toward subjects they believe to be important. Information tied to personal values is perceived as worthwhile, and dietitians should identify patient values, attitudes, and beliefs when assessing education needs to increase the interest of nutrition information. Information that enhances the whole person has value because it affects self concept. Self-maintenance is a basic motivational factor for most persons (Frymire, 1985).

Because the changing health care environment requires greater patient involvement throughout the continuum of care, successful outcomes of nutrition education intervention will depend on patient motivation. Dietitians can help generate interest in nutrition to increase patient motivation and thus improve the quality of care.

NUTRITION EDUCATION AND COUNSELING

How can the busy practitioner realistically hope to identify and meet the learning needs of each patient? Dietitians know the fundamentals of learning theory, motivation, and patient assessment. They learn to develop behavioral objectives, select instructional materials, and communicate scientific principles to individuals and the public.

Nutrition education and counseling require a paradigm shift to meet the challenges of today's health care market. Today, dietitians are more apt to succeed if they assess and document patient learning needs; integrate the outcomes of assessment with instructional and behavioral strategies that promote quality care; provide individualized, comprehensive, and effective instruction; and document the outcomes of nutrition education intervention.

Assessing Learning Needs

Nutrition education intervention begins with identification of learning needs, learning ability, and readiness to learn that is specific for each patient. Learning needs assessment includes identification of the patient's cultural and religious barriers, desire and motivation to learn, physical and/or cognitive limitations, degree of literacy, and language barriers. The values and beliefs of the family must also be included as part of the assessment in addition to the family's ability, as appropriate, to learn (Joint Commission, 1995).

Not all patients will be ready or able to learn in the acute care setting, especially with the ongoing trend toward shorter lengths of stay. It is the dietitian's responsibility to determine who needs instruction, when instruction will be given, the amount of information that must be taught, and who the postdischarge sources of referral will be. Because of physical (pain, medication, fatigue), psychological (emotions, attitudes), cognitive (literacy, knowledge), and socioeconomic (culture, religion, education) factors that may be present, instruction in the hospital should often provide only "survival guidelines" (Ruzicki, 1989). More complete information should be provided through outpatient follow-up.

Individual assessment must be an ongoing process resulting from communication with and observation of the patient, the patient's family members, and other health care providers. The patient's ability to participate actively in decisions affecting his or her health care begins with delivery of effective instruction. A denial of fundamental information is a denial of basic patient rights. Patient education allows hospitalized persons to share the power related to their care (Hartmann & Kochar, 1994) with health care providers. Ultimately, patient compliance is not as important as patient involvement (Webber, 1990).

Methods of Instruction

Nutrition education is a process of assessment and intervention that teaches application of scientific facts about and principles of the relationship between diet and health to food practices (American Dietetic Association, 1990). The goal is health maintenance and/or improvement.

As mentioned earlier, most dietitians teach using the instructional methods that they encountered as students. This instructor-controlled method is called direct instruction because it leads learners through a systematic presentation of information sequenced from basic to more complex concepts. Direct instruction is useful for beginning and low-ability learners. It assumes that learning occurs when the instructor clearly explains what the learner should know and then demonstrates the steps related to the learning task. Basic components of this method include the following (Bennett, 1986):

- development of learning goals that are understood by the learner
- sequenced and organized assignments
- provision of clear and specific examples and explanations about the material to be learned
- use of instructional methods such as questioning or inquiry to verify comprehension of the material
- provision of practice opportunities to reinforce and demonstrate learning

Many different methods of instruction can be employed to teach nutrition. These include lectures, discussions, projects, demonstrations, experiments, and gaming methods. Each has strengths and weaknesses, and careful consideration of the learning situation will lead to adoption of the most effective methods for groups and individuals.

The lecture is the most widely and perhaps inappropriately used method of instruction. It is appropriately used to provide basic information to large groups of people. As an instructional method, it is nonthreatening, inexpensive, efficient, and instructor controlled. Its weaknesses include the following: It does not enable the learner to provide feedback about what is learned, learning is unimodal (auditory), and the format is formal and may be boring because it does not elicit learner participation. It is not an appropriate method for teaching skills or higher level objectives in the cognitive domain.

Discussion includes panels, debates, instructor inquiry, and case studies. Strengths are the increased learner participation, which often leads to increased interest; the informal learning environment; multimodal (auditory and verbal) instruction, which enhances memory; and the ability to teach objectives in the upper level cognitive and affective domains. Weaknesses are the requirement for learner preparation before the discussion, the tendency for more verbally expressive or confident personalities to dominate discussions, the need for more time, size limitations for groups if all learners are to participate, and the need for a moderator to facilitate the direction of discussion.

Projects, demonstrations, and experiments are methods that motivate and enhance learning because of the real-life multimodal (tactile, visual, auditory, and verbal) experiences offered, active participation, and teaching of higher level cognitive objectives. Weaknesses include the greater amounts of time required to complete projects, increased costs from equipment and space, and the inherent limitations on group size.

Many different gaming methods (e.g., role playing, case studies, and scenarios) may be appropriately used to teach critical thinking and problem-solving skills, higher level cognitive objectives, and application of theory to practice. The active participation by learners and multimodal style lead to improved memory of what is learned. Weaknesses are that these methods are time consuming, require smaller groups, and may incur higher costs if equipment is needed (Even, 1987).

Materials of Instruction

The materials of instruction include the learning environment as well as the teaching materials. In many hospitals and clinics, the learning environment (the architectural and arranged structures) is less than ideal. Poorly arranged or inadequate furniture, dim lighting, and obstructive pieces of equipment and furniture create an environment that does not support learning. There is often little privacy, and dietitians must often compete with other health care providers for patient time and attention.

Selection of appropriate teaching materials leads to more effective instruction. Learning is enhanced when instructional materials are interesting, challenging, appropriate for the level of the learner, and appropriately designed and have content related to the purpose of the instruction. Instructional materials include all printed and nonprinted materials, learning resources, and planned activities (O'Neill, 1988).

Instructional materials enhance learning in many ways. First, they provide visual reinforcement for information that is disseminated orally. Second, they provide repetition of instruction each time the information is read, watched, or listened to. Third, they can be used to save instructor time when given before instruction and can lead to more productive and individualized instruction by giving the patient time to process new information and generate questions.

Printed Materials

Because so many types of printed materials are available today, dietitians should begin the selection process by assessing the learning needs of their target audiences. This should be followed by an identification of needs that can best be met by printed materials. Finally, dietitians should locate available material to determine whether it meets the identified needs. If it does not, appropriate learning materials should be developed (Mercurio, 1993).

Written materials are the most commonly used instructional materials. Effective written materials must be appropriate for the target audience in content and design. Appropriateness is determined by writing style (formal or informal), definition of terms used (technical or general with specific examples), typeface, layout (one column or multiple columns), amount of white space on the page, use of illustrations, use of common rather than exotic foods in displays, and methods used to describe data (tables, bar graphs, or pie charts; Shepherd, Sims, Davis, Shaw, & Cronin, 1994). As the United States grows as a diverse society, the content of materials becomes a more important factor to consider. Important content features include respect for cultures, values, and traditions; relevance to needs and interests of individuals; attractiveness; and persuasiveness (Rice & Valdivia, 1991; Rudd & Comings, 1994).

Another issue affecting material selection is readability and patient literacy. Almost 23 million Americans are not able to read and comprehend the written instructions that lead to health improvement (Gibbons, Reed, & Holt, 1992), and 18 million are functionally literate, possessing reading and comprehension skills between the fourth and eighth grade levels (Ruud, Betts, & Dirkx, 1993). The average citizen reads at the eighth grade level (Gibbons et al., 1992) despite more than 8 years of formal education. Some studies have reported an inability of participants to comprehend materials that span the fourth to eighth grade levels (McCabe, Tysinger, Kreger, & Currwin, 1989).

Nutrition educators, however, should not assume that low-literacy adults are uninformed, unaware, or unintelligent. Instead, educators must recognize that these adults have less general knowledge (which limits information and comprehension), poor vocabularies, and weak decoding skills (needed to interpret the meaning of words). Effective materials for low-literacy adults provide information that relates to experience. These materials use concrete, specific terms rather than abstract and conceptual terms. Finally, the ideas presented progress from basic to more complex (Ruud et al., 1993).

Much has been written about the use of readability formulas to estimate the grade levels of written materials. Readability formulas are useful in some settings, but their usefulness in the evaluation of health material has been questioned because health information differs from general reading material. Typically, the grade level of written material increases as the length of individual words and sentences increases. When readability formulas are applied to health information, however, several interesting facts are noted. First, different reading levels often are identified within the same piece of information. Second, materials with higher reading levels have been wrongly discounted for low-literacy adults. The problem relates to the fact that low-literacy adults are often able to comprehend the messages in materials with higher reading levels because the more commonly used medical terms, such as *cholesterol*, are readily understood (Hopkinson, 1993; Meade & Smith, 1991). Third, because readability formulas approach reading mechanistically, they do not account for the influence of human elements: motivation, interest, attractiveness, culture, and experience. Fourth, because reading is an interactive process, comprehension is enhanced when there is a good fit between the learner and the reading material. Nutrition educators should keep these important points in mind when selecting instructional materials because readability formulas do not consider any of these in the evaluation process (Meade & Smith, 1991).

Audiovisuals

A variety of nonprint media is available to enhance the effectiveness of instruction. Some of these include audiocassettes, videos, and computers. Educators should select instructional media based on appropriateness, needs of the target audience, accuracy of the information presented, cost, space, and ease of use. Dietitians should prepare learners in advance by identifying the goals of the instructional material, developing personal learning/behavioral goals with each learner, and describing important details that should be observed or considered (Ruzicki, 1989).

Audiocassettes have been used to provide information to patients about general procedures. Surprisingly, Webber (1990) showed that 92% of patients listened to the cassettes with family and friends rather than while alone. With this in mind, dietitians should include the same family members in follow-up instructions (Ruzicki, 1989).

Closed-circuit television, a centralized system of transmitting videotaped programs, is effective as a method of providing baseline information. Television viewing, however, must be followed by personal contact and instruction to reinforce learning. Patient familiarity with television makes it a valuable supplement to other methods of instruction (Nielsen & Sheppard, 1988). For short-term knowledge gains, videos are as useful as traditional instructional methods, and they help practitioners manage time more efficiently (Webber, 1990). They are especially helpful in long-term care and clinic settings because they can be given to patients to review and reinforce concepts taught between education sessions.

Computer Applications

The latest technology used for patient instruction is computers. Computers have been used to develop tutorials, drills, problem-solving activities, simulations, role playing experiences, and games. They can also be used to provide educators with baseline information about patient knowledge, practices, and beliefs to tailor information to meet individual learning needs. Tailored messages produce greater behavioral change than standardized materials because patients remember the details and read the materials more thoroughly.

Some computer programs are designed on the basis of behavioral models that provide educators with information about target areas. Educators can use the information to assess nutrition status and knowledge from multiple variables and can design comprehensive programs for target audiences. In addition, computer networks can be used to link patients, dietitians, and other health care providers together to improve communication about diet-related issues. Also, computer-generated data can be stored to develop patient profiles and identify education needs in target groups.

If adoption of computers is considered for patient education, the following points should be kept in mind: The program should be easy to use; instructions should be kept simple; printed, personalized feedback should be provided for users; computer interaction should be followed by interaction with a health professional; and computer experts and health professionals should work together to develop instructional materials. Despite the many advantages of computers, this technology is not widely used, nor has the potential for time saving been realized. The education uses and benefits of computers need further investigation (Skinner, Siegfried, Kegler, & Strecher, 1993).

Promoting Behavioral Change

The goal of nutrition counseling is to change behavior. For intervention to be effective, dietitians must identify behaviors to change, behaviors to adopt, and behaviors that will be affected throughout the change process (Glanz & Eriksen, 1993). Positive patient outcomes occur when behavior change occurs and is sustained.

Because a clear relationship has been established between behavior and health, comprehensive education programs must address behavioral as well as cognitive issues. People are systems. This means that their observed behaviors (outputs) are not random reflexes to stimuli from internal and/or external factors (inputs). Rather, behavior results from interactions among life-long experiences: knowledge, behaviors, attitudes, and beliefs. Behavior changes when individuals become aware of their inappropriate responses and use successful strategies to develop new ones. Change is rarely easy, and for this reason "microchanges" with smaller impacts on the total system are less stressful than "macrochanges." They are also easier to make and therefore will be more easily adopted (Anon., 1993).

Dietitians are nutrition experts. They are qualified to provide comprehensive nutrition care (E.R. Monsen, 1989), which begins with assessment of nutrition and education needs. Education intervention is a program with distinctly different goals from those of nutrition intervention, however. For too long, nutrition education and counseling have been underdeveloped components of the nutrition care process. Overall, health program development and evaluation have received inadequate attention from health care providers (van Ryn & Heaney, 1992). Dietetics, like other health professions, has not documented the outcomes of education intervention. Patient education has been an activity conducted within the scope of the nutrition program rather than a planned program with identified outcomes to be measured.

As nutrition educators and counselors, dietitians should use behavioral theories to guide program development. Theory guides the evaluation strategies and types of evaluation used. Program development begins with identification of measurable goals and desired outcomes. The next step is to compare the outcomes from different behavioral theories with those desired in the program. This step should be followed by an investigation of construct validity to evaluate the evidence supporting the behavioral theory. Finally, there should be a match between the main points of the theory and the personal values and interests of the practitioner. Because theories are used to explain how individuals relate to the world around them, dietitians must identify theories that complement their own belief systems (van Ryn & Heaney, 1992).

Educators know that knowledge and skill acquisition alone does not lead to behavioral change (Hartmann & Kochar, 1994). In health care, educators have been frustrated by poor patient compliance and their own inability to provide sufficient motivation for change. Perhaps this low rate of success is due to the use of a faulty instructional model. In the traditional health care model, the patient is a passive recipient of advice from an "expert" (Dobs et al., 1994). Improved rates of success may be found when educators choose more appropriate instructional and behavioral models.

Nutrition education intervention is most effective when it identifies factors influencing food intake and when a behavioral model is used to provide a theoretical framework for program design and evaluation. For example, the stages of change model proposes a dynamic, nonlinear progression through five behavioral stages. Each stage identifies different learning needs that must be considered. A failure to recognize the stage of change or to identify learning needs results in ineffective instruction (Glanz et al., 1994).

Patient and Family Involvement

It is no longer possible for health care providers to ensure quality care through diagnosis of illness and provision of medical treatment (Ruzicki, 1989). Today's patients are key players in their medical treatment, recovery from illness, and management of postdischarge care. One reason why patients have become more involved with the care process is dissatisfaction with the prescriptive, paternalistic, traditional model of health care. This is especially true for the younger, more educated person confronted by decisions that do not require medical expertise. Patients also seek greater involvement when decisions are related to their personal values and attitudes (Thompson, Pitts, & Schwankovsky, 1993).

Historically, barriers in the hospital environment, organization, and programs have prevented patients from actively participating in their care. The goal of patient education has been to develop a cognitive understanding of illness and treatment rather than to promote behavioral or psychosocial change. Consequently, there has been little change in patient life style (Giloth, 1990).

Giloth (1990) suggests that reduction of barriers in the physical environment may enhance learning and that hospitals should consider the following:

- Create a comfortable, homelike environment by adjusting lighting and using soothing colors and materials.
- Provide opportunities to personalize rooms and living spaces by use of bulletin boards and so forth.
- Develop room arrangements that optimize privacy, and allow patients to wear their own clothes as much as possible.
- Provide lounges and kitchens for socializing, and encourage use of the kitchen to prepare food for patient consumption, if possible.
- Encourage family involvement throughout the facility, and change rules to expand hours of visitation.
- Prevent confusion and information overload by simplifying forms and streamlining procedures.
- Provide movies, tapes, and relaxation opportunities.
- As much as possible, allow individualization of sleeping, medication, and test schedules.
- Reduce staff stress to promote a healing, healthy environment for all.

New behaviors will probably be adopted if patients and their family members have opportunities to practice newly acquired skills under the supervision of health care professionals before discharge (Ruzicki, 1989). As the length of hospital stay continues to shorten and the acuity level of hospitalized persons increases, more patients will face the need to manage some aspect of their care after discharge.

This challenge must be met by education programs that involve the patient and family members and prepare them for care delivery (Giloth, 1990).

The most effective program is one that is integrated throughout the process of care. Active patient involvement encourages learning and personal responsibility, and several strategies can be used to create an interactive environment. First, encourage patient questions from the time of admission, set learning goals, and use Socratic inquiry to establish baseline knowledge and skills. Second, develop checklists for the patient to enable his or her participation in monitoring progress and learning, and keep these at the bedside. Third, use flow sheets and discharge plans that provide space for the patient to write comments, identify goals, and evaluate and document comprehension; planning, assessment, and evaluation should be a shared responsibility. Fourth, provide chalkboards, notepads, or other writing materials in the patient's room to encourage questions. Fifth, use teaching materials that involve patients; games (crossword puzzles, case studies, sample menus, etc.) stimulate memory and recall and provide practice opportunities that reinforce learning (Giloth, 1990).

To meet Joint Commission approval, health care providers must now assess and document learning and medical needs to provide patients and/or families with relevant instruction. Factors to be considered in the education process are staff resources (time, opportunity, and teaching ability) and patient resources (learning style, readiness, baseline knowledge and skills, motivation, and ability to learn). Research has not identified the most effective program type, but it has concluded that involved patients are more satisfied than those who are not (Ruzicki, 1989). Many patients and family members are reluctant to ask questions or seek help, and for this reason they may not have their health care needs met. Professionals must develop strategies to draw patients and their family members into the process of health care (Grieco, Garnett, Glassman, Valoon, & McClure, 1990; Thompson & Weisberg, 1990).

Patient learning centers have been used successfully to prepare patients and their family members to meet the responsibility for medical care upon discharge. Learning centers provide opportunities to learn information, practice and demonstrate skills, and receive feedback about performance from health care professionals. They are learning laboratories where patients and families practice medical care under careful supervision. The goal of such centers is to promote patient compliance and behavioral change. Goldstein (1991) summarized the benefits of learning centers as follows:

- There is a nonthreatening environment to practice development of new knowledge and skills.
- There is access to equipment and tools needed to simulate life after discharge.

- Teaching may be individualized for patients' and families' needs.
- Because teaching is a planned and coordinated effort, staff resources are better utilized and integrated.
- The learning center is especially effective for those returning to communities with limited services and resources.

In addition, patients are able to assume more control and direct their learning efforts. Increased comfort with new information and tasks develops patient competence. As skill performance improves, there is increased compliance with the plan of care (Sumpmann, 1989).

Special Considerations for Adult Learners

Most of this chapter has focused on identifying and meeting the learning needs of patients in acute care settings. Those in long-term care and rehabilitation centers, however, also have learning needs. Some of these patient groups may present special challenges to the dietitian because of advanced age or mental or physical disability. Because this is a growing population, their needs deserve special attention.

With age comes an expectation that memory becomes less sharp and the ability to learn lessens. Healthy adults, however, can continue to learn and change their behavior with each advancing decade. The use of appropriate instructional materials may overcome some of the age-related physiological changes, such as diminished visual acuity and loss of peripheral sight, decreased tolerance to glare and ability to adapt to changes in lighting, diminished ability to hear, slowed response time, and increased time required for information processing and retrieval. Age-related psychological changes, such as depression and anxiety, may also require attention to avoid interference with learning.

Older learners require multimodal instruction that stimulates multiple senses: vision, smell, touch, hearing, and, if possible, taste. A thorough assessment of learning needs and interests enables selection of appropriate materials and instructional strategies (Kicklighter, 1991).

Memory Deficits

We remember something when the right amount of effort is put forth at the right moment. In elderly persons, declining memory may result from a failure to put forth the appropriate amount of effort in situations. Memory is affected by the presence of both acute and chronic health problems. Dietitians must be sensitive to individual needs and excuse patients from scheduled learning sessions when illness is the current concern.

Finally, memory is tied to self-concept and age-related change in mental speed. Older persons experience change in attention span, which is expressed as increased distractibility, sensory changes in sight and hearing, and increased difficulty with identifying critical information. Educators can improve the quality of instructional effort by teaching in a quiet, private place with few distractions. Speech should be slower than usual, and more attention should be given to clear diction, rate of speech, and volume. Instructional materials should be bright and simple with clear pictures. They should be given to the patient to serve as visual reminders of nutrition information.

Instruction should begin with an identification of current knowledge and behavior. Once the baselines have been established, new information should be tied to what is familiar. Dietitians can help patients remember what they learn by teaching them to practice automatic recall. There are three steps. First, teach information using context cues, pictures in the memory that tie information to time and events. Second, rehearse the newly acquired information to maintain the memory. This may be done orally or through the use of various instructional games and activities. Third, use spaced recall, which involves remembering specific information at predetermined, timed intervals. As information is recalled and remembered, increase the time interval before repeating the request for recall (West, 1991).

Adults in long-term care or rehabilitation centers may also have impaired vision, hearing, or speech. They may have physical, emotional, social, or specific learning disabilities. In these instances, dietitians must adjust the learning environment to accommodate the disability and be aware of the side effects of prescribed medication (e.g., chronic weakness, fatigue, etc.) that may affect learning. Specific teaching strategies will improve instruction for patients with disabilities.

Visual Impairments

Visual impairment is loss of visual acuity, loss of peripheral vision, or progressive loss of vision that affects the ability to function. Impairment may be caused by congenital defects, cataracts, glaucoma, nystagmus, retinal detachment, retinitis pigmentosa, or strabismus, or it may result from accident or injury. Visually impaired persons may exhibit slowed ability to read and comprehend printed information. Exhibit 5–2 provides some suggestions to facilitate learning.

Auditory Impairments

Auditory impairment results from a loss of hearing ability due to congenital defect, deafness, high- or low-tone hearing loss, acoustic trauma, or injury to

Exhibit 5–2 Facilitating Learning for Visually Impaired Adults

- Provide materials to be read before instruction.
- Use audiocassettes for instruction as available.
- Develop outlines using large print (18 pt or larger) to highlight important points from the verbal or audio instruction.
- Read the instruction aloud.
- Face the person when speaking.
- Make instructions short and concise.
- Reinforce information verbally.
- Repeat information as needed.
- Involve other senses, such as touch, in the instruction. For example, use food models for demonstrations.
- Encourage independence and participation.

the ear that results in loss of hearing. Persons with auditory loss often experience difficulty when learning information that is presented orally. They may be unable to integrate oral information and may have trouble following the logic of instruction. Exhibit 5–3 provides some helpful suggestions to assist learning in these individuals.

Speech and Language Deficits

Speech and language disorders result from neurological impairment or physical malformations affecting articulation, fluency, or voice. These include difficulty with using and understanding language (aphasia, dysnomia) and im-

Exhibit 5–3 Suggestions for Educating Adults with Auditory Impairments

- Use an American Sign Language interpreter if this is the usual method of communication. Meet with the interpreter in advance to discuss medical terms and patient needs.
- Maintain eye contact with the patient, and speak to him or her rather than to the interpreter.
- Provide written information to the patient in advance.
- Develop outlines that highlight important points.
- Speak in natural tones.
- Articulate words clearly and slowly.
- Involve as many senses as possible, and utilize different instructional aids, such as food models (tactile) and printed instructions (visual).
- Reduce distracting or interfering sounds.
- Encourage independence and participation.

pairment of the voice (hoarseness, laryngectomy), fluency (stammering, stuttering), or articulation (dysarthria, dyspraxia). The anxiety of having to speak can worsen symptoms. Teaching strategies may include the items shown in Exhibit 5–4.

Physical Disabilities

Physical disabilities result from injury, musculoskeletal and connective tissue disorders, and neuromuscular disorders. Examples include cerebral palsy, head and spinal cord injury, intracranial hemorrhage, cerebrovascular accident, multiple sclerosis, Parkinson's disease, muscular dystrophy, and congenital disorders. These disabilities require adaptation of the learning environment to accommodate a wide range of impairments, such as partial or total paralysis; loss of mobility, strength, speed, coordination, endurance, and dexterity; and dysfunction of speech or other senses. The suggestions given in Exhibit 5–5 can be implemented to improve instructional effectiveness for patients with physical disabilities.

Emotional and Social Impairments

Emotional and social impairments manifest as a range of disruptive or indifferent behaviors. Depression is one of the most common and may appear as hopelessness, despair, helplessness, apathy, inattention, disinterest, irritability, or fatigue. Another common impairment is anxiety, which may manifest as withdrawal, emotional volatility, complaining, constant talking, joking, or other inappropriate interactions. The side effects of medications used to treat these disorders may also result in undesirable behaviors. Exhibit 5–6 provides

---

Exhibit 5–4 Teaching Strategies for Adults with Speech and Language Disorders

- Provide the opportunity for speaking rather than compel speech.
- Evaluate learning and comprehension with written games or quizzes, food models to manipulate, and the like.
- Give extra time for verbal expression and comprehension.
- Ask patients to repeat unclear statements as necessary.
- Assist patients' verbal expression by giving choices rather than requiring open-ended responses.
- Use short sentences.
- Speak using a normal voice and tone.
- Encourage independence and participation.

Exhibit 5–5 Advice for Teaching Adults with Physical Disabilities

- Evaluate physical access, obstacles, and barriers for those with impaired mobility.
- Use tape recorders to record instruction.
- Work closely with appropriate therapists (occupational, physical, rehabilitation) to identify needs.
- Use appropriate strategies for those with speech, sensory, and other impairments.
- For adults who use wheelchairs with mounted tabletops, provide attractive handout materials that can serve as visual reminders of the information covered.
- Encourage independence and participation.

some suggestions for teaching patients with emotional and social impairments (Reasonable Accommodations Faculty Guide, 1995).

Learning Disabilities

Learning disabilities include a range of conditions related to difficulty in perceiving and/or processing auditory, visual, or spatial information. Impairment of reading skills (dyslexia), writing skills (dysgraphia), or math skills (dyscalculia) may be present. Persons with these disabilities do not have impaired intelligence or ability to learn. Adaptation of the learning environment enables improved learning by disabled patients. Dahl and Read (1995) identify considerations for educating persons with learning disabilities (see Exhibit 5–7).

A CASE STUDY

The case that follows may help dietitians incorporate many of the principles covered in this chapter.

Exhibit 5–6 Suggestions for Patients with Emotional and Social Impairments

- Discuss inappropriate behaviors in a nonthreatening manner.
- Do not attempt to diagnose problematic behavior.
- Work closely with appropriate members of the health care team (psychologists, social workers, etc.) to identify needs and strategies.
- Bring other familiar persons into the room during nutrition counseling, if appropriate, to assist and comfort the patient.
- Document observations.
- Encourage independence and participation.

Exhibit 5–7 Considerations for Adults with Learning Disabilities

- Use appropriate strategies to improve visual perception.
- Provide additional support for memory or sequencing difficulties by using concise oral instructions or repetition.
- Teach by using multimodal (seeing, touching, hearing) methods and materials. Ask patients to "show and tell."
- If articulation is a problem, do not require participation in oral discussions.
- Allow extra time during the instruction for those requiring more time to read and process information.
- Eliminate distractions.
- Provide multiple instructions before testing learning.

Source: Reprinted with permission from B.R. Dahl and M.H. Read. Effect of a Nutrition Education Program on the Reduction of Serum Cholesterol Level in Veteran Administration Outpatients. *Journal of The American Dietetic Association*, 95, pp. 702–703, © 1995.

The Patient

J.F. is a 53-year-old veteran of the Vietnam war who has experienced significant bilateral hearing loss due to war injuries. He was admitted to your hospital because of dehydration and weight loss after viral gastroenteritis. J.F. has now been diagnosed with non–insulin-dependent diabetes (NIDDM), and you have been asked to provide instruction before he is discharged tomorrow.

J.F. is 5 feet 11 inches tall and weighs 240 pounds. He is a high school graduate and works as a bookkeeper at a local accounting firm. He does not exercise and currently takes no medications other than a daily multivitamin "just to be on the safe side." He eats three meals daily and snacks on Coca-Cola and salty foods (peanuts, potato chips, etc.) throughout the evening while watching television. J.F. is married, and his wife, a homemaker, is very concerned about his health because of the history of diabetes in his family.

Questions

1. Describe the goals of medical nutrition therapy for NIDDM.
2. Identify your nutritional goals for J.F. based on his medical and nutrition histories.
3. Assess J.F.'s nutrient needs to provide appropriate nutrition intervention. Develop an eating program that will meet his needs and life style.
4. Assess J.F.'s learning needs:
   - Estimate his ability to read and write based on level of education and current occupation.
   - Determine his baseline knowledge of diabetes.

- Identify potential barriers to learning: social, ethnic, psychological, and physiological.
- Identify the factors needed to deliver effective instruction.

5. Develop J.F.'s education intervention.
6. Determine how you will evaluate the outcome of instruction.
7. Identify your plan for follow-up.

Answer Key

J.F. is a high school graduate whose current position requires proficient reading, writing, and computation skills. Therefore, the learning materials and instructional delivery will not need adjustment based on literacy. It will be important to discuss diabetes with J.F. before instruction to discover his knowledge, attitudes, and possible misconceptions about the disease. Because there is a family history of diabetes, he probably possesses an awareness that is above baseline, but he has never followed any therapeutic diet himself.

The acute care environment does not always promote the development of a relationship that will optimize learning. Therefore, the dietitian will need to be flexible and organized and should develop a variety of teaching styles. Without knowing J.F.'s learning preferences, it is best to plan multimodal instruction that will include all learning styles. By involving J.F. actively in the instructional process, the dietitian can identify strong preferences and meet his needs more readily.

Instruction should be planned when J.F.'s wife can be present because, as a homemaker, she is responsible for the grocery shopping and meal preparation. Her expressed concern about J.F.'s health suggests that she will support him as he changes his eating program.

An important instructional barrier to overcome is J.F.'s significant bilateral hearing loss. Hearing losses affect communication, and the dietitian must consider ways to optimize instruction.

The dietitian should begin by providing information for J.F. and his wife to read before the first instructional meeting. This should include a short, written outline that identifies important and personally relevant points in the material. The dietitian should ask both of them to write their questions down before their scheduled appointment.

The delivery of instruction should consider J.F.'s special learning needs. As possible, arrange the meeting in a quiet room free from interruptions, distractions, and background noises. The dietitian should be sure to face J.F. during the instruction and speak slowly, clearly, and naturally.

Materials of instruction should include visuals to reinforce the oral presentation and food models to demonstrate appropriate food types and amounts. During the interaction, the dietitian should rephrase information that is not understood and should listen carefully to J.F.'s responses. As necessary, J.F. should be asked to repeat responses that are not clear. His wife should be kept in a supportive role. The dietitian must make a conscious effort to establish rapport with J.F. rather than his wife.

J.F.'s comprehension of instructions can be measured easily by the dietitian asking him to use the food models and meal pattern to show what he will have for his first breakfast meal at home. It is unlikely that he will be proficient in applying the principles of his new diet after only one meeting. Therefore, referral to an outpatient dietitian or a dietitian at a diabetes treatment center should be arranged before discharge.

J.F.'s prognosis is good if he receives comprehensive nutrition education and intervention. The dietitians involved in his care should document his outcomes and their role in helping him learn to manage his disease.

THE OUTCOMES OF NUTRITION EDUCATION INTERVENTION

In the 1990s, the number of inpatient and outpatient education programs grew. The most common inpatient programs developed were diabetes management, preoperative instruction, prevention of heart attack, cardiac rehabilitation, and nutrition. The most frequently used outpatient programs were diabetes management, nutrition, prenatal education, cardiac rehabilitation, and prevention of heart attack. In all but preoperative instruction, nutrition was a central or supporting topic of instruction.

Nationwide, the number of education programs has continued to grow despite the lack of information about program quality or documentation to support positive program outcomes (Giloth, 1990). The objective of most programs has been to increase patient knowledge, but those promoting skill development may be the most effective (Dobs et al., 1994) and important.

Snetslaar (1989) describes nutrition counseling as among the most challenging and rewarding skills essential to dietetic practice. Dietitians have been challenged to become medical intervention specialists who "promote adherence to a variety of prescribed medical and lifestyle interventions through counseling" (E.M. Monsen, 1992, p. 538).

> It is the position of the American Dietetic Association that medical nutrition therapy is effective in treating disease and preventing disease complications, resulting in health benefits and cost savings for the public. Therefore, medical nutrition therapy provided by dietetics professionals is an essential reimbursable component of comprehensive health care services. (American Dietetic Association, 1995, p. 88)

The Surgeon General's report (Department of Health and Human Services, 1988) found that 8 of the 10 leading causes of death are related to diet and alcohol consumption. Medical nutrition therapy offers numerous benefits to patients receiving acute care, long-term care, rehabilitation, home health, outpatient, and preventive care services. In addition, an objective of *Healthy People 2000* (Department of Health and Human Services, 1990) is to "increase to at least 75% of the proportion of primary care providers who provide nutrition assessment and counseling and/or referral to qualified nutritionists or dietitians" (p. 128). An essential component of medical nutrition therapy is patient counseling, and it will be important for dietitians to document the outcomes of their intervention.

Addressing the topic of outcome assessment, Wilkins (1995) described three types of outcomes to consider: economic outcomes, clinical outcomes, and user satisfaction. According to Wilkins, people in general make health care decisions based on satisfaction and economic issues because they do not always have the knowledge required to assess clinical outcomes. Involvement of patients and their family members and/or caregivers is essential for improving satisfaction. It also contributes to positive clinical outcomes because patients gain a sense of ownership when they are involved in decisions about their care. Table 5–1 shows how the clinical needs and personal preferences of patients can be integrated into the dietitian's screening, assessment, and care planning processes.

When dietitians are asked to instruct patients, or if they determine that instruction is needed, it is not wise to provide the service without first completing an assessment of the patients' needs. It is also recommended either that the education be a part of the standing orders for patient care or that a physician's order covers the service. These suggestions are made to maximize reimbursement, minimize legal difficulties, and ensure that the education provided is individualized according to patients' needs and preferences.

Food and Medication Interactions

The Joint Commission (1995) requires that the patient and/or family member be given appropriate education and training to increase knowledge of the patient's illness and treatment needs and to learn skills and behaviors that promote recovery and improve function. Its standards identify areas of instruction to be potential food–drug interactions, nutrition intervention, and/or modified diets. Food–drug interaction interventions may relate to education, administration, and monitoring. Dietitians should be actively involved in each area and recognize that prevention of food–drug interactions is an important area in need of leadership (Lewis, Frongillo, & Roe, 1995).

Counseling on food–drug interactions has become increasingly important because of the aging of the population and the number of persons with chronic

Table 5–1 Integrating Nutrition Education in Assessment and Care Planning Processes

Activity	Focus for Nutrition Education and Counseling
Nutrition screening	1. Identify high- and moderate-risk patients who may benefit from instruction. 2. Identify the patients who desire nutrition education and counseling. They may be high-, moderate-, or low-risk cases.
Nutrition assessment	1. Pertinent data include: • current knowledge of the diet • barriers to learning (language, emotional, physical, and sensory limitations; sensory, motivation, and cognitive skills) • preferences for education • previous nutrition education efforts and their outcomes • current medications with potential nutrient interactions 2. Assessment includes: • evaluation of baseline knowledge of nutrition and diet • evaluation of learning needs • evaluation of readiness for learning
Care planning	1. Depending on the assessment, care plans can include: • time frame for inpatient and postdischarge nutrition education • suitable content, methods, and materials for education • determination of opportunities for practicing principles taught • involvement of others (family members and caregivers) in the education process for motivation and teaching, when appropriate • obtaining physician orders for nutrition education • plan for education on drug–nutrient interactions • referrals to other care providers to enhance knowledge and application of dietary principles within or outside the facility
Follow-up	1. Monitor and document outcomes of education. 2. Obtain feedback from patients and their caregivers. 3. Adjust nutrition education plan accordingly.

diseases living in long-term care facilities; as a group, the latter require the largest amount of medication. Dietitians should be the professionals who take the lead when evaluating patient medical records for food–drug interactions because they have strong backgrounds in science and communication which enable them to interpret and explain patient needs (Lewis et al., 1995).

Food–drug interactions provide an ideal opportunity for the dietitian, pharmacist, nurse, and physician to work together. For example, dietitians are concerned with food–drug interactions, pharmacists with drug–drug interactions, nurses with medication administration, and physicians with patient management. This type of team effort meets the interdisciplinary vision of the Joint Commission standards and improves the quality of patient care.

Nutrition Counseling

Although the health care model of the future is unknown, the fact remains that fewer dollars will be available to support health care efforts. The future will also yield new health care delivery systems to meet changing consumer needs and expectations. As Baby Boomers continue to age, their numbers will place unprecedented demands on the health care system. In the effort to meet these demands, new opportunities will emerge for dietitians and others in the health delivery system. Those with vision, entrepreneurial skills, and the courage to take risks will seize the opportunity to create new roles (Chernoff, 1995).

For example, dietitians have been encouraged to assume the role of intervention specialists, "clinicians who promote adherence to a variety of prescribed medical and life-style interventions through the health behavior counseling process" (Insull, 1992, p. 551). Diet or diet and drug therapies will be recommended for many Americans in the years ahead (Insull, 1992), and dietitians should be prepared to develop, implement, and evaluate effective education programs.

Anecdotally, medical nutrition therapy saves approximately $3.25 for each $1.00 invested (Derelian et al., 1995). Slowly, dietitians have begun to gather data to show how their services affect care and improve quality of life. Because the education and counseling process leads to measurable outcomes, it should be documented to help justify education programs and provide support for reimbursement. As a component of medical nutrition therapy, nutrition education improves health in numerous measurable ways (Dahl & Read, 1995; Johnson & Valera, 1995; Topping, Humm, Fischer, & Brayer, 1995). Some of these are summarized in Table 5–2. The quality of health care has been measured by evaluating the care process without attention to outcomes. The growing concern over quality should motivate practitioners to develop quality improvement programs that

Table 5–2 Outcomes of Nutrition Education and Counseling

Disease	Outcome	Reference
Hypercholesterolemia	Reduced serum cholesterol levels	Dahl & Read (1995)
Diabetes	Reduced serum glucose Reduced glycosolated HbA$_{1c}$ Decreased use of medication	Johnson & Valera (1995)
Human immunodeficiency virus infection/acquired immunodeficiency syndrome	Improved weight gain/ maintenance	Topping et al. (1995)

document care, measure the outcomes of nutrition education, and provide support for third party reimbursement (Johnson & Valera, 1995).

Research Studies

Studies begin with the development of a research question or hypothesis. This is followed by the development of objectives with measurable outcomes. Data must then be gathered and analyzed. Finally, conclusions are drawn from the data. Often, research results are shared with other professionals through workshops, seminars, and/or written publications so that others can benefit from increased knowledge of the subject.

Two recent studies provide good models to show application of these steps. The first, by Dahl and Read (1995), investigated the impact of nutrition education on serum cholesterol levels of outpatients. The second, by Johnson and Valera (1995), studied the effect of nutrition education on the clinical outcomes of patients with NIDDM. Although the sample sizes were small in each study, sound reasoning and clearly defined objectives produced meaningful results to support dietetic practice.

Some studies have attempted to measure more qualitative outcomes of nutrition education intervention. Trudeau and Dube (1995) investigated variables related to patient satisfaction with nutrition counseling because satisfaction has a positive influence on compliance. They found that patients wanted to be involved with decisions affecting diet, that they responded positively to individualized service, and that dietitians were perceived as change agents rather than information dispensers. The study also found that patients reported a higher perceived value for the information if they believed that they could implement the suggestions made and change their dietary practices.

Another study, by Hauchecorne, Barr, and Sork (1994), evaluated patients' perceptions of the importance of nutrition counseling and its effect on behavior and health. Results showed that patients identified dietitians as emotionally supportive, concerned, knowledgeable, competent, and caring. Nutrition counseling was perceived as beneficial, and patients reported dietary changes after contact with the dietitian.

These few studies need to be followed with more aggressive research to support the dynamic role of the dietitian in education and counseling and to provide data to show the positive impact on quality improvement and positive health outcomes.

CONCLUSION

Dramatic advances are expected in the health care industry in the medicinals used, the process of care, and holistic life style factors. Bezold (1994) states

"New therapies will integrate lifestyle with new medicines. The best dietary knowledge, including individual differences, will be incorporated into these therapies. Dietitians will be needed to advise and direct that integration. There will also be a role for dietitians in developing the protocols that will guide the application of these therapies."

Health care faces a new and uncertain future. The challenges will present new opportunities to all. It is time for dietitians to approach nutrition education and counseling with a new question in mind: What difference will this instruction make?

REFERENCES

American Diabetes Association and American Dietetic Association. (1986). *Guidelines for meal planning*. Alexandria, VA: Authors.

American Dietetic Association. (1990). Position of the American Dietetic Association: Nutrition education for the public. *Journal of the American Dietetic Association, 90*, 107–110.

American Dietetic Association. (1994). *Standards of education*. Chicago: Author.

American Dietetic Association. (1995). Position of the American Dietetic Association: Cost-effectiveness of medical nutrition therapy. *Journal of the American Dietetic Association, 95*, 88–91.

Anon. (1993). Social and behavioral change strategies. *Health Education Quarterly, 1*, S113-S135.

Bennett, W.J. (1986). *What works: Research about teaching and learning*. Washington, DC: United States Department of Education.

Bezold, C. (1994, October). Challenging the future: Shaping food and nutrition choices for a healthier America. Presented at the annual meeting of the American Dietetic Association, Orlando, FL.

Butterworth, C.E. (1974). The skeleton in the hospital closet. *Nutrition Today, 9*, 4–8.

Chernoff, R. (1995). Baby boomers come of age: Nutrition in the 21st century. *Journal of the American Dietetic Association, 95*, 650–654.

Dahl, B.R., & Read, M.H. (1995). Effect of a nutrition education program on the reduction of serum cholesterol level in Veterans Administration outpatients. *Journal of the American Dietetic Association, 95*, 702–703.

Derelian, D., Gallagher, A., & Snetslaar, A. (1995). Letting the outcomes justify the reimbursement. *Journal of the American Dietetic Association, 95*, 371.

Dobs, A.S., Masters, R.B., Rajaram, L., Stillman, F.A., Wilder, L.B., Margolis, S., & Becker, D.M. (1994). A comparison of education methods and their impact on behavioral change in patients with hyperlipidemia. *Patient Education and Counseling, 24*, 157–164.

Dougherty, D., Bankhead, R., Kushner, R., Mirtallo, J., & Winkler, M. (1995). Nutrition care given new importance in JCAHO standards. *Nutrition in Clinical Practice, 10*, 26–31.

Dunn, R., Beaudry, J.S., & Klavas, A. (1989). Survey of research on learning styles. *Educational Leadership, 46*, 50–58.

Even, M.J. (1987). Why adults learn in different ways. *Lifelong Learning, 10*, 22–25, 27.

Frymire, J. (1985). *Motivation to learn*. West Lafayette, IN: Kappa Delta Pi Press.

Gibbons, C.C., Reed, D., & Holt, B.A. (1992). Students learn about adult low literacy. *Journal of Nutrition Education, 24*, 94C.

Giloth, B.E. (1990). Management of patient education in US hospitals: Evolution of a concept. *Patient Education and Counseling, 15,* 101–111.

Glanz, K., & Eriksen, M.P. (1993). Individual and community models for dietary behavior change. *Journal of Nutrition Education, 25,* 80–86.

Glanz, K., Patterson, R.E., Kristal, A.R., DiClemente, C.C., Heimendinger, J., Linnan, L., & McLerran, D.F. (1994). Stages of change in adopting healthy diets: Fat, fiber, and correlates of nutrient intake. *Health Education Quarterly, 21,* 499–519.

Goldstein, N.L. (1991). Patient learning center reduces patient readmissions. *Patient Education and Counseling, 17,* 177–190.

Grieco, A.J., Garnett, S.A., Glassman, K.S., Valoon, P.L., & McClure, M.L. (1990). New York University Medical Center's Cooperative Care Unit: Patient education and family participation during hospitalization—The first ten years. *Patient Education and Counseling, 15,* 3–15.

Guild, P.B. (1989). Meeting students' learning styles. *Instructor, 8,* 14–17.

Guyer, L.K., Roht, R.R., Probart, C.K., & Bobroff, L.B. (1993). Broadening the scope of dietetic practice through research. *Topics in Clinical Nutrition, 8,* 26–32.

Hartmann, R.A., & Kochar, M.S. (1994). The provision of patient and family education. *Patient Education and Counseling, 24,* 10–108.

Hauchecorne, C.M., Barr, S.I., & Sork, T.J. (1994). Evaluation of nutrition counseling in clinical settings: Do we make a difference? *Journal of the American Dietetic Association, 94,* 437–440.

Holli, B.B., & Calabrese, R.J. (1991). *Communication and education skills: The dietitian's guide.* Malvern, PA: Lea & Febiger.

Hopkinson, J.H. (1993). Frequency of use and comprehensibility of health related words in health education literature. *Patient Education and Counseling, 21,* 125–133.

Insull, W. (1992). Dietitians as intervention specialists: A continuing challenge for the 1990s. *Journal of the American Dietetic Association, 92,* 551–552.

Johnson, E.Q., & Valera, S. (1995). Medical nutrition therapy in non–insulin-dependent diabetes mellitus improves clinical outcome. *Journal of the American Dietetic Association, 95,* 700–701.

Joint Commission on Accreditation of Healthcare Organizations. (1995). *1996 Accreditation manual for hospitals.* Oakbrook Terrace, IL: Author.

Kicklighter, J.R. (1991). Characteristics of older adult learners: A guide for dietetics practitioners. *Journal of the American Dietetic Association, 91,* 1418–1422.

Knowles, M.S. (1970). *The modern practice of adult education.* New York: Association Press.

Krasker, G.D., & Balogun, L.B. (1995). 1995 JCAHO standards: Development and relevance to dietetics practice. *Journal of the American Dietetic Association, 95,* 240–243.

Lewis, C.W., Frongillo, E.A., & Roe, D.A. (1995). Drug–nutrient interactions in three long-term-care facilities. *Journal of the American Dietetic Association, 95,* 309–315.

McCabe, B.J., Tysinger, J.W., Kreger, M., & Currwin, A.C. (1989). A strategy for designing effective patient education materials. *Journal of the American Dietetic Association, 89,* 1290–1292,1295.

Meade, C.D., & Smith, C.F. (1991). Readability formulas: Cautions and criteria. *Patient Education and Counseling, 19,* 153–158.

Mercurio, A.R. (1993). Promoting effective use of print materials in patient education. In B.E. Giloth (Ed.), *Managing hospital-based patient education* (pp. 357–377). Chicago: American Hospital Publishing.

Merriam, S.B. (1988). Finding your way through the maze: A guide to the literature on adult learning. *Lifelong Learning, 11,* 4–7.

Monsen, E.R. (1989). The dietitian as the nutrition counselor: The 1989 journal. *Journal of the American Dietetic Association, 89,* 43–44.

Monsen, E.M. (1992). Counseling: Transforming science into art, skills into opportunity. *Journal of the American Dietetic Association, 92*, 538.

Nielsen, E., & Sheppard, M.A. (1988). Television as a patient education tool: A review of its effectiveness. *Patient Education and Counseling, 11*, 3–16.

O'Neill, G.P. (1988). Teaching effectiveness: A review of the research. *Canadian Journal of Education, 13*, 162–185.

Reasonable accomodations faculty guide: Teaching college students with disabilities and accomodating faculty with disabilities (2nd ed.). (1995). University of Florida Americans with Disabilities Act Office.

Rice, M., & Valdivia, L. (1991). A simple guide for design, use, and evaluation of educational materials. *Health Education Quarterly, 18*, 79–85.

Rudd, R.E., & Comings, J.P. (1994). Learner developed materials: An empowering product. *Health Education Quarterly, 21*, 313–327.

Ruud, J., Betts, N.M., & Dirkx, J. (1993). Developing written nutrition information for adults with low literacy skills. *Journal of Nutrition Education, 25*, 11–16.

Ruzicki, D.A. (1989). Realistically meeting the educational needs of hospitalized acute and short-stay patients. *Nursing Clinics of North America, 24*, 629–637.

Shepherd, S.K., Sims, L.S., Davis, C.A., Shaw, A., & Cronin, F.J. (1994). Panel versus novice focus groups: Reactions to content and design features of print materials. *Journal of Nutrition Education, 26*, 10–14.

Skinner, C.S., Siegfried, J.C., Kegler, M.C., & Strecher, V.J. (1993). The potential of computers in patient education. *Patient Education and Counseling, 22*, 27-34.

Snetslaar, L.G. (1989). *Nutrition counseling skills: Assessment, treatment and evaluation*. Gaithersburg, MD: Aspen.

Sumpmann, M. (1989). An education center for patients' high-tech learning needs. *Patient Education and Counseling, 13*, 309–323.

Thompson, S.C., Pitts, J.S., & Schwankovsky, L. (1993). Preferences for involvement in medical decision-making: Situational and demographic influences. *Patient Education and Counseling, 22*, 133–140.

Thompson, R., & Weisberg, S. (1990). Families as educational consumers: What do they want? What do they receive? *Health and Social Work, 15*, 221–227.

Topping, C.M., Humm, D.C., Fischer, R.B., & Brayer, K.M. (1995). A community-based, inter-agency approach by dietitians to provide meals, medical nutrition therapy, and education to clients with HIV/AIDS. *Journal of the American Dietetic Association, 95*, 683–686.

Trudeau, E., & Dube, L. (1995). Moderators and determinants of satisfaction with diet counseling for patients consuming a therapeutic diet. *Journal of the American Dietetic Association, 95*, 34–39.

U.S. Department of Health and Human Services. (1988). *The Surgeon General's report on nutrition and health*. Washington, DC: Author.

U.S. Department of Health and Human Services. (1990). *Healthy people 2000: National health promotion and disease prevention objectives*. Washington, DC: Author.

van Ryn, M., & Heaney, C.A. (1992). What's the use of theory? *Health Education Quarterly, 19*, 315–330.

Webber, G.C. (1990). Patient education. *Medical Care, 28*, 1089–1103.

West, R.L. (1991). The adaptive memory: Maintaining skills in older years. *Outlook on Aging: FLORIDA, 3*, 1–15.

Wilkins, R.G. (1995, October). *Outcome assessment: Your role in documenting the value of medical nutrition therapy*. Presented at the annual meeting of the American Dietetic Association, Chicago, IL.

6

Patient Rights: Case Study of Medical Nutrition Care

Dorothy G. King

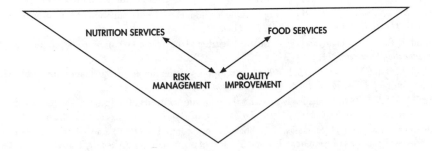

NUTRITION SERVICES   FOOD SERVICES

RISK MANAGEMENT   QUALITY IMPROVEMENT

The World Health Organization and most developed countries, with the notable exception of the United States, perceive health care as a right of all. Neither the U.S. Constitution nor the Declaration of Independence guarantees a right to health care, even though the inalienable rights to life, liberty, and the pursuit of happiness are strongly influenced by proper health care (Annas, 1992). All rights are consequently affected by those who have the power to promulgate policies governing life and death through the allocation of scarce medical resources. Public policy guidelines for medically assisted prolongation of life on the one hand and euthanasia on the other are based on competing values of morals and money.

Professionals in the health care field are in a position to protect and honor the personal rights of their patients. They are encouraged to demonstrate the seven C's of professional responsibility: competence, consent, communication, courage, compassion, conscience, and cost.

A two-part case study is presented in this chapter. In addition to applying the seven C's of professional responsibility, both parts of the case study focus on the dietetic practitioner's role responsibility to establish and implement appropriate *quality* nutrition standards of practice. Although the case concentrates on medical nutrition, underlying concepts apply to food service management as well.

The first step in any controversial discussion is to define key concepts, such as rights and duties. This is not a simple task. The library is filled with scholarly treatises that attempt to define legal and moral rights and corollary duties.

Subtle differences in meaning can translate into enormous differences in decisions and, therefore, behavioral expectations and consequences. Confusion, ambiguity, and strong differences of opinions exist.

Bandman (1978) defines the term *right* as "valid or justified entitlement for making effective claims and demands" (p. 321) and states that "the right to one's domain, whether it is one's body, one's life, one's property, or one's privacy" (p. 51), is based on freedom. The American Civil Liberties Union (Annas, 1992) defines *legal rights* as "claims that would be currently backed by law if the case went to court" and "include the rights of citizenship arising under the Constitution and its Amendments, the laws of the fifty states, and court decisions" (p. 7).

The most fundamental patient right is *safety*. From an ethical and legal perspective, all patients have a *right to a safe* and appropriate diet prescription, diet counseling, and food and nutrient sources in a timely manner (Joint Commission on Accreditation of Healthcare Organizations [Joint Commission], 1995; Krashner & Balogun, 1995). The basic corollary *duty* of all health care providers is expressed by the ancient Hippocratic maxim of non-maleficence: *primum non nocere* ("above all, do no harm"). Dietetic practitioners, like all other professionals, are moral agents and are both personally and professionally accountable for preventable harm to patients (Annas, 1992). Along with the patient's basic right to *safety*, other ethical and legal rights include autonomy (informed consent), privacy (confidentiality), and veracity from care providers.

The concept of *nutrition* care overlaps with, but is separate from, that of *therapy*. The term care as it is used here includes attitudes and behaviors that reflect respect, compassion, and kindness. The opposite would be harm inflicted by mental or physical cruelty, abandonment, or intentional or unintentional neglect. Intimidation of anyone, employee or patient, by the use of degrading or humiliating behavior in public or in private is forbidden. *Humane* care is extolled as seminal for all health care practitioners.

Philosophical content is kept to a minimum. The goal is to stimulate an interest in the need to be well informed and skilled in the ethical and legal analysis of nutrition care dilemmas. The ultimate goal is to encourage active participation by dietetic health care professionals as *patient advocates*. The formula proposed encompasses the principles of integrity and assertive communication skills combined with competence in nutrition science and management delivered with an attitude of respect and beneficent compassion for each person.

Vignette 1 of the case study involves the food and nutrition problems of an alert patient with cancer cachexia and a broken leg. Vignette 2 involves the same patient who slips into a coma one month into the hospitalization and the dynamic interaction among and between the family and the interdisciplinary staff. Both parts of the case focus on the dietetic practitioner's role responsibility to establish and implement appropriate *quality nutrition standards of practice*.

The case study is based on a composite of true stories, with literary license taken to fictionalize the facts enough to protect *patient confidentiality* (Annas, 1992; Gostin et al., 1993). The latter concept is the legal right against an invasion of privacy. Health care information is very intimate and contains a high potential of vulnerability of social harm if this information is exposed without the patient's permission. This ancient medical edict is from the Hippocratic Oath that dictates: "Whatsoever things I see or hear concerning the life of man, in any attendance on the sick or even apart therefrom, which ought not to be noised about, I will keep silent thereon, counting such things to be professional secrets" (Annas, 1992, p.177).

VIGNETTE 1

Stella Günzberg is an alert, articulate, frail, 70-year-old woman admitted to Community Hospital in acute distress with the diagnosis of non–stress fracture of the right femur secondary to disseminated bone cancer. The patient selects her neighborhood hospital to facilitate visitation convenience for her family. Her regular oncologist is not on staff at Community Hospital; therefore, an on-staff oncologist and orthopedist are assigned to cover the case. Her medical record is requested from the original oncologist but never arrives.

Medical History

Medical history includes bilateral radical mastectomy 15 years ago at the Metropolitan Cancer Research Center. During the last 5 years, three different chemotherapies have been given in addition to one experimental chemotherapy protocol administered intermittently for the last year plus radiation. The patient also has a history of obesity (average weight, 180 pounds; height, 5 feet 3 inches) for 40 years, with type II diabetes mellitus of 20 years treated with oral hypoglycemic drugs and diet. She has gradually lost weight over the last couple of years, with rapid loss of 60 pounds in less than one year. Weight on admission is 100 pounds.

Current Medical Treatment Plan

The current medical treatment plan includes traction for leg fracture, radiation to chest and spine for pain control, morphine and other pain medication as needed, Diabeta™ (hypoglycemic medication) before each meal, and an 1,800-calorie diabetic diet.

Social History

Stella Günzberg is a former secretary who has been the sole caregiver of her husband of 45 years since his cerebrovascular accident 10 years ago, which results in hemiparesthesia. A married daughter with six children lives in the neighborhood. Both the daughter and her husband are social workers. Mrs. Günzberg's son, a lawyer, and his family live 300 miles away. One sister, younger by 15 years, lives with her family in the nearby metropolitan area. The sister is a biochemistry professor and has a close relationship with the patient. She routinely accompanied the patient to the oncologist's office at Metropolitan Cancer Research Center for treatment and testing. Despite the patient's state of physical and emotional distress, she is always humble, polite, patient, and cooperative with staff, family, and friends. Mrs. Günzberg's most vocal concerns are for the long-term care of her husband. She drops her head when mentioning the embarrassment she feels for needing help and being physically dependent and sick (Geissler, 1994).

Food and Nutrition History

Self-selected menus imprinted with the heading "Diabetic, Low Sodium, Low Fat" are delivered with the patient's name and "1,800-cal diab" written on the top. The patient is continually frustrated because the items of food that she chooses are often changed without explanation. For example, the patient is not a milk drinker and does not select milk, but it is delivered with every dinner meal. Mrs. Günzberg comments to relatives that she has no appetite and that the dry, tasteless food makes it nearly impossible to eat. She has a dry mouth, which compounds her difficulty in swallowing food, especially meat without gravy.

Mrs. Günzberg's sister asks for permission to contact the nursing supervisor and the dietitian regarding the consistent delays in the delivery of pain medication and the unpalatable food. The patient responds that she does not want to cause trouble for the staff and fears retaliation. At the beginning of the third week of hospitalization, however, Mrs. Günzberg finally acquiesces to her sister's request to contact the dietitian. She recounts today's exasperating incident as follows: Breakfast arrived with dry cereal, a couple of ounces of cream, no carton of milk, plus the usual butter without bread to put it on. She humorously inquires "Am I expected to individually dunk each flake of cereal in the thimbleful of cream? And what am I supposed to do with the butter, spread it on my dry cereal?"

Communication with the Dietitian

The patient's sister is directed by the nurse to the office near Mrs. Günzberg's room that is designated "Food and Nutrition Department." With a warm smile, the patient's sister identifies herself and describes her sister's food problems. She attempts to ease the tension of the complaint by smiling while humorously retelling the breakfast story. The staff member does not smile or identify herself by name or occupation. In a cold, defensive, abrupt manner, she dismisses the breakfast incident by saying that the milk delivery was late. No apology or comment is forthcoming.

The next point that the sister brings up is that Mrs. Günzberg is having major difficulty eating the food because it is tasteless, dry, and difficult to swallow. It also appears ludicrous to the patient and family that she is receiving low-fat, low-salt, tasteless, dry food in light of her recent dramatic weight loss. The dietitian's robotlike response is "Mrs. Günzberg is on an 1,800-calorie diabetic diet. All special diets receive the same menu, and all the food for calculated diets is prepared low sodium and low fat."

The patient's sister then explains to the dietitian that her sister is a mild diabetic, and that other than the immobilization and pain caused by the broken leg, her major medical problem is cancer. Her once robust sister now looks skeletal and feels as if she is starving to death. She needs food for strength and pleasure. The sister asks whether the dietitian has spoken to the physician. The dietitian's response is "The doctor has not contacted me." The dietitian neither acknowledges the seriousness of the patient's food problems nor suggests any possible solutions. The sister walks away frustrated and angry because of the don't care–attitude of the dietitian, who appears not to be concerned about the food needs, desires, or intake of the patient.

Upon returning to Mrs. Günzberg's room, the sister reports that the unidentified nutrition person was uncooperative and hostile and that she strongly recommends the physician be contacted directly with a request for a diet change to regular food. This is done. The oncologist complies with the patient's request. An aide from the nursing department delivers and picks up the regular diet menus. The selection and palatability of the food improves during the patient's last week of hospitalization. No one from the food and nutrition department phones or visits the patient during the entire month.

Medical Chart Documentation

On day three after admission, medical charting on the patient includes one entry from the dietitian who acknowledges the initial diet order by the oncologist as "1,800-calorie diabetic diet." Nursing notes include recording of weekly weighing on a bed scale: weight on admission is 100 pounds, with a total loss of more than 15 pounds during the first three weeks, with stabilization during the final week of hospitalization. The patient is discharged to hospice home care.

Discussion of Case Facts and Issues

The following analysis is predicated on the presumption that this was not an isolated case of neglect that slipped through the cracks of an otherwise well-managed, patient-focused food system. Mrs. Günzberg's cancer-related food and nutrition problems are a common challenge for dietetic practitioners, physicians, and patients. Two of the primary duties of the medical nutrition practitioner discussed below are timely identification of patients at risk for malnutrition in addition to the validation and implementation of an appropriate diet prescription that includes monitoring food intake.

The foundation for ensuring the patient's right to safety is the corollary duty of the dietetic practitioner to be competent. One major source of professional role expectations is the Joint Commission. The continuous quality improvement concepts of the Joint Commission standards require nutrition screening, assessment and/or reassessment, and treatment priorities with ongoing patient monitoring relative to the needs of the patient (Joint Commission, 1995, p. 242).

Case Fact 1

The patient's diagnoses on admission and history of significant weight loss are classic criteria for identification as a patient at high risk for malnutrition. Did Community Hospital have an adequate formal policy for nutrition screening? What role, if any, does the food and nutrition department play in the nutrition screening procedure? Was the food and nutrition department consulted in developing a nutrition screening plan?

From the Joint Commission's recommendation that nutrition care be delivered "as appropriate" by the interdisciplinary team, it is unclear what the dietetic practitioner's specific or unique role responsibility is for continuous quality improvement.

Case Fact 2

The issue of what constitutes an appropriate time after admission for nutrition screening is not controversial in the Günzberg case. The patient was hospitalized in an acute care facility for the unusual length of time of one month.

The American Dietetic Association (ADA) funded a five-year study to establish performance measures (nutrition clinical indicators) in oncology, surgery, and cardiovascular care. In 1993, The ADA Council on Practice Quality Assurance Committee submitted the following recommendations to the Joint Commission: "All [oncology] patients at moderate or high risk are identified by screening and assessed within 72 hours of hospitalization" (Queen, Caldwell, & Balogun, 1993, p. 338). The Joint Commission did not implement the field-tested ADA recommendations. A generic recommendation for screening of malnutrition risk was based on hospitalization of more than five to seven days rather than on specific disease categories (Kushner et al., 1994).

The current Joint Commission (1995) guidelines for inpatient hospitalization indicates the screening by various professionals as follows: The "patient's history and physical examination, nursing assessment, and other screening assessment [must be] completed within 24 hours of admission" (p.103). In contrast, the nutritional status is assessed "when warranted by the patient's needs or condition. . . . The hospital identifies patients at risk for nutrition problems, according to criteria developed by dietitians and other qualified professionals. The hospital refers such patients to a dietitian for further assessment" (Joint Commission, 1995, p. 103). Therefore, it is up to each hospital to determine the criteria for screening and to identify which patients will subsequently receive comprehensive follow-up assessment. The same problem exists for the reassessment guidelines, which state that each patient should be reassessed at points designated by hospital policy.

Standards that are incompatible with quality nutrition care promote a professional dilemma for competent, conscientious medical dietitians as patient advocates. Hospital caregivers must deal with reimbursement constraints, including professional staff downsizing, while simultaneously dealing with a patient population that is significantly sicker on admission and has an average length of hospitalization of less than seven days. Discharged patients therefore are frequently in a more precarious, vulnerable medical state during their posthospital convalescence. Few patients at risk for malnutrition can be identified under these time requirements for nutrition screening.

The Joint Commission is perhaps the most powerful standard setter; its accreditation of health care facilities is used as a prerequisite for reimbursement from Medicare and Medicaid and for state licensure. Background information about this private regulatory agency may shed some light on common complaints against it among health care administrators and professionals, such as excessive expense, confusion due to the frequency of standard changes, and a lack of specificity (which permits too much latitude in interpretation by individual inspectors).

The Joint Commission was established 40 years ago, primarily by physicians. Patients' rights advocate groups, such as the Public Citizen's Health Research Group founded by Ralph Nader, accuse the Joint Commission of conflict of interest, of being industry focused and not patient focused. Support for this accusation includes the following facts. The Joint Commission rarely denies or seriously restricts accreditation of any member facility, including some later found to have serious deficiencies. In addition, physicians have access to a roster of patients who sue for malpractice as well as individuals seeking performance reports by the Joint Commission, but the reverse information is guarded and inaccessible to patients (Anon., 1995, p. 5).

During this century, curricula of American medical schools have not emphasized food and nutrition's impact on health and disease (Frankle, 1976). Although "dietitians are members of the only profession whose sole concern is the nutritional health of people" (Huenemann, 1981, p. 127), physicians have been reticent to acknowledge the significance of the field of nutrition and the profession of dietetics. It is therefore not surprising that the Joint Commission's standards for nutrition care reflect the bias of its core group, physicians.

Case Fact 3

Mrs. Günzberg's medical problems are common reasons for malnutrition. Healing of a major bone fracture requires increased nutrient needs while adequate food intake is hampered by the routine problems of advanced cancer: debilitation, cachexia, anorexia, xerostomia (dry mouth), and hypogeusia (lack of taste) compounded by pain and anxieties (Bloch, 1990). Although the Joint Commission is nonspecific regarding the criteria for nutritionally at-risk status, Mrs. Günzberg's significant weight loss and increased nutrient needs for bone healing meet the multiple criteria provided in general nutrition assessment standards in classic nutrition references (Grant & De Hoog, 1991; Simko, Cowell, & Gilbride, 1984).

Case Fact 4

There was consistent faulty verbal and written communication among the dietetic practitioner and the patient, the patient's family, and the physician. The dietitian's hesitancy to initiate contact with the physician to question or suggest any diet modifications indicated a reactive, nonproactive role perception. Is a passive posture by clinical dietitians based on a lack of medical nutrition competence, confusion of expertise authorization, or personality factors that impede assertive, diet prescription formulation and validation?

Is the frequency of apathy or lack of initiative by medical dietitians a reflection of the degree of confusion on what they perceive as their legal accountability as professionals? Research has consistently exposed serious discrepancies between dietitian role expectations regarding diet prescription responsibility as perceived by dietitians and physicians in contrast to the prudent behavior required of dietitians given the possibility of malpractice litigation (King, 1993). Discrepancies in the mutual role expectations of the interdisciplinary participants and a lack of cooperation or trust are dominant influences that produce intergroup tensions and ineffectiveness, with the logical consequence of hindering safe patient care (Georgopoulos & Matejko, 1967).

The Joint Commission states that "authorized individuals will prescribe or order food and nutrition products in a timely manner" (Joint Commission, 1995, p. 15). Which professional group—physicians, dietitians, or nurses—is authorized to have sole or joint responsibility? Although the answer is not explicitly stated in these regulations, state professional licensing acts generally give physicians sole authority to prescribe medical treatment, which includes both drugs and diets.

Unfortunately, this is not so simple and clear cut. "Interdisciplinary health care providers, physicians, and nonphysicians carry out some identical or similar clinical tasks such as developing diagnoses and formulating treatment plans. The overlap in performing these clinical tasks often makes differentiation unclear. Nomenclature gamesmanship may be the essence of the differences, not the cognitive and behavioral task or skill" (King, 1993, pp. 1269-1270). For example, what is the difference between formulating a nutrition care plan and prescribing a diet prescription or between performing a nutrition assessment and doing a diagnostic nutrition evaluation?

Legally, the terms professional negligence and malpractice are used interchangeably to mean "failure of a professional person to act in accordance with the prevalent professional standards or failure to foresee possibilities and consequences that the professional person, having the necessary skill and training to act professionally, should foresee" (Murchison, Nichols, & Hanson, 1982, pp. 49-50). Malpractice jurisprudence views as harmful conduct to patients both errors of omission (e.g., failing to screen for malnutrition risk or not preventing foreseeable injury from a dangerously incorrect diet prescription) and errors of commission (e.g., serving contaminated food or incorrectly calculating the components of the diet, such as the potassium level for a patient with kidney damage).

The clinical hierarchical role position of the medical dietitian is similar to the professional nurse's relationship to the physician. The nursing literature dismisses the traditional subservient role of the nurse as the "handmaiden of the physician" and promotes the current expanded clinical role of the nurse as a professional colleague of the physician (Bullough, 1980). Likewise, the traditional role of the dietitian could be labeled "kitchen maiden of the hospital." There has been a steady campaign by dietetic practitioners, as with nurses, to transform the medical dietitian to a leadership role as a required consultant who is a professional colleague to the physician (Forcier, Kight, & Sheehan, 1977).

Hassan (1977) hypothesizes that the law may view the clinical dietitian as the "last link in the doctor-nurse-dietitian chain because she/he may well be the last 'qualified professional' who could have circumvented the wrong therapy for the right patient" (p. 357). It is arguable that the dietitian has an even higher level of responsibility for the accuracy of the diet prescription than the nurse does for the drug prescription because "dietitians are members of the only profession whose sole concern is the nutrition health of people" (Huenemann, 1981, p. 127), and they claim to have unique knowledge of nutrition (ADA, 1985, p. 724).

Twenty years ago, federal regulations defined the clinical nutrition standard of practice in the treatment of end-stage renal disease (ESRD). The mandate (P.L. 95-292) stipulated that a qualified dietitian, in consultation with the attending physician, is responsible for assessing the nutrition and dietetic needs of each ESRD patient and for recommending therapeutic diets.

Nurses, unlike dietetic practitioners, receive extensive required education in the ethical and legal duties of their profession. The diet prescription is analogous to the drug prescription. Common sources of litigation against nurses for unintentionally causing harm to patients include giving the wrong medication, giving the wrong dosage, or using the wrong means of administration for a specific drug. The error may originate in following foreseeably dangerous physician orders or carelessly following a physician's prudent prescription.

The federal ESRD regulations had been long standing at the time New York State ESRD facilities were surveyed and yet two thirds of the responding dietitians perceived legal immunity for the dietitian for two hypothetical lethal scenarios involving blindly following a physician's foreseeably dangerous diet order. However, more than 75% of the nurses, in contrast to the opinions of the ESRD dietitians and physicians, perceived the dietitian as being equally accountable as the nurse under similar circumstances. The study concluded "To protect both the professional and the patient, extensive education in dietetic jurisprudence is warranted" (King, 1993, p. 1272).

The 1981 ADA role delineating report elaborated the appropriate and actual role responsibilities of the clinical dietitian more specifically than the federal ESRD regulations and designated clinical decision-making tasks such as "select[ing] appropriate methods of feeding [and] select[ing] appropriate sources of specific nutrients (e.g., food, food products, [and] nutrient solutions)" (Baird & Armstrong, 1981, p. 11).

Twenty percent of 728 responding physicians in a study by Schiller and Vivian (1974) indicated that the dietitian should follow the physician's diet orders without question or adaptation. More than half, however, believed that the physician is not directing adequately the nutrition care of hospitalized patients and that dietitians should assume an assertive, key role and take the initiative in making or changing diet orders (Norwich Eaton Pharmaceutical, 1982). A nearly autonomous dietitian role was suggested by nine of the ten members of a panel of dietetic experts who indicated that only the dietitian should prescribe the appropriate diet regimen based on the physician's diagnosis and general orders (Scialabba, 1973).

Physicians admit to fragmented and inadequate education and expertise in normal nutrition and medical nutrition therapy (ADA, 1994; Schiller & Vivian, 1974). Paradoxically, Butterworth (1974), in exposing iatrogenic malnutrition as the "skeleton in the hospital closet," identified a major cause of this condition as the "unclear diffusion of responsibility for patient care and ineffective communication and interaction between the attending physician and the dietitian" (p. 7). Even so, Butterworth and Blackburn (1975) expressed the traditional view that "only on his [the physician's] signal can the special skills of nurses, dietitians, pharmacists, and consultants be brought to bear on the problem at hand" (p.10).

Case Fact 5

The dietitian portrayed in vignette one demonstrated severe deficits in her verbal communication with the patient and the patient's sister. Identification by name and occupational title was not provided for the patient's sister. The patient was not contacted before or after the sister's visit to the food and nutrition office. There are ethical, legal, and etiquette issues to be analyzed in the communication problems of the dietitian. The model Patients' Bill of Rights Act highlights the importance of a gracious, civilized, full disclosure means of communication (Annas, 1992). This act states that patients have

- the right to considerate and respectful care
- the right to information, including the names, positions, and functions of any hospital staff providing care
- the right to complain without fear of reprisal
- the right to have their rights available in any language beside English if it is spoken by 5% or more of the facility's patients

Communication deficits of staff need to be identified and education on effective communication skills is necessary. Interdisciplinary seminars and workshops on effective conflict resolution are highly recommended. Polite, civilized person-to-person, telephone, and written communication is both a right and duty of all.

Case Fact 6

Mrs. Günzberg was alert and friendly, spoke and read English, and did not have any physical or emotional barriers to communicating verbally or in writing with the staff. This is in contrast to the many groups of patients who have communication obstacles, such as illiteracy, inability to understand written or spoken English, or temporary or permanent physical and/or mental impairments (e.g., dementia, severe retardation, coma, persistent vegetative state, stroke, or amyotrophic lateral sclerosis). Mrs. Günzberg expressed common fears: fear of pain, fear of financial burden of medical costs, fear of who will physically take care of her dependent husband, and fear of starving to death.

Mrs. Günzberg's attitude and behavior are consistent with those described in the psychosocial literature as a "good patient" by hospital staff; they are cooperative, undemanding, respectful, and accommodate to hospital routines easily. In contrast, "the 'bad patient' role has often been described as a behavioral pattern that insists on exerting his or her autonomy and is likened to a consumer-rights role" (Faden, Beauchamp, & King, 1986, p. 371).

Case Fact 7

In addition to Mrs. Günzberg's potential for articulate communication, she had an assertive, concerned, available family member to act as her advocate. The dietetic practitioner's response to the patient's sister was similar to the description by Chenevert (1994) of "health professionals [who] sometimes protect themselves against ego attack by developing a cool, detached, 'professional' exterior" (p. 19). They are burned-out professional zombies: "their bodies are warm but their hearts are cold, and their minds are frozen" (p. 49). Instead of viewing family members as support systems for both the patient and the staff, they too often view families of patients as inconveniences.

Being overworked is a typical source of professional burn-out. A cartoon at a luncheon counter shows a stressed waitress telling the customers that she's "all peopled out." Stress management seminars and workshops for health care workers are highly recommended on a prophylactic and treatment basis. As the patient needs personal contact, so do the professional and nonprofessional employees (Maslach, 1982).

Case Fact 8

There was inadequate dietitian documentation in the medical record of the patient's initial and ongoing nutrition status, nutrition care plan, monitoring response to the care plans, and problems. The concrete data on weight changes were taken and recorded by the nursing staff. Accurately documenting each nutritional high-risk patient's ongoing nutrition care needs and response to the nutrition care plan is a legal requirement. The medical record is the major source of legal evidence and is essential in responding to malpractice accusations of violations of standards of care that allegedly have caused harm to a patient (Cross, 1988). Documentation of the nutrition care plan, the food provided, and the patient's ongoing response to this care is also critical for meeting accreditation regulations.

Case Fact 9

Mrs. Günzberg was a mild diabetic; her priority nutrition problems were cachexia and inadequate food consumption. The use of a multirestricted menu and food may have been convenient for the food service department but was counterproductive to meeting the patient's needs for palatability and intake. The ADA (1992) emphasizes maximizing oral intake of food choices by liberalizing dietary restrictions of the terminally ill.

Kane and Caplan (1990) identify "three enemies" of personal autonomy for nursing home residents as the three R's: routine, regulation, and restricted opportunity. These three R's can also be applied to routines and regulations that result in clinical staff being isolated in an office, circling items on menus, or correcting self-selected special diet menus to conform to nonindividualized American Diabetes Association exchange list patterns in lieu of visiting patients and monitoring their nutrient intake. There may also be a communication gap between the clinical nutrition staff and the food management staff. Do they discuss problems from a cost-effective basis that emphasizes patient satisfaction? In the present case, it was a double waste of food and not meeting the patient's nutrition needs to send milk to Mrs. Günzberg routinely as a dinner beverage. The low-sodium, low-fat cheeses were neither palatable nor necessary. The patient may have benefitted from instruction on the importance of calcium and other nutrients for bone healing and exploration of high-calcium food substitutes for milk that would have been acceptable to her. This is an example of following the exchange list to the letter and missing its spirit or purpose. If the patient does not consume the food, the paper-perfect nutrition pattern is moot.

Paperwork is supposed to be a realistic representation of care given, care that is tailored to the patient's individual medical needs and food preferences. Diligence is often needed so that paperwork does not take precedence over actual patient contact. Processing menu information into actual food is a logical imperative. The goals of quality nutrition care require a balance between the essential paperwork and patient contact.

Case Fact 10

Although the patient was in an advanced stage of a terminal illness, her desire to prolong life could be inferred from her participation in the experimental drug protocol. In addition to the importance of providing acceptable food to support physical strength and avoid the added discomfort of bed sores, the importance of food as a potential source of pleasure appeared to be undervalued by the dietary department.

VIGNETTE 2

This scenario is a continuation of vignette 1 involving Mrs. Stella Günzberg. The facts are the same except for one critical medical difference: The patient lapses into a coma instead of being discharged to home hospice care. This vignette emphasizes a fundamental legal and ethical right of patients—the right to medical informed consent—and the conflicts that can ensue when surrogate decision makers debate whether nutrition support is futile treatment or mandatory humane care. This case illustrates the complexity of this kind of tube-feeding controversy by presenting different medical, legal, religious, and personal points of view.

Advance Medical Directive

Upon admission to Community Hospital, in accordance with federal legislation, Mrs. Günzberg receives a packet of information that includes an advance directive (also called living will, health care proxy, surrogate decision making, and durable power of attorney for medical decisions) and educational material created by a private organization called Choice in Dying. The Patient Self-Determination Act of 1990 requires all hospitals, long-term care facilities, hospices, health maintenance organizations, and so forth that receive Medicare and Medicaid reimbursement to have written policies and procedures on advance directives. Each health care facility is required to provide written information to each patient or facility resident concerning the rights under state law to make decisions concerning medical care, including the right to accept or refuse medical treatment or surgical treatment and the right to formulate an advance directive; and it must be documented in the individual's medical record whether the patient or facility resident has executed an advance directive (Annas, 1992; Anon., 1991).

Several days after admission, a nurse identifies herself as a patient educator from the hospital and inquires whether Mrs. Günzberg would like to discuss advance directive information. The nurse explains that the purpose of these written documents is to guide medical treatment decisions should Mrs. Günzberg no longer be able to communicate her preferences. Mrs. Günzberg politely nods in the affirmative.

The nurse educator assures the patient that signing the document is voluntary and reminds her that decisions should not be made under duress. She can change her mind and revoke her instructions as long as she can communicate.

The document would be a written directive of her choice, based on her values and religious beliefs, to undergo full treatment or forgo treatment under the limited medical conditions indicated. The nurse reviews the medical conditions specified on the document (e.g., final stage of dying, severe and irreversible dementia, or irreversible coma), as well as the kind of life-sustaining medical interventions that are sometimes referred to as heroic, invasive, aggressive, or futile under these limited medical conditions (e.g., cardiac resuscitation, mechanical ventilation, renal dialysis, antibiotics, or artificial nutrition and hydration; Brody & Halevy, 1995). The nurse explains that personal instructions can be added to the advance directive (e.g., "I do not want to be placed in a nursing home" or "I want to die at home"). She also explains that choosing to forgo heroic medical measures does not deprive the patient of other appropriate nursing care and pain control. These noninvasive comfort-care measures are referred to as palliative care by the hospice philosophy of humane care for the final physical stages of dying (Choice in Dying, 1996). The nurse asks whether there are any questions. Mrs. Günzberg responds adamantly that she does not want "tubes" but is hesitant to sign anything without consulting her family. She warmly thanks the nurse at the conclusion of the conversation. Medical records documented by the nurse educator state that the patient has received the written advance directive material with discussion. The patient declines signing the document and indicates that she wants to consult her family. The nurse's note indicates the patient's "no tubes" declaration.

During the second week of hospitalization, the following conversation takes place among Mrs. Günzberg, her sister, and her daughter. The sister notices the advance directive documents on the table and inquires about them. Mrs. Günzberg is emotional when she says that she "doesn't want tubes."

The daughter, in direct contrast to the rest of the family, observes a strictly orthodox Jewish lifestyle. She passionately tells her mother that, according to Jewish law (halakha), there is a prohibition against doing anything that might hasten death and that all persons of Jewish faith are required to do everything to maintain life (Abraham, 1990; Feldman, 1986; Meir, 1982). Mrs. Günzberg is demonstrably upset by her daughter's admonition not to indicate on the advance directive that she does not want tubes. The daughter promises to bring her mother a copy of the Halakhic Living Will which designates a surrogate decision maker in addition to a specific rabbi who will advise on medical decisions according to orthodox Jewish law and custom. The document is given to Mrs. Günzberg but she does not sign or complete it.

Medical Status

At the end of four weeks of hospitalization, the patient lapses into unconsciousness and is transferred to the intensive care unit (ICU) that is in a different wing of the hospital. Although Mrs. Günzberg is breathing spontaneously, she is in a deep coma. Her eyes are closed and there is no response to either auditory stimuli or painful physical stimuli, such as pricking with a needle. She scores 3 on the Glasgow Coma Scale, signifying that she is in the deepest coma possible. Results from a battery of tests rule out metabolic abnormality, such as a diabetic coma. Computed tomography (CT) and magnetic resonance image (MRI) scans confirm a diagnosis of metastasis to the brain. The sole source of nutrition and hydration is intravenous 5% dextrose in water.

Three days after the onset of the coma, the patient is transferred from the ICU to a room on the same floor. The oncologist and neurologist inform the family that the patient's cancer has spread to her brain. She is not expected to regain consciousness before death, which is probably imminent. The son hastily bids farewell to his comatose mother and returns to his out-of-state residence. The rest of the family, excluding the husband, maintain a rotating 24-hour vigil with the patient.

Health Team Collaboration

At the end of the second week of coma, the ICU dietitian, a new staff member, expresses three points of discomfort. First, the patient has lost excessive weight during her current hospitalization (current weight, 70 pounds; weight on admission, 100 pounds; usual weight, 180 pounds; height, 5 foot 3 inches) and is receiving inadequate nutrients from the intravenous dextrose solution. Second, the patient did not die in a few days as predicted by her attending oncologist. This brings question to the accuracy of the prognosis. Third, the patient does not have an executed advance directive indicating her decision to forgo nutrition support under the present medical conditions. The dietitian contacts the attending physicians and the nurses and expresses strong sentiments that the patient should be tube fed soon because she cannot sustain life on the dextrose infusion. Discussion of the case reveals strong feelings and differences of opinion among the interdisciplinary team.

The oncologist and the neurologist concur with each other that according to the objective medical data Mrs. Günzberg's disease is irreversible and severe and, in their opinion, the tube feeding constitutes futile medical intervention whereas the dextrose infusion is used to make the family comfortable (Brody & Halevy, 1995). Although Community Hospital does not have any of the three prognosis scoring systems, the Acute Physiology and Chronic Health Evaluation (Knaus et al., 1991), the Simplified Acute Physiology Score (Le Gall, Lemeshow, & Saullnier, 1993), and the Mortality Probability Model (Lemeshow et al., 1993), attending physicians are reasonably certain that the patient will die imminently of the underlying disease (cancer), regardless of what is done for her. Although enteral feeding will not cause the comatose patient discomfort, it will not improve the quality of life during the dying process. The hospital's option to take this position is supported by the American Medical Association's (1996) statement "it is not unethical to discontinue all means of life prolonging treatment, including nutrition or hydration, for the terminally ill or persistent vegetative state patient" (p. 426). Legal agreement with this position is presented in the 1990 Supreme Court case *Cruzan v. Harman*, in which medically supplied nutrition and hydration (nasogastric tube, gastrostomy tube, parenteral nutrition, and so forth) were considered medical treatment.

One of the ICU nurses reads aloud the information from the Günzberg chart note written by the nurse educator. Although the patient did not complete a written advance directive indicating her preference to commence or forgo a feeding tube under these medical conditions, there is a notation that the patient expressed a "no tubes" wish. The ICU nurse concurs with the physicians. She says that the feeding tube is contraindicated based on medical data of imminent death in addition to the patient's oral statements requesting "no tubes." She suggests that the dextrose infusion be discontinued because the hydration is prolonging the dying process, which would otherwise be expected to occur within ten days. It is her opinion that the American Nurses Association (1988) code for nurses would not view this case of not tube feeding as one of neglect or abuse. In addition, anecdotal observations by hospice caregivers report that dehydration can have potentially beneficial effects by reducing the patient's secretions, thus decreasing breathing problems, vomiting, and incontinence; and that dehydration usually leads to death through hemoconcentration and hyperosmolality with subsequent azotemia, hypernatremia, and hypercalcemia, all of which produce a sedative effect on the brain just before death (Schmitz & O'Brien, 1986). The depth of Mrs. Günzberg's coma precludes the possibility of pain or suffering from the absence of food and insufficiency of fluid.

The ICU dietitian restates the other members' viewpoints, expresses respect for the logically based opposing opinions of the interdisciplinary team, and agrees to reflect on their views about enteral feeding as unwarranted, futile medical treatment (Rusk & Miller, 1993). She then proceeds to present an analysis of the dilemma as she perceives it. First, even with the noblest of intentions combined with state-of-the-art tests that help predict medical outcome, prognosis is an uncertain clinical art. Physicians use the terms terminal and futile based on notoriously variable and arbitrary criteria (Bursztajn, Feinbloom, Hamm, & Brodsky, 1990). The fact remains that the patient has been lingering for weeks, not days as predicted. The patient did not die "on time."

Second, the ICU dietitian expresses her views of a professional duty of dietetic practitioners as a professional group to avoid or intervene in malnutrition for patients as appropriate and states that palliative care does not automatically preclude enteral or parenteral nutrition support. The latter is rarely used for hospice patients because it is expensive and skilled labor intensive. Mrs.

Günzberg would not require any restraints to maintain the intubation. If the patient does not expire in a matter of days, the outcome of withholding fluid and nutrition support, theoretically, would produce death by dehydration and starvation. It would constitute feeding neglect and abandonment of the patient. Although there is a vital parallel between eating and breathing, in that both food and air are essential to life, there is a significant difference between forgoing or removing a feeding tube and the ventilator. Removal of the ventilator neither intends to cause death nor guarantees death for the comatose patient (Meilaender, 1984). For example, in the 1976 landmark New Jersey Supreme Court case of Karen Ann Quinlan, contrary to medical prediction the patient did not die when weaned from the respirator. The patient resumed spontaneous breathing and was physically maintained in a persistent vegetative state for nine years by good nursing care and enteral feeding. The decision to allow the patient to die or let nature take its course is passive euthanasia because death is accelerated by withholding food and fluid. The intent of forgoing or withdrawing food and fluid is to cause death.

The ICU dietitian expresses apprehension about the current atmosphere of health care decisions that are based on financial and utilitarian motives rather than the welfare of individual, vulnerable patients. She articulates her fear of the "slippery slope" of euthanasia. The danger of abuse of the "silent patient is not theoretical but real." Silence may result from the disease itself or the more subtle influences of social, economic, cultural, racial, or personality factors (e.g., the poor are not used to speaking up for themselves, especially in the intimidating atmosphere of the health care delivery system; Golanta, 1995). The legal and moral principles of informed consent can also be distorted by the personality styles of those involved: the stereotypical authoritarian health care professional and the passive, disenfranchised patient (President's Commission, 1982).

Over the last decade, there has been a flood of media reports perpetuated by emotionally dramatic court cases promoting the slogans of "the right to die" and "death with dignity." There is reason to suspect that this aggressively marketed campaign is intended to manipulate both health care professionals and the public to accept "the obligation to die" in a timely manner that financially benefits the government and the health care industry. The individual's legal right of medical informed consent assumes that the patient has the option to request, and not just refuse, resuscitation and other life-prolonging technologies. The current push is for hospitals and insurance companies to have the power to make unilateral medical decisions based on profit incentives rather than the preferences of the patient or family (Capron, 1991; Miles, 1992).

The ICU dietitian concludes by expounding on the third factor: personal conscience. Her conscientious objection stance is founded in her Catholic pro-life convictions (Catholic New York, 1992) that euthanasia is immoral because it is killing by not feeding the sick. Even if the goal of feeding is symbolic, the basic provision of nourishment and fluids is a fundamental matter of human dignity. The President's Commission (1982) warns "A decision to forego such treatment is awesome because it hastens death" (p. 45).

Family Discussion with the Interdisciplinary Team

The interdisciplinary team agrees to consult with the family. The attending physicians reiterate their professional opinion that the tube feeding is futile treatment. The oncologist admits that he did not know the patient before the current hospitalization, that her previous medical record is unavailable, and that he did not discuss termination of treatment issues with her.

The patient's sister speaks with strong feelings in her voice that according to what Mrs Günzberg said on numerous occasions, she did not want "tubes" and would be humiliated to be a "vegetable." The sister says that the patient's son, an attorney, has notified her that he will sue the hospital for any medical expenses incurred after insertion of a feeding tube. Although Mrs. Günzberg did not designate anyone as her surrogate medical decision maker, she did give her son power of attorney for financial decisions because of her husband's mental and physical inability to sign checks and handle financial matters. The son is concerned that if his mother's condition is prolonged because of the feeding tube, it will have a serious impact on his father's future financial security.

Based on their respective religious convictions, the daughter and the ICU dietitian concur that Mrs. Günzberg should receive food and fluid by tube.

The husband is agitated and somewhat confused. There is evidence that he may be decisionally impaired. He is in denial about his wife's impending death from cancer and her coma being irreversible. He blames the medical system for his own health impairments and those of his wife. He refuses to discuss selling their car and speaks of Mrs. Günzberg returning home to drive him to the store. He is outraged at any discussion of not feeding his wife.

Clergy and legal counsel are sought, and the case is referred to the institution's ethics committee for immediate review and recommendations. The last resort would be judicial intervention.

Discussion of Case Facts and Issues

Case Fact 1

The advance directive is based on the patient's right to informed consent for end-of-life medical treatment options and encompasses the common-law right of self-determination and a constitutional right to privacy. Mrs. Günzberg received written and verbal information about advance directives from the nurse educator and her daughter. Like the majority of the population, the patient did not sign the documents. Both lawyers and ethicists agree that informed consent is not a signature but rather an educational process. Health professionals tend not to understand the process, however, and in actual hospital practice it "means no more than the empty formality . . . of obtaining a signature on a consent form" (Faden, Beauchamp, & King, 1986, p. 277). Many believe, except in rare cases, meeting the standards of true informed consent is an illusion and a hoax.

The sister and the nurse-educator's information are evidence that the patient gave oral advance directive wishes of refusing "tubes." The courts have accepted oral evidence alone as clear and convincing evidence of whether the patient would or would not want tube feeding under current medical conditions. Oral statements are, of course, more difficult to authenticate (Meisel, 1995).

A review of the following essential components of the informed consent process (disclosure, comprehension, voluntariness, competence, and consent) is intended to shed some light on the difficulty in obtaining authentic informed consent:

- Adequate disclosure and comprehension of relevant, understandable medical information as it relates to the specific patient's diagnosis and includes alternative treatments and nontreatment options with their statistically anticipated risk-benefit consequences.
- Voluntariness by the patient. There are significant differences in the communication objectives and style of persuasive advice or education and that of threatening coercion (psychological manipulation), or biased, fraudulent manipulation of medical information presented or omitted. The latter is forbidden (Faden, Beauchamp, & King, 1986; President's Commission, 1982).
- Patients' capacity to comprehend the relevant medical information for the decision at hand is "the ability to deliberate in accordance with his or her own values and goals, and the ability to communicate with caregivers" (Hastings Center, 1987, p. 7). The legal doctrine of patient competence for medical treatment authorization is not to be confused with the level of medical knowledge necessary for professional competence. Although patient capacity is usually an informal clinical determination, technically, patient competence is a formal legal designation by the court. "Absent a judicial determination, the law presumes competence in adults" (Hastings Center, 1987, p. 7).

Many aspects of this doctrine are troublesome. Can a person be depressed and/or mentally ill and still have the decisional capacity to direct his or her medical treatment (Powell & Lowenstein, 1996; Sullivan & Youngner, 1994)?

Who decides for children, for the never competent, and for the pregnant incompetent?

There are several elements of the informed consent process that are questionable in the Günzberg case: comprehension and adequacy of information, as well as voluntariness. There was evidence of the patient's ambivalence and possible lack of thorough understanding of the options and consequences of not tube feeding. The nurse educator and the sister did not pursue an in-depth discussion of the "no tubes" request by the patient. Several years ago, the sister witnessed the patient's disturbing level of claustrophobia during a brain CT scan. One can consider that Mrs. Günzberg's claustrophobia may have influenced her fear of tubes on the face. Did the patient know that a gastrostomy tube would not involve the face and could provide her with the hope of a miracle that would give her more time with her family? One can assume a highly motivated will to live by her decision to undergo painful experimental chemotherapy. However, on the other hand, the patient may have used the "no tubes" as a simplified way of saying "pull the plug." Maybe she was too physically and emotionally exhausted from the whole ordeal of illness and treatment to discuss the matter further. Another common problem is the ineffective control of pain for terminally ill patients and its intolerable and depressing consequences. Was this a significant factor during her hospitalization?

It is rare that patients truly understand the medically sophisticated implications of their treatment options. To look at this variable, one is encouraged to discuss the personal opinions of physicians and nurses (especially those in emergency care specializations) about advance directive issues. Have they signed an advance directive? What do they want for themselves? For their family? This professional group has the medical expertise and experience to understand the ramifications of, what is to the lay public, abstract concepts of quality of life and end-of-life biomedical technological possibilities.

The issue of voluntariness needs to be addressed in the Günzberg case. Did she passively capitulate to her daughter's religious argument? Was her daughter coercive? Ideally, the ethic of patient autonomy and the legal doctrine of informed consent provide for "the locus of decisional authority to remain with the individual patient" (Blustein, 1993, p. 6). Mrs. Günzberg appeared to have what Briles (1994) describes as an accommodating conflict resolution style; she did not assert her own claims to power.

Case Fact 2

Mrs. Günzberg neither completed an advance directive nor designated a health care proxy authorized to carry out her wishes. Because of its highly controversial nature, the statutes of many states require that the health care proxy include specific provisions that allow the agent to withhold or withdraw feeding tubes.

If the patient is unable to communicate his or her wishes, and has not executed an advance directive, which members of the family are given a voice in the end-of-life treatment decisions (Veatch, 1993)? Who decides for those who have not expressed an opinion and have no next of kin? What are the role and level of authority of the physician? Does the physician in charge have de facto surrogacy for the surrogateless incompetent patient? Does the patient's designated surrogate decision maker have authority over the physician? Who has the final word?

"There is much ambiguity as to the legitimate ranking among the next of kin as to who has the authority to decide to forgo treatment or to demand treatment against a medical opinion of 'futility'" (Veatch, 1993, p.13). Almost half of the states have statutes authorizing surrogate decision making by ranked ordering of the next of kin for patients without advance directives (Choice in Dying, 1996). On a pragmatic rather than a formal legal basis, "The family member who favors a course supported by the physician is likely to be the designated surrogate. Moreover, whoever is chosen by the clinician will be the recipient of the wrath by the not chosen, hardly making for a good family support system for a difficult time to come" (Veatch, 1993, p.14).

Both federal and state constitutions have recognized that a competent individual has a "liberty interest" (in contrast to a fundamental right) to forgo or withdraw life-sustaining treatment. That right does not cease when the patient is no longer competent. Different states, however, require different standards of proof to establish what the patient would want. For example, New York and Missouri require the highest standard of proof called "clear and convincing evidence" rather than the less stringent standard of "preponderance of the evidence" (Gostin & Weir, 1991).

Components of the legal doctrine of substituted judgment include the following:

- the patient's written or orally expressed "informed" preferences
- the patient's religious convictions as they relate to refusal of treatment (e.g., a doctrine of the Jehovah Witness religion forbids blood transfusions among their believers)
- the emotional and or financial impact on the family
- the probability of adverse side effects of the treatment
- the prognosis with and without treatment

The reasoning given for the legal presumption in favor of family choice when the patient is incompetent is that the family members "ordinarily have deep and detailed knowledge of one another's lives, characters, values and desires; intimacy of family life encourages and is partly constituted by the unguarded disclosure of one's most private thoughts and deepest feelings" (Blustein, 1993, p.12).

The wisdom of Solomon would be helpful in handling the family dynamics of contested cases. It would also be naive not to mention the potential for self-interest or abuse within families. Conflict among families is not new; love and beneficence are not necessarily the foundations of family decisions and relationships. Money and/or menacing memories may contribute to hostility-based decisions by family members that affect the patient. Attempts to discover motives are complicated and time intensive. The Cruzan case concludes that the federal constitution does not require states to defer to the patient's family (Pollock, 1991). The use of the courts to solve these questions is a last recourse because of the expense and emotional toll on the family and professionals.

The ICU dietitian utilized an assertive, diplomatic communication style to pursue with perseverance an ethical and legal resolution to the professional and personal dilemma of fulfilling her perceived duty as a patient advocate and of satisfying her conscience. The patient's daughter and the ICU dietitian were vitalists, conscientious objectors to euthanasia. They based their position on a divine source of authority and did not recognize the opposing opinions of the American Medical Association or the Supreme Court. In addition, the dietitian had a special professional resistance to participating in hastening death by withholding or withdrawing food and fluid, especially in the absence of written information stating the patient's preference. There is compelling evidence that Mrs. Günzberg's next of kin, her husband, is decisionally incapacitated by his stroke. The conflict can best be described as a clash of medical facts and religious faith.

According to The ADA (1992), the dietetic practitioner should set realistic nutrition goals for the terminally ill adult on the basis of an individual, ongoing assessment. When oral intake is possible, the dietitian is urged to use creative, liberal measures to increase the pleasure of food. However, the quantity of food and nutrient intake, as measured by meeting the recommended dietary allowances, may be less important during the final days of life than providing emotional support for the patient and family (Food and Nutrition Board, 1989; Sims, 1996).

Conscientious objection to passive or active euthanasia by individual health care professionals is acknowledged and respected by the American Dietetic Association, the American Nurses Association, and the American Medical Association. When either physicians or health care facilities object to carrying out the patient's advance directive on religious or moral grounds, the care of the patient is transferred to another physician or facility (Grant & Forsythe, 1987).

Although ethicists and legal scholars debate the theoretical constructs of informed consent and patient autonomy, it is the physicians who facilitate passive and active euthanasia. There is increased concern by the public that the decisions are based more on the physician's values and conscience than on the values and opinions of the patient (Hodges, Tolle, Stocking, & Cassel, 1994; ten Have H.A.M.J & Welie, 1992; van Delden, Pijnenborg, & van der Maas, 1993).

"Despite the clear guidelines, empirical research has shown that many factors prevent [physicians'] adherence to patients' preferences about care at the end of life" (Fried, Stein, O'Sullivan, Brock, & Novack, 1993). In a study of relatively noncontroversial scenarios describing critically ill and comatose patients who previously indicated in a living will their wish to forgo life-sustaining treatment, almost 50% of a national group of internists (N = 485) indicated their ambivalence or unwillingness to withdraw life support. There was a statistical correlation between age and religion of the physicians and their clinical behavior. Younger physicians were more likely to withdraw or forgo life support. "Jewish and Catholic physicians [were] more active than Protestants in their treatment of critically ill patients" (Christakis & Asch, 1995, p.370).

There is passionate debate in the United States about the prospect of legalizing active euthanasia as "physician-assisted suicide." It is wise to reflect on the Dutch legal policy and practice of physician-assisted euthanasia. Although there are vast differences in the criteria for this practice, Dutch physicians use a paternalistic view in determining when not to treat and when to hasten the patient's death, assuming that death is near and the patient is clearly suffering grievously (van Delden, Pijnenborg, & van der Maas, 1993). The latter occurs even when the patient has not requested that the physician end his or her life. Rendering treatment against the patient's designated wishes is likewise traditional in the United States. There is increased public concern that reimbursement is a bigger motivator than the conscience of medical decision makers. Economic reward is shifting from trends of overuse of very expensive medical technology to financial incentives to underuse of biomedical technologies (Meisel, 1995).

Case Fact 3

Although the physicians and Mrs. Günzberg's son are in agreement, one cannot underestimate the influence of legal threats by the patient, family, or staff to encourage "active listening" by the physician and the facility administration. The case might have played out differently had the son and the physicians not been in agreement.

CONCLUSION AND RECOMMENDATIONS

Dietetic practitioners have a professional duty to be active patient advocates. To accomplish this, we are encouraged to study and apply the seven C's of professional responsibility: competence, consent, communication, courage, compassion, conscience, and cost, and apply them to the daily analysis of nutrition care of patients.

The Günzberg case dramatically portrays the potential for confusion and conflict because of differences in perceptions and priorities of concerned parties. Each patient is an individual with his or her own unique combination of medical facts, problems, and interprofessional, interpersonal, cultural, and institutional influences.

Vignette 1 discussed dietetic practitioner competency, and communication issues of clinical decision making and legitimate role expectations. Assertive group participation may be needed to challenge inappropriate regulatory standards for institutional nutrition care. With the current emphasis on the "bottom line" profit, more energy needs to be given to validating the cost effectiveness of appropriate nutrition care, the economic impact of iatrogenic malnutrition on morbidity and mortality.

Senge (1990) provides an insightful, inspirational approach to maximizing management communication. The key to more effective creativity is "creative tension, the tension between vision and reality" (p. 226). If dietetic practitioners are to be effective leaders, they need to speak up courageously, with diplomacy, knowledge, and respect—respect for self, respect for the patient, and respect for the profession. We are encouraged to promote moral and morale building techniques of camaraderie, "esprit de corps . . . foster a one-for-all and all-for-one feeling" (Chenevert, 1994, p. 154). All health care providers can be inspired by the nursing code of ethics: "The nurse acts to safeguard the client and the public when health care and safety are affected by the incompetent, unethical, or illegal practice by any person" (Gorlin, 1990, p. 261).

Vignette 2 discussed the dynamic interaction of facts, feelings, faith, and financial considerations in the clinical decision of whether to forgo life-prolonging nutrition support for a terminally ill, comatose patient. Similar decisions are made for approximately 50% of hospital deaths (Smedira et al., 1990). The debate presented the competing interests and value judgments expressed by members of the Günzberg family and the interdisciplinary staff on the moral and medical permissibility of forgoing tube feeding as a means of passive euthanasia. Who decides under which conditions a tube feeding is optional medical treatment verses mandatory humane care?

Professional groups, governments, and corporations do not commit unethical, inhumane acts of abuse: people do (Blyer & Thralls, 1993). Groups of individuals who make decisions and policy make up organizations, and their behavior as role models and their written policies are important incentives for good or bad organizational behavior. The true ethical test of a society and its health care system is how the most vulnerable, disenfranchised patients or subjects—

those without financial resources, those with communication barriers, minority groups, and those without family or friends to negotiate the system in their best interest—are treated.

REFERENCES

Abraham, A.S. (1990). *The comprehensive guide to medical Halachah*. Jerusalem: Feldheim.

American Dietetic Association. (1985). Standards of practice for the profession of dietetics. *Journal of the American Dietetic Association, 85*, 723–726.

American Dietetic Association. (1992). Position of the American Dietetic Association: Issues in feeding the terminally ill adult. *Journal of the American Dietetic Association, 92*, 996–1004.

American Dietetic Association. (1994). Position of the American Dietetic Association: An essential component of medical education. *Journal of the American Dietetic Association, 94*, 555–557.

American Medical Association, Council on Ethical and Judicial Affairs. (1996). Persistent vegetative state and the decision to withdraw or withhold life support. *JAMA, 263*, 426.

American Nurses Association Committee on Ethics. (1988). Guidelines on withdrawing or withholding food and fluid. *BioLaw, 2*, U1124–1125.

Annas, G.J. (1992). *The rights of hospital patients*. Totowa: Humana.

Anon. (1991). *Medical Ethics Advisor, 7*, 1–16.

Anon. (1995, February). JCAHO releases reports for accredited facilities: Consumers should be interested but skeptical. *Public Citizen's Health Research Group Health Letter*, p. 5.

Baird, S.C., & Armstrong, R.L. (1981). *Role delineation for entry level clinical dietetics 1980: Summary and final documents*. Chicago: American Dietetic Association.

Bandman, B. (1978). Option rights and subsistence rights (pp. 51–61); The human rights of patients, nurses and other health professionals (pp. 321–331). In E.L. Bandman & B. Bandman (Eds.), *Bioethics and human rights: A reader for health professionals*. Boston: Little, Brown.

Bloch, A.S. (Ed.). (1990). *Nutrition management of the cancer patient*. Gaithersburg, MD: Aspen.

Blustein, J. (1993). The family in medical decisionmaking. *Hastings Center Report, 23*, 6–13.

Blyer, N.R., & Thralls, C. (Eds.). (1993). *Professional communication: The social perspective*. Newbury Park, CA: Sage.

Briles, J. (1994). *The Briles report on women in healthcare*. San Francisco: Jossey-Bass.

Brody, B.A., & Halevy, A. (1995). The role of futility in health care reform. In R.I. Misbin, B. Jennings, D. Orentlicher, & Dewar, M. (Eds.), *Health care crisis? The search for answers* (pp. 31–40). Frederick, MD: University Publishing Group.

Bullough, B. (1980). *The law and the expanding nursing role*. New York: Appleton-Century-Crofts.

Bursztajn, H.J., Feinbloom, R.I., Hamm, R.M., & Brodsky, A. (1990). *Medical choices, medical chances: How patients, families, and physicians can cope with uncertainty*. New York: Routledge.

Butterworth, C.E. (1974). Iatrogenic malnutrition—The skeleton in the hospital closet. *Nutrition Today, 9*, 4–8.

Butterworth, C.E., & Blackburn, G.L. (1975). Hospital malnutrition. *Nutrition Today, 10*, 8–18.

Capron, A.M. (1991). In re Helga Wanglie. *Hastings Center Report, 21*, 26–27.

Catholic New York. (1992, April 2). Nutrition and hydration: Moral and pastoral reflections, pp. 18–20.

Chenevert, M. (1994). *STAT: Special techniques in assertiveness training for women in the health professions.* St. Louis: Mosby.

Choice in Dying. (1996). *Right-to-Die Law Digest.* New York: Author.

Christakis, N.A., & Asch, D.A. (1995). Physician characteristics associated with decisions to withdraw life support. *American Journal of Public Health, 85,* 367–382.

Cross, A.T. (1988). Legal requirement of private practice medical records. *Journal of the American Dietetic Association, 88,* 1272–1274.

Faden, R.R., Beauchamp, T.L., & King, N.M.P. (1986). *A history and theory of informed consent.* New York: Oxford University Press.

Feldman, D.M. (1986). *Health and medicine in the Jewish tradition: L'hayyim—to life.* New York: Crossroad.

Food and Nutrition Board. (1989). *Recommended Dietary Allowances.* 10th ed. Washington, D.C.: National Academy Press.

Forcier, J.I., Kight, M.A., & Sheehan, E.T. (1977). Point of view: Acculturation in clinical dietetics. *Journal of the American Dietetic Association, 70,* 181–184.

Frankle, R.T. (1976). Nutrition education for medical students. *Journal of the American Dietetic Association, 68,* 513–519.

Fried, T.R., Stein, M.D., O'Sullivan, P.S., Brock, D.W., & Novack, D.H. (1993). Limits of patient autonomy: Physician attitudes and practices regarding life-sustaining treatments and euthanasia. *Archives of Internal Medicine, 153,* 722–728.

Geissler, E.M. (1994). *Pocket guide to cultural assessment.* St. Louis: Mosby.

Georgopoulos, B.S., & Matejko, A. (1967). The American general hospital: A complex social system. *Health Services Research, 2,* 76–112.

Golanta, G. (1995, April 3). Withholding care from patients: Boston case asks, Who decides? *New York Times,* pp. Al, B8.

Gorlin, R.A. (1990). *Codes of professional responsibility.* Washington, DC: Bureau of National Affairs.

Gostin, L.O., Turek-Brezina, J., Powers, M., Kozloff, R., Faden, R., & Steinauer, D.D. (1993). Privacy and security of personal information in a new health care system. *JAMA, 270,* 2487–2489.

Gostin, L.O., & Weir, R. (1991). Life and death choices after Cruzan: Caselaw and standards of professional conduct. *Milbank Quarterly, 69,* 143–173.

Grant, A., & De Hoog, S. (1991). *Nutritional assessment and support.* Seattle: Authors.

Grant, E.R., & Forsythe, C.D. (1987). The plight of the last friend: Legal issues for physicians and nurses in providing nutrition and hydration. *Issues in Law & Medicine, 2,* 277–296.

Hassan, W.E., Jr. (1977). Legal issues facing dietetic practice. *Journal of the American Dietetic Association, 70,* 355–360.

Hastings Center. (1987). *A report by the Hastings Center: Guidelines on the termination of life-sustaining treatment and the care of the dying.* Briarcliff Manor, NY: Author.

Hodges, M.O., Tolle, S.W., Stocking, C., & Cassel, C.K. (1994). Tube feeding: Internists attitudes. *Archives of Internal Medicine, 154,* 1013–1020.

Huenemann, R.L. (1981). Leadership and quality in nutritional care: Our role in today's world. *Journal of the American Dietetic Association, 78,* 124–128.

Joint Commission on Accreditation of Healthcare Organizations. (1995). *1996 Accreditation manual for hospitals.* Oakbrook Terrace, IL: Author.

Jones, J. (1976). *Bad blood.* New York: Basic Books.

Kane, R.A., & Caplan, A.L. (Eds.). (1990). *Everyday ethics: Resolving dilemmas in nursing home life.* New York: Springer.

King, D.G. (1993). Interdisciplinary perceptions of the dietitian's legal responsibility for lethal dietary prescription errors for patients with end-stage renal disease. *Journal of the American Dietetic Association, 93,* 1269–1273.

Krashner, G.D., & Balogun, L.B. (1995). 1995 JCAHO standards: Development and relevance to dietetic practice. *Journal of the American Dietetic Association, 95,* 240–243.

Knaus, W.A., Wagner, D.P., Draper E.A., Bergner, M., Murphy, D.J., Harrell, F.E., Zimmerman, J.E., Bastos, P.G., Sirio, C.A., & Damiano, A. (1991). The APACHE III prognostic system: Risk prediction of hospital mortality for critically ill hospitalized adults. *Chest, 100,* 1619–1636.

Kushner, R.F., Ayellow, E.A., Beyer, P.L., Skipper, A., Van Way, C.W., II, Young, E.A., & Balogun, L.B. (1994). National Coordinating Committee clinical indicators of nutrition care. *Journal of the American Dietetic Association, 94,* 1168–1177.

Le Gall, J., Lemeshow, S., & Saullnier, F. (1993). A new simplified physiology score (SAPS II) based on a European/North American multicenter study. *JAMA, 270,* 2957–2963.

Lemeshow, S., Teres, D., Klar, J., Avrunin, J.S., Gehlbach, S.H., & Rappoport, J. (1993). Mortality probability models (MPM II) based on an international cohort of intensive care unit patients. *JAMA, 270,* 2478–2486.

Maslach, C. (1982). *Burnout—The cost of caring.* New York: Prentice-Hall.

Meilaender, G. (1984). On removing food and water: Against the stream. *Hastings Center Report, 14,* 11–13.

Meir, L. (1982). Code and No-Code: A psychological analysis and the viewpoint of Jewish Law. In A.E. Doudera & J.D. Peters (Eds.), *Legal and ethical aspects of treating critically and terminally ill patients.* pp. 90–97. Ann Arbor, MI: American Society of Law and Medicine.

Meisel, A. (1995). Barriers to forging nutrition and hydration in nursing homes. *American Journal of Law & Medicine, 21,* 335–382.

Miles, S.H. (1992). Interpersonal issues in the Wanglie case. *Kentucky Institute of Ethics Journal, 2,* 61–72.

Murchison, I., Nichols, T.S., & Hanson, R. (1982). *Legal accountability in the nursing process.* St. Louis: Mosby.

Norwich Eaton Pharmaceuticals. (1982). *The RD and the MD.* New York: Author.

Pollock, S.G. (1991). Identifying appropriate decision-makers and standards for decision. *Law, Medicine & Health Care, 19,* 63–65.

Powell, T., & Lowenstein, B. (1996). Refusing life-sustaining treatment after catastrophic injury: Ethical implications. *Journal of Law, Medicine & Ethics, 24,* 54–61.

President's Commission for the Study of Ethical Problems in Medicine and Biomedical and Behavioral Research. (1982). *Making health care decisions: The ethical and legal implications of informed consent in the patient/practitioner relationship.* Washington, DC: Government Printing Office.

Queen, P.M., Caldwell, M., & Balogun, L. (1993). Clinical indicators for oncology, cardiovascular, and surgical patients: Report of the ASA Council on Practice Quality Assurance Committee. *Journal of the American Dietetic Association, 93,* 338–344.

Rusk, T., & Miller, D.P. (1993). *The power of ethical persuasion.* New York: Viking.

Schiller, M.R., & Vivian, V.M. (1974). Role of the clinical dietitian. *Journal of the American Dietetic Association, 65,* 284–287.

Schmitz, P., & O'Brien, M. (1986). Observations on nutrition and hydration dying in cancer patients. In J. Lynn (Ed.), *By no extraordinary means: The choice to forgo life-sustaining food and water* (pp. 29–43). Bloomington, IN: Indiana University Press.

Scialabba, M.A. (1973). *An analysis of role functions and competencies of nutritional care dietitians and dietetic technicians for use as curriculum inferences.* Unpublished doctoral dissertation, University of Pittsburgh.

Senge, P.M. (1990). *The fifth discipline: The art and practice of the learning organization.* New York: Doubleday Currency.

Simko, M.D., Cowell, C., & Gilbride, J.A. (1984). *Nutrition assessment: A comprehensive guide for planning intervention.* Gaithersburg, MD: Aspen.

Sims, L.S. (1996). Uses of the Recommended Dietary Allowances: A commentary. *Journal of the American Dietetic Association, 96,* 659–662.

Smedira, N.G., Evans, B.H., Grais, L.S., Brais, B.H., Cohen, N.H., Cooke, M., Schecter, W.P., Fink, C., Jaffe, E., May, C., et al. (1990). Withholding and withdrawal of life support from critically ill. *New England Journal of Medicine, 322,* 309–315.

Sullivan, M.D., & Youngner, S.J. (1994). Depression, competence, and the right to refuse lifesaving medical treatment. *American Journal of Psychiatry, 151,* 971–978.

ten Have H.A.M.J., & Welie, J.V.M. (1992). Euthanasia: Normal medical practice? *Hastings Center Report, 21,* 34–38.

van Delden, J.J.M., Pijnenborg, L., & van der Maas, P.J. (1993). The Remmelink study: Two years later. *Hastings Center Report, 23,* 24–27.

Veatch, R.M. (1993). Forgoing life-sustaining treatment: Limits to the consensus. *Kennedy Institute of Ethics Journal, 3,* 1–19.

Cost Containment and Revenue Enhancement

Michele M. Fairchild

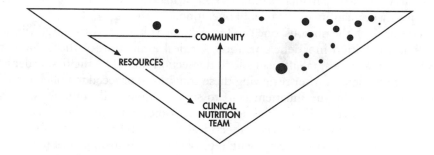

Health care in the 1990s presents one of the greatest challenges to dietetic professionals in more than three decades. To thrive in an era of cost containment/reduction, multiskilling of health care workers, elimination of familiar job descriptions, and a new alphabet soup of MCOs, PPOs, TPAs, and HMOs, not to mention an ever-faltering indemnity option, requires a creative practitioner who demonstrates peripheral vision to succeed professionally in a fluctuating health care system.

Whether clinical nutrition managers are entangled in the decision-making process of establishing a new patient care system that applies a shared governance philosophy or a matrix system, the institutional objective to reduce the operating cost of patient care services is a reality. The role of the dietetic professional in an operational redesign facility is the opportunity of a lifetime, providing a forum to showcase the multifaceted educational background and training of a dietetic practitioner. Thus with the reduction in the number of health care professionals at the patient's bedside, which is a primary institutional organizational goal of the 1990s, contributions to the financial objectives abound for the entrepreneurial dietetic practitioner.

Dissecting the clinical nutrition section of a food and nutrition department into two distinct operating units, this chapter explores the numerous cost reduction methods that can be employed to promote greater operating efficiency.

271

INPATIENT COST CONTAINMENT MEASURES: MANPOWER OR MATERIALS?

A rule of thumb to remember while one is undergoing a cost reduction program is that deprivation is the last outcome of such an effort. As a matter of fact, synergistic energy and an adrenalin rush result when managers discover the magnitude of the department's internal cost savings measures that never reduce the quality or quantity of the overall operation.

To start with the obvious, one can focus on the volume of forms used within a clinical nutrition inpatient operation. Critical evaluation of the computer hardware and clerical talent available to the section should be the first order of business assessment. After reviewing these conditions, proceed to collecting all the forms used by the inpatient staff to support their daily functions. This would include forms used by dietetic technicians, diet assistants, diet clerks, and dietitians. To ensure that an accurate critical evaluation occurs, it is important to form quality evaluation teams with representatives from all professional and technical job classifications. In reviewing the absolute need and value of each piece, these teams should proceed by initially force-ranking the forms to determine the destiny and value of each.

Team discussion should ensue about the potential for consolidating as many forms as possible to eliminate the vast majority. Remember, when this process is delegated to the user group, the users' empowerment in the redesign process results in group consensus and timely implementation. Concerns that are expressed by them in this process typically result in the team's desire to revert back to the familiar and to retain all that is familiar to them. Their charge must be clearly stated, however, with specific parameters given to ensure that the goal will be accomplished (e.g., reduce the number of forms by at least half, and redesign all the forms that will result in greater work efficiency). Because the team is probably looking at the actual use and functions of these forms for the second time since they were developed and has no hidden administrative agendas, the team will be able to accomplish this task successfully. The final acceptance of a redesign team effort should rest with the clinical nutrition manager, who did not participate in the quality team process.

One pointer for the clinical nutrition manager who establishes quality teams is to remember that team meetings should be no longer than 1 hour. The teams should be self-directed and have a team leader appointed by team members and an agenda written for each session. Availability of time in the course of the staff members' day is always a critical element of concern, but with increased operating efficiency and a commitment to the process, the team should understand the essential operating rules of self-evaluation/analysis. A specific time period should be defined for each team function, and multiple, short evaluation meetings should be held to maintain the group's momentum. Consideration should be given to establishing a warm-up activity for each meeting that would be led by one of the team members on a rotating basis. This would serve to divert the focus away from the tasks that members were performing before the meeting and refocus their attention on the task now at hand. These warm-up sessions do not need to take more than 10 minutes and represent the best investment that could be made to ensure group efficiency and effectiveness.

Once the teams have completed this process, the clinical nutrition manager should critique the teams' recommendations and provide constructive feedback for team consideration if the original charge has not been adequately met. Once the objective is met, then the production of the new forms should be scheduled. Typesetting costs have continued to increase exponentially over the years, so that a department computer would pay for itself, on average, in less than 1 year (contingent on the section's overall printing volume). Today's word processing software packages are versatile and include form and manuscript capabilities at a reasonable cost. Thus any clerical support individual with word processing skills would be able to produce camera-ready copies of forms for printing.

Negotiating Printer Bids

Much to the amazement of any manager is the fact that there is always room for competitive bidding. Today's economic environment fosters competition among printing vendors. Therefore, in collaboration with the institution's purchasing department, a formal, sealed bidding process should be pursued. The placement of form printing out for bid should consist of no fewer than three formal submissions, but more would inspire greater competition among the printers. Consideration should also be given to any in-house printing operators (i.e., the institution's copy center or print shop) to compare more adequately the cost effectiveness of these operations in relationship to the competitive pricing of outside vendors. After these sealed bids are formally opened with the purchasing department agent, a cost analysis spreadsheet should be prepared.

The outcome of this process should be at least a 35% cost reduction in the overall cost of printing, in addition to the reduction already achieved in having consolidated forms. A typical scenario could result in as much as $20,000 to $30,000 in overall savings with the elimination of typesetting costs by optimizing the use of clerical staff's talents and establishing a competitive price war among printing vendors. The purchasing department should be consulted to verify the existence of a rebate program consisting of local vendors in group purchasing programs of which the institution is a member, which could add another 3% to 10% off the new competitive price if the vendor that is awarded this new bid is a participating member.

Menus

In today's competitive managed care environment, menus contribute a large portion of the annual printing budget. Typically, institutions today change their menus at least twice within the fiscal year, accounting for a large amount of staff time aligned to this tedious but essential function. In an effort to ensure that all materials and staffpower are utilized effectively, a menu management guide is an added resource tool for use by the staff. This menu management guide outlines all the menu correction methods to be employed, the acceptable patient specials, kosher meals available, standard portion sizes used in serving, fresh fruit rotation list, acceptable diet restrictions to be placed on each respective color-coded menu, routine diabetic meal patterns, lists of foods high in various nutrients (depending on the institution), and any other resource material that will promote consistency in staff performance. This reference manual would be most complete if it included the order of meal service, cut-off times for trays, and an estimated tray delivery schedule. This menu management guide could be called a menu glossary because it is not taking away the staff's judgment but rather providing the needed resources to support their tasks.

The preparation of this guide would be in conjunction with the menu revision; the guide would be three-hole punched to fit into a 1-inch, three-ring binder, thus allowing for future updates or revisions. Although it may be felt to be time consuming for the manager, it is extremely cost effective in a number of ways after initial production, returning the investment threefold to the department. Staff participation is strongly encouraged in this area as well because they will identify areas requiring clarification that have consistently surfaced over the years.

Actual menu development should be evaluated as a new project at each revision. Consider the menu jacket and the number of colors used. Is the message from the department read? What size is the menu, standard printer production size or nonstandard? Are diets color coded, and is this necessary? What is the unit cost for each perforated menu printed, and how many of these menus are wasted each day when the diets are changed? Additional consideration should be given to those automated systems that produce another menu ticket after the patient has completed the color-coded menu; are there menu coding sheets that are also used to do menu production sheets or to generate other computer data? All this adds cost to the average patient rate for the department. Where does one begin in reevaluating potential cost savings from managing menus?

Consider the menu jacket and size first. Does the facility need as many specialty diet menus under managed care, with its reduced lengths of stay, as was once the standard? Is color coding for patients or the tray line staff needed? Does the colored menu jacket increase patient satisfaction, or are there other, more vital issues that are more valued by patients (e.g., getting what they ordered, timeliness of tray service, hot and cold menu choices, etc.). Value must be added today with more sophisticated consumers, and we must capture their needs appropriately. Choose a standard size menu, reduce the designs and colors used, minimize the number of actual menus, and, last but not least, type menus in house to eliminate typesetting costs.

Competitively bid out menu printing, and reduce the number of menus held in storage to no more than 6 months' worth, but get quotes for annual usage. This allows for maximum value and flexibility. The menu choices today no longer support numerous selections of culinary excellence but rather basic fare that is familiar to and predictable by patrons. Thousands of dollars can be saved in this category with ingenuity on the part of the menu management team.

Another factor that has been incorporated recently is a limited or nonselect menu for patients whose lengths of stay are less than 7 days. These will produce sizable savings in food cost, but to ensure patient satisfaction one must reevaluate the tray look, or the amenities used on the tray. Marketing such a program change will be crucial to organizations' success. Consistent and well-chosen menu items will also influence patient satisfaction. Maintaining effective communication with the nursing staff and conducting a focus group session will provide invaluable safeguards to successful implementation.

Formulas

All institutions have a nutrition committee or therapeutics committee that reports to the medical board. What has this committee done for the food and nutrition department lately? If enteral and infant formulary products are managed by the food and nutrition department, then why should anyone outside the department manage the budget? The nutrition committee should have medical and nursing representation that reflects all the various patient care specialties of the institution and allies who will assist in effecting policy changes where necessary. The committee can identify each major enteral formula category required for patient care, identify the specific attributes of each product required, and break these out by the ounce or milliliter to ensure consistency in the comparative analysis. Other considerations may be the service provided by vendors, printing of the new formulary for housewide distribution, the use of product reference books, the location of the distribution warehouse relative to the institution, and emergency delivery options. These products should be put out to a competitive bid for at least 2 years (if not 3 years). One vendor may wish to include free pumps and a reduced price for intravenous sets and bags. The committee should review the all-in-one feedings and modules in relationship to better pricing and staffpower availability (they are not always cost effective) and review, with the purchasing department, various manufacturer rebate programs that are available to the institution that may provide a competitive edge for the department in the process. It is important not to make any assumptions. A close evaluation of all pricing options will reveal some interesting savings to the institution and provide a greater efficiency in utilization of possibly costly feeding modalities.

Physician education will be a key element to success in implementing a consolidated formulary, and the nutrition committee members will play an essential part in the overall success. Consider developing a nonstandard formulary ordering form that the physician will have to complete before securing a formula that is currently not available, with the caveat that this will be a charge to the patient because a product is already available in house that provides for those needs. The going may be rough at first, but the savings far outweigh the challenges presented by limiting formulary choices, and the nutrition committee will assist in resolving difficult issues. Exhibit 7–1 presents an example of how one department put such a program together to cut expenses and limit the number of formulas offered.

Exhibit 7–1 Establishing a Cost-Effective Formulary

"Our new formulary was implemented in June of 1995," says Melissa Hansen, nutrition support dietitian at New Hanover Regional Medical Center in Wilmington, North Carolina. This 628-bed facility has an average of 35 tube fed patients per day. Along with two other dietitians on staff, Maria Stasios and C. Havrila, Hansen pioneered the effort at her hospital and involved other disciplines in the process by presenting a proposal to the Pharmacy and Therapeutics Committee.

The first step was to thoroughly review the scientific literature for justification to retain, add, or delete products. This information was compiled into a detailed proposal justifying a decrease in the formulary from 17 to seven enteral products.

"The information was presented to the committee in an easy-to-read chart form to facilitate evaluation of the data and to simplify comparison of the present system to the proposed formulary," reports Hansen. "Our proposal resulted in quick approval and praise from administrations and physicians. I think doing the background research and presenting the material as we did greatly contributed to our success."

"Physicians and administrators always seem to be interested in what the 'other guys' are doing," says Hansen. So nutrition support dietitians and pharmacists from hospitals greater than 500 beds across the state of North Carolina were surveyed to determine the composition of their formularies and this information was included as well.

Once the plan was approved, memos and pocket formulary cards were distributed and the dietitians began to monitor costs.

"During the first quarter after implementation, our enteral product costs decreased by 35%," says Hansen. "I continue to chart costs each quarter and expect to demonstrate an annual savings of $42,000 per year. Overall, it's been real positive. If they forget about the

continues

Exhibit 7-1 continued

formulary items, the dietitian calls them directly and this has improved the relationship we have with physicians." Hansen has found the physicians to be very understanding and frequently thank the dietitian for making an effort to contact them.

"Since beginning the system," says Hansen, "we've had very few problems come up. Out of more than 300 physicians, one requests an item that we discontinued. If a non-stock item is ordered, it is not sent automatically to the patient unit. Our policy is that the dietitian in charge of the floor goes up to review the case and tries to recommend something that is on the formulary list." In cases where the need for a non-stock item is verified, it is made available.

No negative feedback has come from the nursing department at New Hanover Regional Medical Center. The dietitians provided a pocket reference for physicians, and sent timely memos to the nursing staff regarding the change. They are considering the addition of the formulary list to the diet manuals which are located on each floor. "As with any new system, some still can't remember exactly what is on the formulary, or the lists get lost, so we get some occasional calls. But, there have been no major problems so far."

"Our pharmacy used to distribute all enteral feedings. Now, they only carry the more expensive elemental formulas and our department distributes all others," says Hansen. "The pharmacy staff was thrilled about the new system because they saved storage space and time."

Hansen stresses the need for continued research on the part of dietitians for objective reevaluations of the formulary. As recommended diet therapy for the different disease states change, so should formula composition. "The companies that sell commercial supplements will continue to sell their products as long as people are buying them," she says, "so it's up to dietitians to keep abreast of current research to be sure their formularies are on-line with it."

Source: Adapted from Establishing a Cost-Effective Formulary, *Hospital Food & Nutrition Focus*, Vol. 12, No. 7, pp. 1, 4–5, © 1996, Aspen Publishers, Inc.

Kardexes

When was the last time the staff reconsidered the use of Kardexes? How much do these Kardexes cost in comparison to a standard 1-inch, three-ring binder? Are colored flags used to tag Kardexes, and are more of these flags found on the floors of the institution than in the Kardexes? Routine evaluation of these issues can help to contain costs.

Reconsider the standard computer sheets available on each patient or service of patients daily. Is more information needed than what that is providing? Do the dietary technicians and dietitians all need to have the same information available in each of their patient care record sheets or cards? If a Kardex is attached to a patient screen sheet, what are the real costs and savings associated with these forms today now that managed care has patients in and out, often, within 3 days? Is it time to change the systems?

These are all hard decisions to make, but they are essential when one considers staff reductions or efficiencies. For the dietitian, consider a standard 8½ × 11 sheet that can be typeset by the department and three-hole punched for standard notebooks. Empower the staff to design such a form with essential information that is not duplicated anywhere else in the department. Consider what patient care information the diet technicians or nutrition assistants are collecting and how useful it is in their daily operations. Can this be a 3 × 5 inch card that can be printed in house, or can they work off a general computer printout that is routinely available through the institution's patient care computer system? The benefits of flagging the Kardexes without color tabs may be great; if this cannot be done, consider reducing the number of flags to a minimum. If Kardex holders are eliminated, a probable $500 annual savings on the holders alone could be achieved, not to mention the savings from eliminating the special cards that are rapidly turned over with reduced lengths of stay. Many area hospitals have realized more than $5,000 in annual saving when they have reconsidered their patient information systems; is this in your cards?

Formula Usage Sheets and Nonformulary Requisitions

How many full cases of formula go to patient units daily? How many full cases of formula are used each week? What type of feeding tubes and formulas are used on each service, and for what length of time? If the team members cannot answer these questions, then they probably can save money in this category also. The team should develop in-house, two-part formula case usage forms to be used as an identification form to attach to the case, with the second copy remaining in the department for weekly submission and tabulation. This method will help in maintaining an accurate inventory and reducing shortages. Another benefit is that unnecessary inventory (or "money on the shelf") will not be held. It takes all the guesswork out of routine functions while saving money in the process.

It is important to maintain an awareness of the various feeding administration methods used by physicians for their patients. This useful information will assist in defining bid specifications on feeding tubes and in managing employees' work demands. It may also provide the clinical manager with the opportunity to evaluate the appropriateness of feeding methods used in an effort to ensure that the least expensive treatment modality is applied. These statistics would be supportive in quality improvement monitoring in assessing the overall care management process.

One may think that these tools create more work for the staff and result in less efficiency, but this is quite contrary to the outcome. The department is passively generating documentation on the utilization of both supplies and staffpower. The forms can be preprinted to simplify the collection and recording of information using a check-off system for the items needed or used. Managers can also avoid unwarranted formula shortages over the weekends with such a system while eliminating the need to send expired product back for credit.

Office Supplies

How many pencils, pads, paper clips, staples, and forms do staff members use each year? Developing a supply ordering system for these routine supplies can save both money and manpower by coordinating the requisitions to a monthly distribution. Develop an order form for standard supply material that is typically requested, and have a space for name and service covered. Then designate a certain day each month for submission and filling of supply orders. Designate a pick-up location, and do not allow the staff to stockpile supply materials on their services.

Develop a computerized spreadsheet with the unit costs of the supplies, and tabulate these costs monthly. On a quarterly basis, managers should distribute a cost-to-date summary sheet delineating the total cost for supply usage by service. This will provide a frame of reference for the staff to manage their supply costs better and to reduce a considerable expense that typically goes unnoticed. Another added benefit to this system is that it will prevent a large volume of unanticipated traffic into the main office, which typically reduces the productivity of the secretary in assisting individuals with their last-minute office supply needs. Thus the system becomes predictable for ordering, collecting, and expending.

Diet Manual Development

Depending on the size of the facility, one can consider the following questions carefully when determining which diet manual to use. Is the institution large enough, with enough specialty practitioners, to warrant writing an individualized diet manual? If not, then one can consider adopting another institution's or the American Dietetic Association's diet manual. Consider the degree of uniqueness of the patient population, in addition to staff time and interest, to justify developing a separate manual. There are few unusual attributes associated with a diet manual that would necessitate this major undertaking. Of course, it will be essential to seek approval from the nutrition committee and medical board before adopting another institution's standards. Armed with the cost savings of doing so, one can be successful in obtaining this approval in writing.

If the choice is to develop a diet manual in house, recognize that it is a gratifying reward for the staff to influence the standards of patient care management. With strict deadlines and support, where necessary, one can effectively type a manual in house and submit a camera-ready copy to be printed. Typesetting and layout costs can be put out for competitive bidding to numerous vendors. A standard three-ring binder with a computer-generated graphic on the cover can look as professional as silk screening but will return a sizable cost savings to the department. Stitched or glued hard covers should not be used because the entire book will have to be reprinted for even small changes. Consider scheduling a meeting to have staff insert the typed diet manual sheets into the binders themselves; this will save between $1 and $3 per book in printing costs.

Patient Acuity

It is essential to collect patient acuity data on a routine basis. The method does not have to be complicated, and the benefits are many. Consider the methods used for screening patients, which determine the overall distribution of staff members' daily workload. Choose 1 day per quarter to tally the severity of illness for all patients in the house on that day. Then summarize this tally per dietitian service, and ascertain the complexity of work required of each dietitian.

Consider the shortened lengths of stay for the patient population, and determine where some patient services might be "consultation only" because these patients are not critically ill and generally stay less than 3 days. Also, rearrange the coverage of staff according to where their efforts would be better utilized. This may result in actually freeing up a staff member to provide additional outpatient coverage where an increase in utilization has been evidenced recently. The use of dietetic technicians in some facilities can relieve the overburdening of dietitians and place the workload at the appropriate level among the staff. It is imperative that this review be conducted quarterly because managed care continues to reduce the length of hospitalizations.

Standards of Practice

Standards of practice are not a luxury but a necessity. They should be developed by a clinical team and approved by the nutrition committee. Define all references that will be used in determining weight standards and calculating protein, calorie, and other nutrient needs. Define the growth charts that will be used for the pediatric population, and determine whether head circumferences will be an integral part of assessment determinations. Identify the various protocols to be used along with amputation standards or burn surface calculations.

Clearly spell out all the parameters that will be employed by the staff in performing their assessments. This can then be communicated to the medical and nursing staff, and it will act to maintain consistency among all staff members.

The question often arises as to where clinical expertise comes into play versus when assessment procedures should be standardized. Standard procedures will not in any way preclude the use of judgment in managing patients, but allows the other members of the clinical team and case manager to know where and how these determinants were made. They will also assist in defining expected outcomes and serve as a foundation in the development of critical pathways. When these parameters are written, the integrity of the practitioner is greatly enhanced, because managers can quantify how and why they have made recommendations. These standards could be printed in a reference manual for all staff to carry with them throughout their day or have readily available in their offices. They will eliminate the various reference sheets or cards cascading from lab coat pockets. Do not forget to include the facility's laboratory standards, the recommended dietary allowances, and the institution's accepted abbreviations for the ultimate completeness.

Career Apparel

Are uniforms or laboratory coats provided for staff members? There may be savings here. With the nutrition assistants, diet technicians, or dietary aides, decide what purpose the uniform serves. If there is flexibility to redefine the purpose of the uniform, consider business suits for the staff. This will serve as a statement about the essential roles that these individuals play in the patient care process. It establishes a business look in what may appear as a sterile environment. Involve the staff in the selection process, keep the suits simple, determine whether pants will be appropriate for the team members, and check with purchasing to determine whether there are contracts with vendors to ensure competitive pricing. Patients may respond more positively to people in suits and may perceive them as having more authority or responsibility.

OUTPATIENT SERVICES AND REVENUE ENHANCEMENTS

With the federal government clamping down on hospitals, it will be important to review the institution's guidelines on unrelated business expenses before embarking on any novel ventures. You may be able to cut costs and increase revenue by becoming more involved in the process. The example found in Exhibit 7–2 shows how this can be done. If there is flexibility in the system that fosters an entrepreneurial spirit, then consider which account will be used for depositing income. If at all possible, identify a separate account to track this

Exhibit 7–2 Hospital-based Nutrition Counseling

The first rule for managing outpatient nutrition care, says Deborah Konkle, is to have a reliable system of scheduling patient visits. Konkle, who is in charge of outpatient nutrition at Boston Regional Medical Center, feels that it is important to keep records of the number of scheduled visits and rate of "no-shows" and cancellations. She knows that when follow-up reminders are made via telephone or mail, the rate of no-shows decreases. "To assess the value of the reminders," says Konkle, "you can cost out the amount of time to make them versus the time that is wasted when people are not reminded and forget about their appointments." At Boston Regional Medical Center, dietitians are equipped to do other direct care activities if patients miss their appointments. "We do telephone consults for our home health care clients or early intervention consults during this time," she says. Konkle explains how she fills the gap with other reimbursable activities if appointments are missed.

Before their appointment, a secretary asks patients to complete a background questionnaire and a written three-day food record. These documents are the first step in creating a paper trail that is designed to satisfy the reimbursement criteria of third party payers. Historically, the patient documentation process is quite labor-intensive. Konkle worked with physicians to come up with a plan to expedite this process. About a year ago the physicians said "we don't need all the details, just use bullets or lists of what you want us to know and what the patient should do." As a result the process was streamlined.

Konkle tries to keep abreast of the trends in the industry. Proper coding, she feels, is essential for maximizing reimbursement. She advises that dietitians spot-check the accuracy of codes and billing to insure optimum reimbursement. "About three years ago," she says, "our bills started to include CPT-4 codes because failure to use these codes could have prompted many payers to deny coverage." The CPT-4 codes are used by physicians and other health care professionals for office visits. When the dietitians from Boston Regional Medical Center work in physicians' offices, the established patient codes are used for everyone because they are already in the physicians' system. The services are billed to third party payers using the hospital's provider number. "The key to implementing CPT-4 codes for our ambulatory care patients is to ensure that the essential components of patient assessment are properly documented," says Konkle. She now uses the term medical nutrition therapy more to describe the services provided to maximize reimbursement.

The hospital does the billing for ambulatory nutrition services but Konkle believes in getting involved in the coding process. "I have worked with the staff in medical records and patient accounting to make sure they do it properly," she says. Simple things like the wrong reimbursement or diagnosis code might jeopardize reimbursement. "In our department, we post all of the charges so we can keep a tighter lid on the charges generated and greater accountability in the system," she says. She has learned that hospitals may be billing less optimally because no one is aware when an error is made. Learning about coding and reimbursement can help dietitians to secure their positions. Being able to talk about net revenue generated by their services is a powerful tool in today's downsizing environment.

Source: Adapted from For Sale: Hospital-based Nutrition Counseling, *Hospital Food & Nutrition Focus,* Vol. 12, No. 4, pp. 1, 4–5, © 1996, Aspen Publishers, Inc.

revenue more accurately. With these essentials clearly defined, the following can be considered.

Speaking Engagements

It is best to identify a master form that allows the clinical nutrition manager to collect data needed to prepare a presentation to any group with goals and objectives clearly defined. Include the contact, name, address, and telephone number. Whether or not an honorarium is being paid, one should construct one portion of the form to include a cost analysis section to determine the profitability of the event. This will aid in determining fees to be charged or provide the needed data for justifying how much money was indirectly given back to the community by the institution delivering these programs. Another section should address the outline of the presentation, handouts used (these should be attached for future reference), and an evaluation section for the presenter to complete at the end of the session. The last of these is important in determining future relationships with organizations because they may not have marketed their program and had low attendance or were completely disorganized and took more time than was allotted, reducing productivity in other areas.

An ongoing education series with the same individuals might also be beneficial. When this is done, be sure to know what was discussed previously and what participants were given so that this is not left to guesswork or a former staff member's memory. Maintain this information in a large reference notebook for all to retrieve. This will also be useful if the department needs to justify its efforts in this area. Nothing in life is free, and practitioners must define their worth and recover expenses for all events. Group sessions are cost effective and even more so if the groups provide the space and do the marketing for an event. These days, each food and nutrition service that represents an expense to the organization must produce revenues to cover salary and overhead expenses to remain a player in a managed care environment.

Educational Materials

It is important to define volume and housewide use of educational materials given to patients. Consider a policy for inpatient instruction based on reduced lengths of stay and patients' readiness for learning. This last fact presents a challenge in meeting standards of the Joint Commission on Accreditation of Healthcare Organizations, but reference sheets with outpatient appointments will support long-term patient compliance and comprehension. Therefore, the amount of information contained in the educational material should reflect the majority of the patients' educational comprehension level and be age appropriate.

Consider multiple uses for these materials across the diets and make them interesting, or there will be wasted time and money. Although some practitioners have developed many effective pieces, if they are not filed clearly and carefully, again it will be money lost. Maintain a directory of materials, and date them. These directories can also be modified to serve as an order form for issuing to the patient floors. Consolidate where the bulk of these materials will be filed as well as who will file and approve them for consistency in delivering a unified message to clients. Have the inpatient staff order their materials monthly, as they do their office supplies. This affords the opportunity to keep lower inventories and predict usage from year to year.

All educational materials should also be costed out by service and added to the cost of conducting counseling sessions or lectures. Value added must underlie any and all efforts. If a service cannot be quantified, then it should not be done. If the institution is large or if it collaborates with other regional or area institutions, one can achieve a timely development schedule with increased volume and reduced unit costs. There is always the possibility of selling material to other institutions, but before a marketing campaign is developed, the benefits of this effort should be reviewed in relationship to time, money, and staff availability.

Salary Cross-Charging

Depending on the configuration of the outpatient facility, clinical nutrition managers may have the potential to charge the dietitian's salary back to a medical department. With the increase in team approaches and physician group practices, the cost of the dietitian's time when assigned to office practices can be covered. Add an administrative fee to these charges because there is time spent in developing contracts and managing. Relief coverage is an added value of these groups.

Educational materials should also be included in the general rate, which would mean determining an average cost and factoring this into the hourly rate. If reference manuals are to be included in these arrangements, consider these as a separate, one-time charge. Opportunities abound in this area under managed care, and outcomes are critical for acceptance into health maintenance organizations, preferred provider organizations, and independent practice associations. Care managers will only approve a defined number of counseling sessions, and they want to know what to expect and why.

Health Fairs

Food and nutrition activities can be one of the featured highlights at health fairs in the state because they create opportunities for interactive endeavors.

While planning health fairs, be sure to establish a fee structure to recover at least salary expenses. Unless the institution is sponsoring the event or wants to be prominently featured at any of these fairs, there should not be a booth fee of any sort because the information provided will be an invaluable part of each participant's experience.

Satellite Nutrition Clinics

Dietitians do not have to limit their business within the walls of their institution. They can go into the community and expand their roles. Space can be rented, preferably within physician groups practices where both office space and clerical services can be shared. Parking in the community is never an issue and patients want convenience and familiarity. Dietitians can travel to different physician group practice suites to be where the patients are while functioning as a member of the medical teams. The same principles apply to the fee structure in these settings.

The Managed Care Department

The clinical nutrition manager should be known to the administrator and case managers in the department of managed care. This is vitally important to ensuring the inclusion of nutrition services into contractual arrangements. If nutrition is not known or valued and is not represented accordingly with standards and outcomes, dietitians will be out of the game. The various agreements do not always necessitate a clearly defined nutrition entry, but such an entry must be considered in general capitated agreements. If this does not happen at the outset of these agreements, then an amendment is highly unlikely to be approved in the near future.

Managers need to reassess their professional position and the rapport that has been established by dietetic staff members with physicians and nurses. Are they considered invaluable members of the patient care team? If there is any doubt, define carefully and quickly the actions that can be taken to reverse this position. If the state has produced a cost savings document articulating the advantages of nutrition services to the overall care plans of patients, there will be an advantage. Do not only consider the third party payers because the Medicaid and Medicare groups are a market niche to be reckoned with today and in the future. They, too, have choices, and it is imperative that practitioners understand the ground rules of these factions in the new health care arena, which differs in each state.

Media

Is the institution aggressively advertising and marketing its services using the mass media? With administrative approval and the assistance of the public information department, dietitians can obtain a weekly radio or television slot to increase the community's awareness of the profession and the institution. Of course, these efforts would not add to the institution's budgeted expenses because dietitians would be invited to speak on the plethora of nutrition topics that consistently confuse the consumer. These activities do not have to interfere with the actual work schedule because they can be scheduled before and after a typical 8-hour workday. A picture is worth a thousand words, so television is the preferred forum. The example presented in Exhibit 7–3 will serve to inspire clinical nutrition managers to get more involved with the media and other community programs that can generate income for their departments.

Other good sources for information are found in the "Suggested Readings" list at the end of this chapter. By integrating institutional and community services dietitians can expand their horizons beyond the imaginable.

Exhibit 7–3 "Seamless" Health Care

"When I first joined staff in 1970, I was one of two dietitians here," says Kay Larsen, director of nutrition services at Gundersen Lutheran Medical Center in La Crosse, Wisconsin. Larsen now employs 17 registered dietitians at this facility which has an average patient census of only 180. In addition, she coordinates her efforts with one dietitian employed in their eating disorders unit and another in their teen health program. In her quiet but persistent manner over the past 25 years, she has successfully and subtly infiltrated the community by offering nutrition services on many fronts.

Larsen feels that the changes in the health care environment present more and more opportunities for dietitians and that their education prepares them well for the change. "If we don't welcome change and take advantage of the opportunities, we will become 'dinosaurs of nutrition delivery,'" she says.

The 500 Program is perhaps the most well known program from Gundersen Lutheran Medical Center. Dietitians work with chefs in a variety of community settings to develop healthy meals that do not exceed 500 calories. Consumers look for these meals because they are approved by Larsen's staff who are clearly considered to be the nutrition experts. Clients include restaurants, grocery stores, convenience stores and university food services.

"Our Nutrition and Lifestyle Center serves the local fitness and racquet club," says Larsen, "and local corporations use our nutrition, weight management, wellness, and cafeteria programs." Counseling is also provided to high risk, home health clients. Their prevention service involves risk identification and nutrition referral.

Twice a week, on the local ABC affiliate, TV watchers learn about nutrition as they see One Minute Morsel which is filmed in a studio right in the hospital. This program promotes very positive public relations at a time when maintaining a competitive edge is extremely important.

continues

Exhibit 7-3 continued

School districts also employ the dietitians. Services range from teaching nutrition in the classroom to menu consultation and analysis. For university food services, menu analysis is also provided along with a wellness program and nutrition consultation for sports teams.

Other clients include HMOs, managed care companies, nursing homes, and intervention for AIDS patients both in the hospital and through home visits. There is a Sports Medicine Clinic which involves dietary counseling as well.

And, if one may think that this is not enough to occupy the dietitians' time, contracts are also in effect with a local college for teaching and training students and interns who surely benefit by seeing one of the most progressive community outreach programs in the country today.

Over the years, Larsen has established her credibility; and as a result, she continuously receives support from her administration. The profit margins for her various programs vary, but on the average, she says, "we at least break even." Although some programs, like the "One Minute Morsel," do not generate tangible income, they succeed in establishing interest in the hospital's programs and work well as marketing tools. As a result, Larsen's administration encourages the development of such programs which benefit the facility in other ways.

"Departments in the hospital," says Larsen, "used to work in little microcosms, all by themselves; and they really did not invade anyone else's turf. But finally, we see the walls are coming down, and we are seeing an interdisciplinary approach to patient care. To me this is most exciting!"

Source: Adapted from Seamless Health Care: Dietitians Find Their Niche, *Hospital Food & Nutrition Focus*, Vol. 12, No. 7, pp. 1, 6–7, © 1996, Aspen Publishers, Inc.

SUGGESTED READINGS

Baber, A., & Waymon, L. (1992). *Great connections: Small talk and networking for business people* (2nd ed.). Manassas Park, VA: Impact Publications.

Barker, A., Arensberg, M., & Schiller, R. (1994). *Leadership in dietetics: Achieving a vision for the future.* Chicago: American Dietetic Association.

Conner, R., & Davidson, J. (1987). *Getting new clients.* New York: John Wiley & Sons.

Cox, T. (1993). *Cultural diversity in organizations: Theory, research & practice.* San Francisco: Berret-Koehler.

Crosby, P. (1984). *Quality without tears: The art of hassle-free management.* New York: McGraw-Hill.

Desatnick, R. (1987). *Managing to keep the customer: How to achieve and maintain superior customer service throughout the organizations.* San Francisco: Jossey-Bass.

Fitzenz, J. (1993). *Benchmarking staff performance: How staff departments can enhance their value to the customer.* San Francisco: Jossey-Bass.

Helm, K. (1995). *The competitive edge: Advanced marketing for dietetic professionals* (2nd ed.). Chicago: American Dietetic Association.

Hyatt, C. (1990). *Shifting gears: How to master career change and find the work that's right for you.* New York: Simon & Schuster.

Quinn, J., Anderson, P., & Finkelstein, S. (1996). Managing professional intellect: Making the best from the most. *HBR, 74*(2), 71–80.

Ramacitti, D. (1990). *Do it yourself publicity.* AMACOM.

Reichheld, F. (1996). Learning from customer defections. *HBR, 74*(2), 56–69.

Schiller, M., Miller-Kovack, K., & Miller, M. (1994). *Total quality management for hospital nutrition services.* Gaithersburg, MD: Aspen.

Seglin, J. (1990). *The McGraw-Hill 36 hour marketing course.* New York: McGraw-Hill.

Shott, S. (1990). *Statistics for health professionals.* Philadelphia: W.B. Saunders.

Management of Food Services

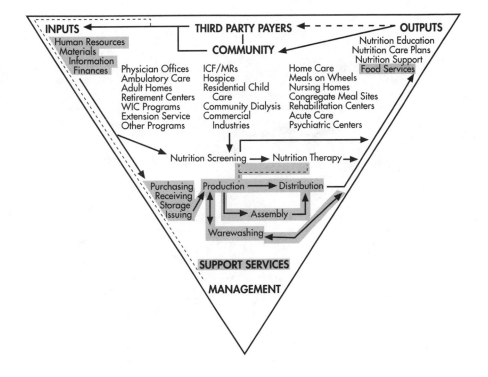

8

Trends in Purchasing

Thomas J. McCann and Jacques W. Bloch

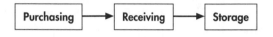

Purchasing ⟶ Receiving ⟶ Storage

In the managed care environment, hospitals and other health care facilities are under pressure to increase revenues and reduce costs. As a result, they are continuously looking for new ways of doing business. Food service often plays a major role in a facility's strategic plans for marketing its health care services. In addition, because most of the revenues generated from food and nutrition departments are from food rather than from clinical services, sound purchasing practices are of paramount importance to success. Food service purchasing represents 5% to 7% of a health care facility's supply budget, and it is often looked at as a source for cost containment. Now that the entire industry is being mandated to use resources more judiciously in terms of both supply and labor, the most effective and efficient use of these resources is required to succeed in the new health care financial environment.

These trends are complicated by the fact that food and other supplies are commodities that continuously change: Their prices change, their availability changes, and their character changes. Therefore, the buyer is presented with major challenges today. Recent trends and issues of importance to the buyer for food and nutrition departments are presented in this chapter.

CHANGING PERCEPTIONS OF QUALITY

Thus far in the 1990s, customers' food choices have been influenced by many trends in the marketplace. Health care food services are competing with the influences of the local fast food chains, convenience stores, and theme restaurants. They are serving a clientele that is more familiar with fast food than in the past. At the same time, managers are forced to be competitive with outside food service establishments without the lower price advantage they had in the past.

The level of customer satisfaction is also more important now than in the past as a result of the competitive health care environment. The quality of food is evaluated by customers based on the way it looks and tastes, its temperature, and the manner in which it is served. Customers want all their expectations to be met when they assess quality. Careful menu planning and proper selection of food can greatly affect the quality ratings of the food and nutrition department.

Trends in Patient Menu Design

The menu and its therapeutic modifications have always been looked at as a basis for teaching patients about nutrition. With the increased focus on patient satisfaction, it is clear today that patients will no longer accept many of the items that traditionally have been placed on menus. Either the foods are too bland, or they do not resemble the foods that patients are used to eating at home or at the local fast food restaurant. For optimal patient satisfaction, health care menus must reflect the clientele's personal food preferences. These preferences vary with age, cultural and ethnic background, religion, activity level, and many other factors. The preferences of patients and other customers are commonly reflected in the successful commercial food services in the region, so that menu planners and food buyers can learn a great deal by looking on the outside.

Budgetary constraints and the focus on patient satisfaction have made practitioners in health care facilities look closely at the traditional menu systems offered. Trends in menu planning are currently going in many different directions. Some cost-conscious operators are converting from selective to nonselective menus in an effort to streamline food and labor costs. Some are converting to the spoken menu to avoid paperwork and increase direct patient contact. With this type of system, the menu items are recited to patients, all at once, from appetizer to dessert. Patients accept the entire menu or are offered some standard alternatives for the foods they dislike. This normally occurs on the same day the menu is served, and food production is based on forecasted amounts. Nonselective menus provide the opportunity for food service personnel to produce and serve fewer items, so that efforts can be focused on getting a few things done right rather than many things done half right. From a purchasing and materials management point of view, the advantages are numerous.

In other settings, cycle menus with limited choices are being replaced with restaurant style menus that offer many choices in the hopes of pleasing the palate of many patients and customers. With the increase in competition in the health care field, menus are expected to be higher on administrators' agendas because they represent an important component of customer satisfaction.

A Blueprint for Dietary Operations

Regardless of the type of menu that is used, successful food service managers realize that menus are blueprints for all dietary operations. They determine the number and types of activities performed by most staff members as well as the sequencing of these activities. For the most part, menus and recipes dictate the costs of the operation and the ease of the purchasing.

With these factors in mind, it is clear that a team approach is best for the menu planning process. An effective team comprises the department director, clinical nutrition manager, production manager, chef or lead cook, and buyer. Persons representing the tray assembly and meal service functions should also be included, along with others who have an insight into the food preferences of patients and other customers. In some settings, it is even possible to include patients, family members, and other customers on the planning team. The buyer's responsibility as an active team member is to provide unit costs for all menu items and alternatives that are readily available for quality improvement and cost containment or reduction.

PURCHASING ETHICS

The buyer is considered an agent of the facility for which he or she is buying. Legal responsibilities are automatically generated with this arrangement. Policies and procedures should be available to set guidelines for the purchasing function. These guidelines will indicate that the buyer is the legal agent for the department, and his or her loyalty is with the facility. This requires that the buying agent avoid conflicts of interest when dealing with vendors and all other contacts. Policies should indicate the latitude for accepting free services from vendors that are currently selling to the facility. They should address illegal practices such as accepting gifts, kickbacks, "payola," and other monetary and nonmonetary "freebies."

Situations will undoubtedly arise that are not covered directly by policies and procedures. At such times, one should use acceptable and ethical personal judgment to make decisions or bring other members into the decision-making process. Practices that should be avoided include the following:

- giving confidential information to a supplier's competitor
- buying supplies without a legal bid system when superiors suggest a vendor
- allowing quotes to be shared between bidders
- pressuring vendors to lower prices through veiled threats
- accepting higher quotes without justification

- accepting "freebies" from vendors
- allowing vendors to sponsor parties or meetings
- allowing vendors to have influence or change a decision after an award has been made
- giving the impression that larger quantities are under consideration when only a small order will be placed
- having the entire purchasing, receiving, and payment system in the hands of one individual or department

GOALS OF THE BUYER

A wise quotation from the early 19th century English writer and art critic John Ruskin (Kelly, 1976) is worth repeating here:

> It's not wise to pay too much, but it's worse to pay too little. When you pay too much, you lose a little money, that is all. When you pay too little, you sometimes lose everything, because the thing you bought was incapable of doing the thing it was bought to do. The common law of business balance prohibits paying a little and getting a lot, it can't be done. If you deal with the lowest bidder, it is well to add something for the risk you run, and if you do that you will have enough to pay for something better.

Meeting Production Needs

Today, the modern kitchens in health care facilities are actually production operations similar to those found in the manufacturing industry. Raw materials are fabricated into finished products. The menu is the factory's production order, and the recipe is the factory's production specification. The purchasing function is the supporting component of the manufacturing process. It is an important management activity that should be monitored no matter who is doing the different parts of the job. A person knowledgeable about food should at least be involved in developing the specifications and monitoring the outcomes of the purchasing function. Departmental costs are directly related to the purchasing function. Poor quality and unnecessary expenses can result if purchasing is not done properly.

Many large facilities have central purchasing departments that order food and other supplies for most of the departments. This can work for food services if certain guidelines are followed. First, the food service experts should write specifications. Copies of these specifications should be made available to vendors with which they customarily do business. Specifications ensure that quality is maintained. They should include how the product is packaged, grades, and other quality standards that are acceptable. Many references are available to managers for writing specifications, and some of these are listed at the end of this chapter. In addition to specifications, the amount, date, and time of delivery need to be identified. A separate segment of this chapter deals directly with specifications.

Second, the buyer should feed information back to the department about market conditions; vendors' offers, especially "specials" for the week; items overstocked by the vendor; items of lower cost suggested by the vendor; and factors that may increase costs, such as cases where the written specifications might be hard to attain and a premium price would be charged as a result.

Third, the food service director must consider the knowledge and expertise of the buyer and his or her ability to acquire products that meet production needs. There is little sense in having menus or recipes that require products that one is unable to obtain routinely or that have a tendency to cost more each time there is a market shortage.

The fourth essential consideration in a decision to use centralized purchasing is the flexibility of the buyer. Inevitably, situations come up when orders must be changed or items added. Last-minute requisitions may have to be filled, unexpected catering functions may be mandated by administrators, and other circumstances may occur that require flexibility so that customer satisfaction can be achieved.

Quality at the Best Price

Whether buying is done centrally or by the individual food service department, the goal is always to suit the needs of production as specified in each recipe. Recipes for stews, for example, would not need the same fine-quality tomatoes as those for salads. A lower-grade tomato product could be used. The production manager or chef should be on the material specifications committee, or its equivalent, to advise the buyer what the products will be used for and which grades are suitable. This could result in significant savings to the facility. The chef would know whether chopped nuts, for example, which are less expensive than whole nuts, could be used for baked products because they are chopped up anyway. The production manager knows product yields, so that this person could best identify the fat content of meats used in recipes for roasting. The higher the fat content, the greater the cooking loss, so that the wrong choice could result in a false economy.

Using price alone as the prime reason for purchasing a food item could be costly. Value should be considered first as one selects the most suitable item at the least cost for the recipe or tries different items that do not compromise the quality of the recipe but lower its cost. In using value analysis, one would follow a product through the production process and determine the yields and quality that are expected. The goal is to improve value continually by buying a more suitable item for the same or lower price. This, of course, is an ongoing process. Some questions to ask to determine the best fit are as follows:

- What value does this item add to the recipe? Will the recipe have the same taste without this ingredient? Will another, less costly ingredient maintain the quality of the recipe?
- Are the costs of all ingredients in line with the overall cost of the product? Adding saffron to recipes, for example, makes for a costly product. Special mushrooms do the same. Are these specialty ingredients worth the cost?
- Will a more costly food product result in a lower volume usage compared with a less costly product? Small amounts of a pure flavoring extract, for example, might be needed to obtain the same flavor as large amounts of an artificial one. The overall cost may be less. One might need fewer pounds of a strong cheese versus a mild cheese to obtain the same overall flavor.
- Will other types of new products substitute for what traditionally is used? Soup bases have replaced stock pots in most kitchens found in health care facilities. The use of fully prepared salads has replaced the cooking and deboning of chickens and turkeys for chicken salads in many kitchens as well. Artificial seafood products have replaced scarce ones, such as crab legs. Tiny salad shrimp are used in most salads instead of larger shrimp, which must be deveined and chopped. Frozen or canned vegetables usually can be purchased at a better price than fresh vegetables, and less labor time is needed to prepare them for cooking. Knowledge of the products available on the market can decrease both food and labor costs. Careful analysis of quality and consumer satisfaction is important to include when these decisions are made.
- Can using the manufacturer's established specifications reduce costs? Use of the manufacturer's specifications, as opposed to one's own standards, will allow the buyer more latitude in finding products at lower prices. *The Meat Buyer's Guide* (National Association of Meat Purveyors, 1992), for example, shows institutional meat purchasing specifications (IMPS) that are universally followed for the cutting, grading, and purchasing of standard cuts of meats. One simply orders a meat product by its IMPS code. Because the cuts are carried by all vendors, prices are more competitive. Using special cuts or a butcher who cuts meat especially for one institution might be a costly practice.
- Will there be a benefit from cooperative buying or a prime vendor arrangement? Cooperative buying could lower prices and improve services

because there is bargaining strength in numbers and better prices would result from larger volume. Prime vendor arrangements ease the purchasing task and provide many other services that could benefit the facility.

- Will other vendors sell for less? Search the area market, and check references of other vendors. Sometimes they will sell at a lower price than established vendors in attempts to pick up a new account. If so, they must be monitored for price increases thereafter because vendors often "low ball" first orders to get additional business.

- Can the product be purchased less expensively ready-made than if it is made on-site? Products such as lasagna, stuffed shells, and manicotti are labor intensive when produced on-site. Frozen or canned vegetables can usually be purchased at a better price than fresh vegetables, and less labor is required to prepare them for cooking. While one is dealing with the "make versus buy" decision, three major issues need to be addressed: comparative nutrient composition, customer satisfaction, and real savings in the sum of labor, food, and supply costs.

- Will a more expensive food product enable an increase in pricing and perhaps even a greater profit margin? For example, specialty foods, brand names, or gourmet foods may have a higher food cost, but for cash operations they may also have a higher perceived value to customers. Value analysis therefore should include consideration of the food cost as a percentage of sales price with labor and other costs factored in.

PURCHASING METHODS

The traditional method of purchasing, where the buyer calls different food distributors, gets quotes, determines which distributor is priced fairly, and calls back to place the orders, is rapidly changing. Over the past several decades, there has been an increase in group purchasing, the process whereby institutions join forces in their purchasing efforts for increased buying power, which can lead to lower prices. In addition, as a result of market conditions, many individual specialized purveyors are being forced to change by adding more products to their lines. Because they are already experiencing the cost of delivery to an institution, the more products they have available, the more they will benefit.

One recent survey (Scott, 1993) covered 50 suppliers in the nation that had contracts with 10,941 independent and system hospitals, representing 1.6 million acute care beds and 6,686 nursing homes and other sites. It was found that the 10 largest suppliers of health care products reported data that accounted for more than 80% of total volume. This represented a 5% increase from the previous year. Small vendors are merging with larger chains to service accounts with larger purchasing volumes in larger geographical areas. Many facilities now use prime vendors, from which they receive the majority of their foods and supplies. In addition, manufacturers are now willing to sell directly to customers when volume is high. This cuts out the "middle man" and brings better pricing to the institution.

For the most part, health care customers are happy to deal with a limited number of suppliers because they cut their deliveries from many to one. Food delivery trucks are now designed to have separate freezer and refrigerator compartments where different food items can be stored. One delivery receipt, one payment, and one record entry all save time.

Another trend in the industry is that suppliers are trying to provide more than just the traditional delivered products. To attract customers, they are offering value-added services. These services range from help with menu planning to computer assistance for inventory control, purchasing, and recordkeeping. Computerization improves the purchasing process because of better forecasting methods, which enables more precise order quantities. Some vendors are electronically connected to their customers through electronic data interchange (EDI) for automatic ordering based on inventory levels. Suppliers are offering consulting services on design, layout, and equipment. They often provide nutrient analysis programs for menu planning and many other food service activities. Such services enable food service managers to be better informed about which products will fill their needs at a competitive price. Directors should take advantage of the services that are being offered to lower purchasing costs and improve quality of the products produced. Caution must be exercised, however, to ensure that unreasonable costs for these services are not built into food and supply prices and that the services provided are really needed by the institution.

Purchasing processes include informal buying, group purchasing, purchasing alliances, prime vendors, buying clubs, and just-in-time (JIT) purchasing. Each has its advantages and disadvantages. Most facilities use a combination of these to accomplish their buying, and they usually do this on a competitive bid basis.

Informal Purchasing

Informal purchasing entails calling vendors for price quotes over the phone or placing an order when suppliers call on the buyer. It is also called noncontract buying. Although this method enables the buyer to learn about the various products that are available, routine face-to-face contact with suppliers takes quite a bit of the buyer's time. Another pitfall of this method is when representatives push for orders, which could make the purchasing experience stressful. This tends to encourage impulse buying as well because suppliers often receive orders for items that are not always needed. In addition, friendships that could influence the buying process are all too likely to develop when this type of purchasing is practiced.

Phone orders are more common with informal purchasing. Most of the daily perishable items, such as milk and bread, are ordered in this manner. Fruits, vegetables, meats, and fish are usually purchased this way in smaller facilities. When frozen foods, grocery items, and supplies are included, it is helpful to get monthly quotes from suppliers by mail to decrease the time used each week to collect bids. If possible, one should take at least three phone bids if they are available. It is the easiest method as far as steps in the purchasing process are concerned, and the steps can be delegated so that no one person is responsible for all steps. It makes for a better controlled buying procedure. Figure 8–1 shows an example of a form that can be used for informal purchasing.

To ensure quality, the person who reviews bids and determines orders should do so by basing decisions upon the lowest cost for each specification that is identified. After filling in the bids from vendors, this person circles the lowest unit cost and then places the orders. There are only three conditions that would cause the lowest bid not to be accepted:

1. The supplier has a history of not being able to provide the proper amounts of the item required and tends to "short" the facility on the day of delivery.

Item*	Specifications	On Hand	Par Level	Amount Needed	Supplier 1	Supplier 2	Supplier 3

*List items by category and group by delivery date to expedite inventory and purchasing activities.

Figure 8–1 Sample form for informal buying.

2. The supplier has a history of not meeting the specification for a particular item, even though the supplier submits a bid.

3. A supplier would receive an order with such an unusually low volume that it would not be worthwhile for the supplier to make a delivery. Many suppliers have minimum order amounts to discourage this practice.

Group Purchasing

Group purchasing is usually organized by like facilities (health care institutions, schools, correctional facilities, etc.), or an outside agency can coordinate the program for many facilities. The purpose is to secure merchandise at lower prices through volume buying. Most group buying agencies receive a percentage of the total dollar volume purchased by each participating facility to cover their administrative costs from the vendor. Compared with individual bid buying, this method normally saves money, especially for the smaller institutions involved. The participating facilities benefit from an increased capability to evaluate alternative suppliers and products. Figure 8–2 demonstrates this capability and the amount of research that typically goes into the selection of suppliers for joint purchasing corporations. Needless to say, this is why group purchasing has become popular. For example, in the study reported by Scott (1993), it was found that the volume of goods and services purchased through group contracts increased by 14% in 1992 alone.

One problem with this method is that the participating facilities sometimes feel like "house accounts," without a salesperson to offer alternative products and value-added services. Another problem is that some facilities find difficulty in setting up reasonable delivery schedules with designated suppliers because many accounts are serviced in the same geographical area. Resolving this problem is difficult at times because the buying agency has little control over the suppliers' delivery schedules.

Once the facility agrees to join a buyer group, there may be pressure to remain in the group despite unresolved problems that may occur. After the facility joins the group, some difficulty might occur when suppliers are dropped for a week or more. Also, because there are so many facilities in the group, agreement upon certain standardized specifications is sometimes a problem. To make this a workable program, the participants must develop specifications that are acceptable to all. Cooperation and communication are the basis for success, and when these occur there are many advantages. The system must have a vehicle in place to deal with potential problems effectively and efficiently. Figure 8–3 shows one common technique for doing so.

Participating in group purchasing saves much time in evaluating sources of supply, gathering information on price and market conditions, testing samples,

SUPPLIER CAPABILITY REPORT

JOINT PURCHASING CORPORATION
1865 Broadway, New York, New York 10023

Return to_____

This is a guide to determine basic capability and should be used when inspecting a supplier's facility or when interviewing a supplier representative on a visit to Joint Purchasing Corporation.

Name of Firm _____ Telephone _____

Main Office _____ Address _____

Principal Sales Contact _____

Type of Organization: ❑ Proprietorship ❑ Partnership ❑ Corporation ❑ Public ❑ Private

Affiliated Concerns or Branches (Please list names, locations, interest, or operation)

_____

_____

_____

Initial contact made by: ❑ Letter ❑ Visit ❑ Other _____

Products Offered to Joint Purchasing Corporation:

_____   _____   _____

_____   _____   _____

_____   _____   _____

Total Sales—19___ $_____

Has the Company ever supplied member agencies of the Joint Purchasing Corporation?

❑ Yes ❑ No When _____

What agencies? _____

What percentage of your business is now with Joint Purchasing Agencies?   _____%

Annual Volume to Joint Purchasing Corporation   _____%

Financial Rating: D&B_____ Other_____ Principal Customers _____

Trade Policies: Method of Selling: ❑ Direct ❑ Distributor ❑ Other _____

Prices: Do you offer ❑ list and discount ❑ net selling prices, or ❑ cost plus

Union Affiliation? ❑ Yes ❑ No Name of Union(s)_____

Union Agreement Dates from _____ to _____

_____

Union Agreement Dates from _____ to _____

Brief Description of Union Relations: _____

Number of Employees: Managerial & Administrative____ Production____ Quality Control____

Production Control____ Engineers____ Office & Other____ Total____

continues

continued

Brief Description of Buildings:

Manufacturing— Type of Construction _____ Square Feet_____

Office—   Type of Construction _____ Square Feet_____

Storage—   Type of Construction _____ Square Feet_____

Capacity at which now operating:_____%

Number of Shifts   ❑ 1 shift   ❑ 2 shifts   ❑ 3 shifts

Hours per Shift per Week: _____   _____   _____

Machinery & Equipment:

Quantity	Description	Manufacturer	Age	Condition
_____	_____	_____	_____	_____
_____	_____	_____	_____	_____
_____	_____	_____	_____	_____
_____	_____	_____	_____	_____

Special Facilities: Training _____

                    Research _____

                    Other _____

Inspection Equipment: _____

_____

_____

Testing & Laboratory Facilities: _____

_____

_____

Remarks (Attach facilities photographs, brochures, organization charts, etc.) _____

_____

_____

Date_____ JPC Representative _____

Figure 8–2 Sample supplier capability report. Courtesy of The Joint Purchasing Corporation, New York, New York.

and interviewing sales people. Many groups also offer added value by conducting vendor's expositions, seminars, and arranging field trips.

Purchasing Alliances

In the late 1970s and early 1980s, many of the small local, state, and regional group purchasing organizations found that they could get even better discounts if

JOINT PURCHASING CORPORATION
1865 Broadway, New York, New York 10023

Date_____ Time_____

JPC Agency: _____

Telephone Number _____ Fax Number _____

PROBLEM REPORT—FACSIMILE TRANSMISSION
(If it is important to you, it is important to us)

The food department was seriously handicapped in discharging its responsibilities
because of unsatisfactory food or supplier delivery.

(Give complete detailed explanation—BE SPECIFIC!)

Date of Delivery: _____ P.O.#_____ JPC Contract Number_____

Name of Vendor: _____

Nature of Problem: _____

_____

_____

_____

Do you have any suggestions? _____

_____

_____

Please deliver this document to: Name of Buyer
                                     JOINT PURCHASING CORPORATION
                                     1865 Broadway, New York, New York 10023

Figure 8–3 Sample problem report. Courtesy of The Joint Purchasing Corporation, New York, New York.

they joined forces in larger regional or national organizations, which eventually came to be called hospital purchasing alliances. Although these alliances were primarily involved in purchases of equipment and supplies, they soon saw the need for consulting services in the industry and began to offer a variety of plans. According to Montague (1995), approximately 35% to 45% of the business that large purchasing alliances do involves the purchasing component. Some of the larger ones in the country include VHA, Inc., AmHS, Inc., Premier Health Alliance, Inc., SunHealth Alliance, UHC, Inc., and COHR, Inc.

These alliances, as well as the group purchasing organizations, are being challenged by the large multihospital systems and health care networks, which are finding that they may be able to achieve volume discounts on their own, without the help of group purchasing corporations or alliances. As mergers continue in the industry, some feel that the trends will reveal increases in direct purchasing by health care systems and networks because they will be large enough to do their bidding for themselves. This threat to some of the larger alliances has caused them to work even harder to expand the scope of their services. VHA, for example, now even offers some of its participants a chance to collaborate with other hospitals on managed care contracting.

Based upon these trends, it is important for the food service manager and buyer to understand that their work and the suppliers with which they do business are only a small part of a much larger picture in an industry that is changing at a rapid pace.

Prime Vendors

There has been a trend toward the use of prime vendors in recent years because of the consolidation of many small purveyors into larger companies that offer a full line of products. To enter into a prime vendor agreement, suppliers usually require a contract for 2 years and a commitment to spend at least 70% to 80% of the estimated budget on their products. Discounts are also usually based on percentages over the 70% to 80% minimum. As the percentage increases, so do the discounts. One may also be able to get a discount for receiving products on pallets during off hours. Whatever makes the prime vendor spend less to service one's account can usually be negotiated to reduce prices.

Cost-plus contracts are common with prime vendors. These types of contracts are based on the manufacturer's costs to the distributor plus a set percentage. This type of contract should be audited to make sure that the costs are truly based on the manufacturer's charges per product to the prime vendor and that everyone involved fully understands and implements the contract.

One major advantage of using prime vendor contracts is that they eliminate the time and effort of the daily bidding process. Requisitions to many different vendors are not necessary, and this could save a substantial amount of time. Another advantage of a prime vendor that has at least 70% of a facility's volume is that the sales representative has a greater stake in keeping customers happy. This person's commission is certainly larger from a prime vendor account than from non–prime vendor customers. Losing such an account would therefore be a much greater monetary loss.

One of the disadvantages, or at least a temporary problem, might be if the prime vendor does not have the capability to fulfill all the facility's requirements. Testing the prime vendor's stock and adjusting menus to minimize stockouts and special order items are always advisable. Using regular items that the prime vendor stocks for other customers will reduce "shorts" and make life a lot easier. As with other purchasing methods, it is suggested that prime vendors be given specification lists for all products that are normally needed. This will enable the supplier to acquire products in the correct amounts used exclusively by a facility. Often, large prime vendors have different grades of the same products available, so that it is important to make sure that the grade specified matches the grade received. For example, a product of prime grade should not be delivered and charged when an economy grade product is ordered for pureed items or casseroles.

Prime vendors usually have more services available than just food and supply products. Computerized reports on usage are one of these value-added services. Other possible services include the following:

- rebate tracking and automatic submission of rebates directly to manufacturers
- health care allowances, which are off-invoice rebates sometimes offered specifically to nonprofit customers by manufacturers
- inservice seminars geared toward continuous training of health care employees on a variety of topics
- marketing ideas to promote cafeteria and vending sales
- market forecast newsletters to keep customers informed about the availability of food products
- newsletters containing new recipes and menu items
- information regarding trends in food tastes by the public and research in the field
- electronic order entry and price checks of needed supplies
- management reports on buying trends
- reports showing patterns of purchases and types of merchandise received for different time periods
- annual food shows and demonstrations to learn new products and ways of using them (most prime vendors have a chef on staff for demonstrations and recipe development)

A note of caution: The costs of all these extra services are built into the price that is paid for products. It is therefore important to make sure that the facility is not paying for services that the food service operation does not need.

Prime vendors are generally computerized in their operations. EDI will of course be a benefit when orders are placed with these vendors. Many will provide a computer for the account if there is none available. Training for the system is usually provided as well, along with periodic reports of purchases, which are useful for financial reports.

Buying Clubs

Buying or "price" clubs are a relatively new form of purchasing for commercial food service facilities. Target groups are usually large families and small food service establishments. There is a membership cost up front for the use of these services, and cash payment is sometimes required. Wholesale packaging of products is common, such as number 10 cans and gallon sizes. Advantages to using a buying club include convenience, quick access for emergency supplies, good pricing, and ample product selection. Large health care facilities could use these clubs for last-minute catering requests or special products not carried by institutional suppliers and to meet last-minute needs, such as those discovered late on a Friday afternoon.

Just-in-Time Purchasing

Along with EDI, JIT purchasing is being used more and more in food service operations. According to Golden (1995):

> "[JIT] purchasing is a production tactic heavily adopted by manufacturing firms after the end of World War II. JIT systems purchase in restricted quantities, enough only to produce a specific production run. Suppliers deliver in smaller quantities, more frequently, with lead time to production severely limited. The JIT process requires and creates a partnership between buyers and suppliers." (p. 1)

The case study in Exhibit 8–1 describes how a hospital converted to this type of plan and thereby succeeded in reducing costs.

CHOOSING SUPPLIERS

As already noted, traditional vendors that carry one product line, such as meat, produce, fish, or groceries, are slowly disappearing and are being replaced by suppliers that carry a full line of products. Before suppliers are selected, one should consider the advantages to buying from a main distributor as opposed to dealing with a host of different vendors. Consider on-site expenses first and the fact that the average cost of a purchase order is somewhere between $50 and $85. Service is another concern, especially in the long run. Consolidating purchases and concentrating on service, along with establishing a good relationship with the distributor, will enable one to get better long-term service because more is at stake. Bonds must be forged with a distributor that has a large part of the business. The current view of a supplier is more like that of a

Exhibit 8–1 JIT Purchasing: Case Study

More than 5 years ago, food service management at the 418-bed Sherman Hospital in suburban Chicago began to explore JIT purchasing opportunities. Department staff spent months carefully studying potential effects on just about every aspect of their system. This resulted in the recommendation and a plan to implement a comprehensive JIT purchasing program in the department.

Although each institution considering JIT purchasing will have unique opportunities and requirements, Sherman's staff determined significantly important requirements to maximize successful outcomes. The plan entailed the following:

- *Philosophy:* JIT purchasing would become the nucleus of a total reorganization of the department, and all activities would be predicated upon the JIT philosophy.
- *Prime vendor partnership:* This was the number 1 requirement—a supplier to assist in planning, implementing, and supporting JIT changes.
- *Production systems:* Reengineering needed to include a modified ingredient room for all prepreparation for the cooks' unit, salad pantry, and dessert areas. Prepreparation would be done a day ahead, and patient, employee, and catering menus needed to be rewritten.
- *Equipment needs:* These included computer hardware and software and equipment for receiving, storage, the ingredient room, and production.
- *Diet office:* This system would have to change from hand tallying to forecasting requirements for patient and employee food service.
- *Information systems:* The needs included, but were not limited to, computerized inventory and ordering; a supplier interface capable of on-line, real-time information regarding product availability status; cost analysis; and status of incoming orders. Linkage with the supplier would have to accommodate ordering via EDI. Information for production included forecasts, ordering amounts, assignments for ingredient room and cooks, exploded standardized recipes, and usage monitoring sheets.
- *Ordering systems:* Requirements included a minimum of three deliveries per week from the prime vendor partner. A system needed to be designed for an order to be generated for delivery today and use tomorrow on a systematic, ongoing basis. Deliveries were to be completed before 7:00 a.m. to accommodate last minute lunch and dinner requirements. Invoices that were separated by product category needed to replace shipping tickets and had to include the department's line item chart of account numbers to facilitate payment. Daily production par levels were also required to replace inventory par levels.
- *Space:* Receiving, production, and storage space had to be evaluated. Minimum square footage was determined to support significantly reduced storage and product flow in all areas of the department.
- *Staffing and employee scheduling:* Requirements had to be evaluated because major changes would affect all areas. Scheduling patterns, ordering and receiving flow, production time schedules, and daily task sheets had to be developed and/or revised to accommodate the JIT reorganization.

Since implementation in 1989, many positive outcomes, related directly or indirectly to JIT purchasing, resulted. The prime vendor/JIT partnership resulted in food supply cost savings of 3% to 5% per year. A vendor rebate tracking program increased annual

continues

Exhibit 8–1 continued

revenues ($8,800 current year), and JIT-based purchase penetration returns contributed $5,000 in revenues for 1994. Prime vendor/JIT program value adds included placement of hardware and software for EDI with an interface to download data into the department's management information system. Additionally, programs are available for inservice training, staff development, menu development, product sales analysis, and cost/revenue projections. Under the former competitive pricing and bidding system, the department's supplier base included 50 companies. This was reduced to one primary, a secondary, and eight other suppliers. Real and soft costs associated with competitive pricing, bidding, ordering, handling, receiving, problem resolution, accounting, and check procession have been reduced 50% or more.

Staffing needs were decreased by 5.0 full-time equivalents (1.0 purchasing agent, 1.0 employee in receiving and storage, 1.0 diet office clerk, and 2.0 production workers). This was accomplished through reduction in workloads, job combinations, skill mix changes, and scheduling alterations. Inventory was reduced by 71%, from $58,000 to $17,000 on hand at any given time, resulting in a cash flow enhancement of $41,000. Storeroom space was reduced by 1,050 ft^2 to allow for expansion of the cardiac rehabilitation exercise room for a growing number of clients.

Less measurable, but certainly demonstrated, effects accrued to employee morale. As changes were implemented, non–value added functions were eliminated, systems and work flow became more efficient, and employees' sphere of control and participation broadened as a high level sense of accomplishment evolved throughout the department.

Source: Reprinted from R. Keith Golden. Does Just-In-Time (JIT) Purchasing Really Work? *Hospital Food & Nutrition Focus*, Vol. 11, No. 8, pp. 2, 4, © 1995, Aspen Publishers, Inc.

partner: a firm that will help the facility achieve its goals in providing high-quality customer service at the lowest possible price.

Performance Criteria

Surveys of vendors in the geographical area should be completed by purchasing personnel, and the performance records should be kept for all vendors. Purchasing agents will rarely forget a poorly performing vendor. They can usually give you good insights into a vendor's past performance, which is a lot better than the sales pitch from a company's representative. Here are some questions to ask while identifying performance criteria:

- Does the supplier meet delivery dates and times?
- Does the supplier respond to emergency orders, and how long does this take?
- How many rejections due to nonconformance to specifications occur per month?

- How many late deliveries occur per month?
- What type of phone service is used in the company, and what are the times of operation? Does the company use human operators, electronic mail, and/or fax machines? How are fax orders handled?
- What are the suppliers' practices regarding delivery stoppages due to late payment of bills? Are warning notices issued to the department using their products?
- What is the financial stability of the supplier?
- What is the company's history and number of years of experience in business?
- What is the geographical location of warehouses for 60% of the products you will be ordering? Exactly who will ship products, the distributor or manufacturers?
- How much inventory will the distributor have available for delivery and restocking times?
- Does the supplier have EDI, or will it have this ability in the near future? If so, could the supplier provide the facility with software, hardware, and training?
- Will the vendor allow initial and routine site visits to its facility?

Making Site Visits

While one is making site visits, there are several considerations. First, the general condition of delivery trucks should be evaluated. They should be clean inside and out, and refrigeration machinery should be working properly. Trucks should also be in safe operating condition with back-up buzzers that work.

The order handling processes can be evaluated as well. Identify the flow of products at the site. Assess storage methods, and note whether cases are stacked too high and whether they comply with Occupational Safety and Health Act regulations. Look to see whether perishable products are left out of refrigerators or freezers for lengthy periods of time. Ventilation for staples such as flours and cereals needs to be assessed as well. Evidence of traps, insects, rodents, or conditions that could hatch vermin should be noted. Control records should be available for these potential problems. While one is observing warehouse employees, their uniforms and methods of handling foods and supplies can be identified and their interactions evaluated. The order-taking systems should be explained, and the inventory system should be questioned. Learn how long items are stored and whether the vendor follows last-in, first-out stocking methods. Keep in mind that many of the same quality assessment standards that are used within a health care facility to determine whether foods are handled properly can be applied to the warehouse site for an objective evaluation of food safety. Figure 8–4 shows an example of standards that are commonly used for vendor site evaluation.

Completing Background Checks

To ensure that reliable suppliers are selected, the facility's purchasing department personnel are often involved in the selection and approval process. They normally check the following items:

JOINT PURCHASING CORPORATION

Legend: S = Satisfactory
U = Unsatisfactory

Plant _____ Location _____

Date of Evaluation _____ Guide _____ Evaluation Team ____ ____ ____

		S	U
A. Customer Relations	1. Usually the same person handles a customer's account.	☐	☐
	2. There is a customer service representative.	☐	☐
B. Personnel	1. Friendly, cooperative, and businesslike attitude.	☐	☐
	2. Clean appearance of workers.	☐	☐
	3. Employees smoke only in designated areas.	☐	☐
	4. Adequate lockers and restrooms for employees.	☐	☐
C. Plant	1. Area is clean and free of debris.	☐	☐
	2. All food is properly stored (i.e., at proper temperatures, on shelves or skids, etc.).	☐	☐
	3. Chemicals and cleaning supplies are stored separately.	☐	☐
	4. Storage area is free of uninsulated steam and hot water pipes or other heat- and moisture-producing devices.	☐	☐
	5. Adequate garbage or trash receptacles are available.	☐	☐
	6. No evidence of vermin, insects, or rodents.	☐	☐
D. Refrigerators, Freezers, and Storage Areas	1. Walls, floors, and shelves are free of spills and debris.	☐	☐
	2. Properly functioning thermometers.	☐	☐
	3. Appearance is orderly and neat.	☐	☐
E. Transport	1. Transport vehicles are well maintained, clean, and free of debris.	☐	☐
	2. For refrigerated or freezer trucks, proper temperatures are maintained.	☐	☐
	3. Cargo area for motor vehicles is clean and free of debris.	☐	☐

Figure 8–4 Sample vendor site evaluation form.

- criminal charges pending
- past lawsuits
- the principles of the companies
- compensation insurance
- current bankruptcy proceedings
- past performance with major customers
- discount and payment terms
- methods of billing (i.e., electronically or manually, monthly or as delivered)
- delivery vehicle insurance
- bonding of employees
- compliance with local laws
- union affiliation and duration of labor contracts
- past responses to changes in billing procedures

Communicating Expectations

The needs of the health care facility should be identified before a contract is signed so that suppliers are clear as to exactly what is expected. The more information that potential vendors have about a facility's inventory needs, anticipated inventory turnover, space requirements, specifications, receiving procedures, loading dock availability, and times of other required or mandated deliveries, the more accurate their quotes and services will be. If suppliers have to make assumptions, they may make them to benefit their company, not the facility.

The distributor sales representative (DSR) or salesperson must be given a set of guidelines that the supplier is expected to maintain. This acts to create good partnership relations. For establishing these guidelines, the following recommendations are made:

- Cold calling should be discouraged. Appointments or routine visits should be set up before the contract is signed.
- Telephone access to the DSR should be available during all working hours. Coverage should be assigned to another DSR during vacations or leaves.
- Common courtesy dictates that the DSR should go only to the designated contact person, not the storeroom or cooking personnel.
- Problems should be followed up promptly. Written procedures will avoid problems in the future.

- Follow-up of orders should be done by the DSR, especially on products new to the facility.
- Training in the use of products unfamiliar to the users should be done by the manufacturers' representatives.
- The performance of the DSR will be evaluated periodically based upon these and other necessary criteria. How well the DSR contributes to the goal of enabling the food service operators to serve quality foods while keeping costs at a minimum needs to be a part of the performance evaluation.

Other standards regarding routine communications will also need to be set forth. Such standards are of paramount importance to good relations. It is important to make sure that everyone understands the proper channels of communication. Institutions sometimes have a way of making everyone important in his or her own cell, and crossing over the wrong way may damage relations. It is helpful to all when a communications flow chart is developed for clarification. The facility's representatives must decide who has the authority to send regular or change orders and who has the authority to reject orders. Truck drivers have their own procedures for rejected orders, which usually require a phone call to a dispatcher or warehouse supervisor. Make sure that the most desired procedure is communicated ahead of time and that these procedures are followed by employees of the supplier and health care institution after the contract is signed.

Conducting a Trial

It is probably a good idea to narrow the field to a few good prospects and to give them a trial period, starting with the most promising first. Give the new suppliers several orders for evaluation. Be sure that the DSR is aware of the criteria that will be used for evaluation, and let him or her share in the results of all the surveys while having the opportunity to make corrections, if necessary, before the business relationship is confirmed or severed. Figure 8–5 shows a sample distributor performance report form that can be used for this purpose. It is important that the detailed information from this trial be kept in strict confidence. Even if a supplier does not meet current needs, at some point in the future the facility might find itself in need of the services that this supplier offers, and burning one's bridges may be a mistake.

MATERIALS MANAGEMENT

Materials management functions encompass all the tasks involved in purchasing, receiving, storage, and issuing of products. The personnel involved in this activity in a health care facility are trained in the processes of moving mate-

Distributor:		Period Covered _____ to _____			Date:	
		Excellent	Very Good	Good	Fair	Poor
Product Quality: Damaged products Freezer burn Thawed or refrozen products Dented cans Temperature controls Outdated products Off-specification products Other _____ Other _____						
Service: Timely deliveries Number of rejected deliveries ___ Wrong products delivered Accessibility of sales representative Follow-up on problems Incomplete orders Accuracy of billing Timeliness of corrections Responses to emergencies Notification of price changes Other _____ Other _____						
Description of Outstanding Products and Services:						
Description of Substandard Products and Services:						

Figure 8–5 Distributor performance report form.

rials into and through the institution. These staff members could be of tremendous help with the purchasing of food and supplies, and they should be made firm allies of the food service and nutrition department. Several categories of employees perform materials management activities. Buying agents usually analyze all the bids, and receiving clerks check items in.

There are many guides to the basic principles of materials management, which includes purchasing, receiving, storage, inventory control, issuing, and transportation of products. In this discussion, emphasis is placed on some of the recent advances, such as product identification through value analysis and EDI.

Concepts related to security and inventory control are included because these are two key issues for effective management of materials.

Product Identification

Today there is a great diversity of products in the marketplace and an increasing number of choices in the types of goods that can be used. Food service managers have a choice of fresh and chilled, fresh and cooked, frozen, irradiated, cook and chill, dried, and long-life packaged or canned foods. There are generic and branded foods. Trends that affect the home consumer tend to be carried over to the institutional buyer because consumers feel more comfortable with familiar foods. Menus should be developed to maximize the use of foods that are readily available, of high quality, reasonably priced, and best suited to the food preferences of the population served.

Mass customerization is a new manufacturing idea developed to produce products for individual customers rather than mass produce for many. In food service, this will mean developing methods to produce different food products from basic ingredients and still be cost effective. Patients who are unhappy with the standard menus will be allowed to request other foods, and kitchen personnel will have to develop methods similar to those in a full-scale restaurant to satisfy the customers' needs. The challenge will be for food managers to make their kitchens flexible enough to accomplish this task. This is where purchasing will be a critical function. Foods will have to be purchased to satisfy a new mind set of serving the customer rather than just feeding the patient.

There are three important tools that food service managers can use to identify the products that are best suited to their budgets and the population they serve: value analysis, standards of quality, and purchasing specifications.

Value Analysis

One method of ensuring that the products selected are appropriate is value analysis. This concept can be applied to everything that is purchased, including food, supplies, equipment, and services. Value analysis is the study of all characteristics of a product or service with the ultimate goal of minimizing cost and maintaining or improving quality. It is best if the entire team is involved in value analysis, from the chef to the purchasing agent or buyer. The following method can be used.

1. Identify the customer. Are the customers top executives who desire French style gourmet meals, or are they middle-income patients wanting a meal they can feel comfortable eating with foods whose names they can pronounce? Do the facility's administrators or board members understand the patients' needs as opposed to their own personal needs? Exactly what type of foods and preparation styles do customers really prefer? One can try to answer these questions first to determine the style of menu that will best suit the population served.

2. Prioritize needs. Based on actual costs and budget restrictions, the team determines the financial parameters that will guide the decision-making process. For patient food services, consider the allocated budget per patient day and per meal. For a cash operation, confirm the decision as to whether the operation should be subsidized, break even, or make a profit; if a profit is expected, what profit margin should be attained? From the average meal cost or selling goals, one can then decide what percentage of the menu items should be high and low cost. It is important to consider food, labor, and supply costs.

3. Evaluate current costs. Most computer programs are able to produce a report that shows the cost of all ingredients in a recipe. By adding labor and supplies to this figure, one can obtain the average production cost for all recipes. Some also add costs for overhead and energy expenses. Based on the needs established in the previous step, it can now be determined whether the high-cost recipes are worth producing. Consideration should be given to items that have high customer satisfaction. Avoid the tendency to delete all high-cost items because a monotonous menu might result. Balance high- and low-cost items whenever possible so that the perceived value of the menu can be established at a high level. Some popular high-cost entrees, for example, should probably be maintained for marketing reasons, and they can be balanced by other low-cost recipes.

4. Investigate alternatives. As the team members work through the menus, they can develop a cost standard for each recipe, see where the priorities are, and determine how they can get the most for the money spent. Decisions can be made for each menu item and its component ingredients. Items can be deleted entirely or changed, or new items can be added, until objectives are met. The menu items can even be changed to different days or different meals to cut costs. For example, if a selective menu for lunch and dinner offers one high-cost entree and one low-cost entree at each meal, the tendency for patients to select the high-cost item would probably be greater and more than 50% of the patients could select it. If instead the luncheon menu offered two low-cost entrees and the dinner menu offered the two high-cost entrees, a savings would result. Balancing the menu from a unit cost point of view is a helpful technique to master.

Computers are, of course, helpful in this type of analysis, but if unit costs are known, this process can be accomplished manually as well. Figure 8–6 is a form that can be used to compare the value of different options available for the typi-

Menu Item:		Portion Size:	
	Standardized Recipe	Product A	Product B
Cost for 100 servings			
Raw food cost (all ingredients)			
Labor time			
Labor cost (including benefits)			
Energy cost			
Supply cost			
Total cost per 100 servings			
Total cost per portion			
Product cost percentage (total cost divided by selling price)			
Quality			
Appearance			
Flavor			
Consistency			
Overall			
Average quality score			
Recommendations:			

Figure 8–6 Value analysis of alternative products.

cal "make versus buy" purchasing decision. As shown in this example, when products are sold in a cash operation, potential profit can be included in the analysis. The form includes quality aspects as well.

5. *Project future costs.* Depending upon how extensively one is able to apply value analysis, it is indeed possible to identify the approximate annual cost of a given menu. The team will be able to ascertain which ingredients and recipes are economy products and which ones are expensive products. In the end, this would allow one to come up with an acceptable menu with the best mix of products in an objective fashion.

Standards of Quality

Standards of quality are used by food service managers to identify the characteristics of final products that have been found to be acceptable for their patients or customers. Depending upon the purpose of food evaluation, one has a choice of how quality is determined. One may establish set criteria as the basis for comparison of new products, or one may use the personal preferences of panelists who reflect the target population. One advantage of preestablished criteria is that all panelists objectively evaluate food samples based on one well-known standard. For example, Exhibit 8–2 provides appearance, texture, and flavor criteria for several types of foods.

To do this, one must know the characteristics that are preferred by customers. If the majority of patients or customers do not agree with the criteria that are used, the menu item will be unsatisfactory. For example, in some communities in the south, vegetables must be cooked past the crisp stage before they are accepted. Everyone knows that nutritive value and color both deteriorate when this is done, but the fact of the matter is that patients will benefit more by eating an overcooked vegetable than no vegetable at all. Therefore, the standard should be based upon patient food preferences in such a case. Once the desired characteristics of food products are known, they can be documented and listed on a form that can be used as the basis for routine product evaluation. Such a tool is shown in Figure 8–7 for meat products.

If the personal food preferences of taste panelists are used as a basis for product evaluation, a more generic method can be used for product evaluation. A form can be designed that simply lists the common characteristics, such as appearance, flavor, consistency, and overall acceptability. A Likert type scale ranging from very acceptable to very unacceptable for each characteristic will enable scoring of each food sample. Scores can be averaged for comparative purposes. This system works well when the panelists are actual patients or customers. It can be used in the long-term care setting and conducted at resident council meetings, and it works well for selected cafeteria customers to evaluate new products. Once the preferred products are known, recipes and purchasing specifications can be finalized.

Purchasing Specifications

To serve quality meals, one must use ingredients of a suitable quality. Use of purchasing specifications is the only guaranteed method of ensuring the receipt of products that meet quality expectations. Specifications are best developed by the team that plans menus and recipes. In this way, the ingredients that are selected will ensure satisfactory end products. A specification is simply a statement of the

Exhibit 8–2 Standards of Quality for Selected Foods

Eggs

Appearance—Color of white is opaque white, yolk is bright yellow, and there is no evidence of greening. Portions are uniform in size. Syneresis has not occurred. Product appears moist, not dry. There is no visible oil or fat.
Texture—Eggs are tender, not rubbery. They are completely coagulated but not dry.
Flavor—Eggs are lightly seasoned and have no off or burned flavors.

Poultry Entrees

Appearance—Color is opaque white or natural brown and no red color is apparent, even around bones. Portions are uniform in size. Exterior is golden brown but not burned. Product appears moist, not dry. There is no visible oil or fat. Garnish is edible and appropriate for the dish.
Texture—Poultry is easily cut with a fork, holds together, and is moist.
Flavor—Poultry is seasoned with a pleasant balance of seasonings. It is juicy and does not have an off flavor or burned taste.

Meat Patties and Loaves

Appearance—Color is golden brown with no burned edges. Serving portions are uniform in size. Product appears moist, not dry or wet. There is no visible oil or fat. Garnish is edible and appropriate for the product.
Texture—Patties and loaves can be cut with a fork. They have a definable texture, not pasty or gummy, and have no evidence of meat cartilage, bone, or gristle.
Flavor—Product is seasoned with a tasty balance of herbs, spices, and salt. There is no raw, burned, or greasy taste.

Fish Entrees

Appearance—Color is opaque white or salmon pink. Portions are uniform in size. Exterior is not burned and product appears moist, not dry. There is no visible oil or fat. Garnish is edible and appropriate for the dish.
Texture—Product flakes easily with a fork, holds together, and is moist.
Flavor—Fish is seasoned with a pleasant balance of herbs, spices, and salt. It is juicy and does not have a strong fishy flavor or an off flavor.

Rice, Legumes, and Pasta

Appearance—Color is clear and distinctive. Grains, legumes, and pasta are whole and well formed. Product appears moist but not watery. No oil or fat is visible in the final product. Garnish is edible and appropriate to the product.
Texture—Product is soft and tender but not mushy. Product is moist, not dry. Pieces are individual, not gummy.
Flavor—Product does not have a raw or starchy taste. It is well seasoned but not to excess. Product is free from scorched or burned taste.

continues

Exhibit 8–2 continued

Vegetables

Appearance—Color is clear and bright. Pieces are similar in size, moist, and plump. There is no visible oil or fat. Garnish is edible and appropriate for the dish.
Texture—Vegetables are tender but slightly crisp. All pieces have the same texture.
Flavor—Vegetables have a definite fresh flavor with a tasty blend of seasonings.

Sweet Breads

Appearance—Colors are evenly light to golden brown. Size is no less than 3 inches and no greater than 5 inches in diameter, and thickness is at least 1/2 inch. Icing extends to edges. Fillings, if any, are clear and distinct. Fruits and nuts in fillings and glazes are bite size and of uniform size.
Texture—Crumbs are moist and tender, not doughy. Texture is even throughout. Icing is smooth and creamy.
Flavor—Breads are fresh tasting with no rancid or bitter taste. Breads and icings are slightly sweet, neither too salty nor too sweet.

Source: Reprinted from K. Ruf, *Quality Control, Quality Assurance Manual for Food and Nutrition Services,* © 1989, Aspen Publishers, Inc.

desired charactistics of a product, including any tolerance variations that would be allowed. Specifications can be written for branded products as well, whereby the buyer accepts by brand name. For other foods, performance criteria or U.S. standards can be used. The important issue for developing specifications is to research the products that are available in the area. Products with specifications that are too tight will usually cost more or may be impossible to obtain. Well-written specifications have the following characteristics:

- They are simple to understand and clearly written.
- They include standard products, such as IMPS or U.S. Department of Agriculture grades.
- They identify the market form and type of packaging.
- They state the size of each container in a case.
- They give counts per case or container or sizing of items such as fresh fruits.
- They give weight or other unit on which price will be quoted.
- They use national standards whenever possible.
- They describe temperature standards for delivery.
- They include brand if the product is a branded item or if certain brands are acceptable.

Panelist #_____		Sample #_____	Date_____
	Yes	**No**	**Comments**
Appearance			
Color is pinkish brown to brown for beef, evenly brown for pork, lamb, or veal, with no evidence of green or gray tinge			
Portions are uniform in size			
Exterior is browned but not burned			
Product appears moist, not dry or crumbly			
Visible fat is less than 5% of serving			
Texture			
Product can be pierced with a fork with a minimum of pressure			
Product is firm and moist			
Flavor			
Meat is seasoned with a pleasant balance of herbs, spices, and salt			
Meat is juicy			
Meat does not have any off flavors or burned flavors			
Service temperature			
Temperature, as served, is no lower than 145°F and no greater than 180°F			
Totals			
Acceptability %			

Figure 8–7 Sensory evaluation based upon preestablished criteria: Meat entrees. *Source:* Reprinted from K. Ruf, *Quality Control, Quality Assurance Manual for Food and Nutrition Services,* © 1989, Aspen Publishers, Inc.

- They have availability from several distributors so that the items will draw several price quotes.

For meat, the commodity that takes a substantial part of the food budget, specifications from the *Meat Buyer's Guide* of the National Association of Meat Purveyors (1992) will ensure complete understanding of the exact items that are expected. Other guides are commonly available in the industry.

There are two major advantages of having written specifications for food and supplies. First, suppliers know exactly what is needed. Second and equally important, specifications are used as a basis for training employees to evaluate the goods that are received at the facility. In addition to specifications, the tools that employees need to perform their jobs successfully include copies of purchase orders, large-volume and portion control scales, and other measurement devices such as temperature gauges and instruments for measuring the fat content of meats. Routine quality control audits should be made to ensure that products are properly checked in so that the manager knows that the facility is receiving exactly what is ordered and paid for.

Branded Foods

Branded foods have the ability to raise the perception of a quality service because everyone is familiar with and trusts the brands. When included with menu items, branded items may upgrade the quality of the whole meal presentation. Consumers willingly accept brand names they are familiar with and like. A quick way to upgrade patient tray presentation is to purchase a few branded condiments and prepackaged items. Brand names tend to give food credibility.

There is a trend in the field toward contracting with restaurant and fast food chains that can open up storefronts or branded food outlets inside health care facilities for the purpose of serving employees and guests. Many considerations need to be made when one is planning this type of project. Figure 8–8 shows a form that can be used in considering important points in selecting alternative suppliers for the service.

As with similar projects, a request for proposal (RFP) is normally sent to interested vendors. Their ability to develop a branded food facility reflects their capability, resources, talent, staffpower, and expertise in designing, developing, implementing, and administering the project. Experience in providing concession services in the health care environment is important. Originality and creativity of the RFP response demonstrate the vendor's earnest desire to provide unique services. Plans for capital improvements that are needed and identified in the RFP should also be evaluated. The vendor's commission and price schedules should be submitted and evaluated, and the variety of foods and services that are proposed need to be assessed. Options such as food delivery services and catering are important to consider as well. One should learn and evaluate the sales history of the vendor's other concessions, especially those at similar sites. Visits to these facilities are helpful in determining potential problems, quality, and cost effectiveness. Any promotions or discounts that are proposed

Selected Criteria*	Vendor A	Vendor B	Vendor C
1. Ability to develop project			
2. Experience			
3. Originality			
4. Capital improvement plans			
5. Commissions			
6. Price and variety of food			
7. Variety of services			
8. Sales history			
9. Promotions			
10. Customer satisfaction			
11. Service improvements			
12. Marketing			
13. Ability to work with facility staff			
14. Equal Opportunity Employment policy			
15. References			
Totals			

*Vendors are rated on a scale of 0 to 4, 4 being the highest possible rating. The use of 0 indicates that the criterion was not addressed by the proposal, and 4 indicates that the proposal exceeds the requirements.

Figure 8–8 Proposal evaluation form for branded food outlet. *Source:* Data from the Bronx Municipal Hospital Center, Bronx, New York.

can be evaluated as well. The vendor's recognition of the vital role of satisfaction for hospital staff, visitors, and patients is an essential element, along with the ability to make qualitative service improvements. The vendor also needs to be able to work well with the facility's staff and comply with the policies of the institution.

EDI

As noted earlier in this chapter, EDI represents a significant improvement in materials management. This technology is used extensively in the manufacturing industry for order placement, inventory referencing, and pricing. The electronic placement of orders eliminates phone, fax, and in-person ordering. Most users of EDI find that electronic links with major trading partners help build better working relationships. Errors and wasteful procedures are reduced, and this creates better business relationships between the buyer and seller. Some major features of a trading partner using EDI include the following:

- An inventory master list containing products from all suppliers can be built and maintained. The customer controls the sequence of products.
- The unit of inventory is determined by the user. This flexibility allows an item sold by the pound, for instance, to be inventoried by the case, or vice versa.
- Inventory value can be calculated on demand at any time.
- Costs of products bought could be updated automatically.
- The products that have increased in cost, and how much they have increased, can be determined by generating a cost comparison report, which compares current inventory with a previous one.
- Purchase orders can be created from the inventory and be automatically transmitted to suppliers.
- New items ordered could be automatically added to the inventory file.
- Shelf labels could be printed from the inventory file, and the capability for bar coding exists.
- Product availability could be accessed through the computer before ordering.
- Purchase history reports are available on line from each distributor.
- Access to account status (i.e., how much is owed and for how long) is possible.
- Value-added services could include electronic access to a recipe library, results of nutritional analysis of a manufacturer's product, ingredient lists, and even pictures of the products.
- E-mail can resolve problems with delivery or be used to summon the sales representative for product information.

It is expected that EDI will be used exclusively in commerce by the year 2000. As costs continue to escalate in the health care field, EDI will be used for billing, accounts payable, and purchasing and wherever paper forms are presently being used. This should help contain labor costs and improve accuracy and efficiency of materials management functions.

Security and Control

Whether or not the materials management department is involved in the handling of food service products, it is best when various purchasing functions are shared because this eliminates a tendency for the same person to receive quotes, make the buying decision, receive the merchandise, and make approvals for payment. Spreading out these responsibilities is highly recommended for optimal financial control. This will also reduce the chance of any one person being tempted to engage in any wrongdoing. Appropriate materials management procedures are always written to protect the facility from giving too much responsibility to one employee.

The materials management department is often responsible for recording serial numbers and marking all equipment received. An inventory of assets is normally completed annually to account for property. Food and supply inventories are taken more frequently, and it is a good practice to monitor them closely to determine whether strict controls are being used. Security is the responsibility of all staff members, not just the security department. Food and supplies are always a temptation and require constant lock-up. Theft could increase food service costs considerably.

Kitchen workers sometimes seem to have the idea that they are in their own home kitchens. Strict discipline and control are required for both security and sanitary handling of products. All kitchens should have policies and procedures on theft so that employees know the measures that will be taken should they be found to have unauthorized possession of property on or off the facility's premises. These standards guide supervisors as well so that they are better equipped to act effectively in situations where they suspect or actually observe persons violating the standards.

An age-old problem in kitchens is whether employees should be allowed to eat or take home leftover foods. This issue should be discussed with appropriate individuals from administration, personnel, and security so that a specific philosophy and guidelines can be developed. The universal rules that are established should avoid favoritism and need to apply to everyone—buyers, receiving clerks, food service workers, supervisors, managers, and so forth—to prevent theft. Exhibit 8–3 shows such a policy statement with procedures for implementation.

One alternative to allowing the practice of employee removal of leftover food is to donate it to a homeless shelter, if the food is safe. Regarding the eating of foods on the job, policies should state that employees are encouraged to taste foods to determine whether they are safe and of high quality for customer service but that this is to be done only in small amounts using the proper techniques. Health care managers need to have firm guidelines and to incorporate their content into the inservice training program, obtaining signatures from employees who receive this training. If rules are lax, employees may take food and store it in lockers until the end of a shift, creating problems with vermin. The products that are ordered for patients' service will not be available when needed. To ensure strict inventory control, the supervisor in charge of storage needs to be aware of missing stock and

Exhibit 8–3 Sample Policy and Procedure for Unauthorized Possession of Hospital Property

Policy

Hospital property, food or otherwise, should not be taken from the premises without permission from the director of the department or his or her designee who provides written authorization.

Procedures

1. **Removal of Hospital Property**
   (a) Before any item that belongs to the hospital is removed by an employee, the employee must first get a package pass from the director of food and nutrition services or that person's designee and then show this pass to security when he or she leaves the hospital premises.
   (b) All food or scraps from soiled patient trays or pots are considered potentially hazardous and should be thrown away immediately. Employees are not granted permission to take these foods, even if patients have not completely consumed them.
   (c) Food service supervisors who are in charge of meal service identify foods from the food production, tray assembly, and cafeteria areas that are safe for future food consumption. They are properly dated, labeled, and sealed. Those that can be used within 24 hours in the facility are recirculated in the food service area. Those that will be donated to the homeless shelter are placed in the designated freezer space for pick-up.
   (d) Employees should not give foods, supplies, or equipment that are hospital property to anyone inside or outside the department without written authorization in the form of a package pass or signed requisition.

2. **Supervisory Procedures**
   (a) Supervisors and managers are responsible for ensuring that unauthorized removal of hospital property does not occur. *Unauthorized possession* refers to incidents when a person is found with the item(s) in an area other than his or her assigned workstation. *Unauthorized removal from the premises* refers to incidents when an employee is found leaving the hospital grounds without a package pass for the item(s).
   (b) The procedure to be followed is:
      (1) Ask the person to exhibit the item(s) and tell why it is being transported away from the workstation.
      (2) Ask the person whether he or she has a *package pass* or *signed requisition* for the item(s).
      (3) In the event that the person has no written documentation, ask whether he or she received verbal permission and from whom. Verify the source and ensure that proper documentation is issued.
      (4) If unauthorized possession is determined, ask the person whether he or she is aware of the policies regarding removal of hospital property. Tell the person that it is your job to act on the incident and notify security immediately. Security will interview the person and write an incident report. Obtain a copy of this report.
      (5) In cases where a person is identified as leaving the hospital premises with stolen property, the supervisor should work with the security department to document the incident.

continues

Exhibit 8–3 continued

(6) Confer immediately with the highest level food service manager on duty to determine appropriate disciplinary action. This manager, in turn, will consult with the human resources department, and the employee's history of disciplinary actions, the union contract, and hospital policies will be reviewed for application to this case.

(7) If the manager and/or human resources personnel are not available, confer with the person in charge of security for the day. Issue a notice to the employee, with the union representative present, that tells the employee that he or she is *suspended pending further investigation* and the date to return to the facility to discuss the matter further. Provide copies of this notice for all.

(8) Secure the item(s) that were removed, and write down all the details of the incident, including date, time, location, employee or person involved, job title, work hours on the day of occurrence, full description of the property, and the account of the incident from your point of view and that of the person, witnesses, and other persons involved.

should be routinely involved in minimizing variances between physical and perpetual inventories. The actual variance found each month can be used as a basis for the supervisor's performance appraisal.

In addition to the establishment of security controls, solid waste disposal units should be checked periodically for eating utensils such as forks, spoons, knives, plates, and glasses. It is amazing how much flatware tends to end up in the garbage. Most flatware has a substantial amount of iron in it, so that a magnetic collar around the garbage pails will help catch flatware if it is about to be thrown out. Unfortunately, the magnet does nothing for the plates and glasses. Clear plastic bags are also recommended for garbage. In this way one can see what is inside. Today recycling of metal and glass is being done in most communities. Can crushers and glass cutting machines reduce the volume of recyclable items substantially. Styrofoam can be compressed and baled for recycling. Pulping machines are available to compress and remove the water from most garbage, reducing its volume by as much as 60–70%.

THE POWER OF PARTNERSHIP

Changing consumer values and continued pressure to decrease the cost of labor, food, and supplies present challenges for the buyers of the future. Sound business practices and good communications with the staff members within the facility and with suppliers from the outside will help them achieve their goals. As can be seen in the case study shown in Exhibit 8–4, the team approach can work to develop an atmosphere that fosters success.

Exhibit 8–4 Case Study on the Power of Partnership

Adapting, from a proactive approach, to the continuing revolution in the health care industry, the food service department at Sherman Hospital in Elgin, Illinois, identified the need to reduce the food budget by 3% to 5% during the current fiscal year. This was the fifth year that the department rose to the challenge to identify such reductions. In the absence of budgeting inflationary dollars, however, the reduction realistically had to go even deeper, between 8% and 12%.

The director of support services' challenge was one that is becoming all too familiar to other health care administrators nationwide: How can we reduce costs while maintaining quality, services, and patient satisfaction in this dramatically changing environment? To resolve this dilemma, Sherman Hospital's food service department implemented a strategy that may appear at first to be somewhat risky and unorthodox. The strategy was to expand even further into the open book, open door partnership with its prime vendor, one of the leading suppliers in the country. The partnership had existed for 5 years and remained a catalyst in producing cost-saving initiatives for the department. This partnership was established when staff challenged the traditional purchaser–vendor relationship as obsolete. The long-term partnership had subsequently evolved into an innovative working relationship based on trust, shared objectives, and a willingness to "think out of the box" to arrive at solutions that best address the challenges that currently confront the health care food service industry.

Experience at Sherman Hospital has subsequently proved that it is no longer enough for a vendor to sell and deliver products or for the food service department to control costs by reducing staff or choosing the supplier with the lowest bid. This partnership, equally represented, sets departmental goals, measures outcomes, and seeks out the specific expertise, programs, and services necessary to increase the effectiveness of day-to-day operations while capitalizing on the opportunity for continuous improvement.

Goals typically place strong emphasis on cost reduction, making it logical and essential to enlist the assistance of the prime vendor. The partnership was the basis for the department's JIT program and has continued to be viable, resulting in the latest successful outcome in the area of product selection. Product selection is the systematic process of analyzing the most frequently purchased items and exploring low-cost alternatives of comparable quality. It can work well if the facility is a single, standalone hospital or if it is a part of a health care network or system. It could be as easily implemented in a multiunit organization as in a single one. This process was able to document annual savings of $49,000 in Sherman Hospital, which had previous credible operational results; one can imagine the potential in a larger system.

Sherman Hospital's product selection process began with the formation of a team made up of representatives from the prime vendor and department staff. Leading the team was the director of food and nutrition services. The team agreed at the outset to target all products to review. Every item received an equal amount of scrutiny. Team members recognized the importance of keeping an open mind and avoiding a "can't do that" attitude, which could impair effectiveness and ultimately success.

During two initial planning discussions, a target of $20,000 was established as achievable with aggressive analysis. It did not take long to find potential cost-saving opportunities. Savings were identified in the areas of warewashing chemicals, beverages, center of the plate products, convenience foods, and vegetables. The actual product selection

continues

Exhibit 8–4 continued

analysis took the team members only about 10 hours and resulted in reductions beyond their wildest expectations. A total in excess of $49,000 in potential annual savings was identified. This level of savings represented an 8% decrease in the food service food budget. Subsequent product cutting, trials, evaluations, and customer taste panels confirmed a 99% ability to change product without compromising quality or customer expectations. In addition, the product selection process produced secondary success in the areas of additional inventory reductions and enhanced cash flow, and it maximized the use of remaining budget dollars. At Sherman Hospital, product selection is now a continuous process, keeping staff informed about market fluctuations, menu trends, and seasonality. This enables staff to adjust purchasing patterns and policies routinely.

Food service managers must continue to eliminate the old type of vendor relationships. If a current supplier is unable to assist in cost management initiatives, now is the time to find one with the proper experience and resources. It is helpful if managers bring in someone who will work with them and for them in an environment of trust and cooperation to help redefine new opportunities for achieving your business objectives. In this time of revolutionary change for our industry, we can surely expect cost cutting to continue to be a priority for the foreseeable future. Applying the business management practices to health care food service is an important first step in meeting the challenge. Tapping into the right resources can lead to a quantum leap forward, ensuring the attainment of operational efficiency as well as your budgetary goals. This can all be done simultaneously while maintaining the superior service and care levels that customers require.

Source: Reprinted from R. Keith Golden. The Power of Partnership. *Hospital Food & Nutrition Focus,* Vol. 12, No. 8, pp. 1, 3, © 1996, Aspen Publishers, Inc.

Juran (1989) once said "customers' needs are a moving target" (p. 101), and this especially holds true in the food service industry. Food service managers, their staff members, and their suppliers are forever reacting to the desires of the public. It is their job to keep up with consumer trends. If this is not done, they are doomed to fail. It is indeed possible to see a manager go out of his or her way to provide conventionally prepared meals "from scratch" because they themselves were trained to appreciate good homestyle foods, but their clientele may have no appreciation whatsoever for these efforts because their food values are different.

The facts show that 20 years ago 62% of the average family's food bill was spent at a grocery store to prepare meals at home. This figure has decreased to 50% because many more of the foods purchased in grocery stores are convenience entrees. Cooking at home is becoming a hobby. The buyer's job is to keep up with the ever-changing American palate, trends in the marketplace, and cost containment methods. Only then will the buyer be able to make a considerable contribution toward meeting the challenges that face health care systems of the future.

REFERENCES

Golden, R.K. (1995). Does just-in-time (JIT) purchasing really work? *Hospital Food & Nutrition Focus, 11*, 1–3, 8.

Juran, J.M. (1989). *Juran on leadership for quality: An executive handbook*. New York: Free Press.

Kelly, H.J. (1976). *Food service purchasing: Principles and practice*. New York: Chain Store Publishing.

Montague, J. (1995). Can purchasing alliances adapt? *Hospitals & Health Networks, 69*(16), 30–33.

National Association of Meat Purveyors. (1992). *The meat buyer's guide*. Reston, VA: Author.

Scott, L. (1993, Sept.). Buying groups seek compliance. *Modern Healthcare*, pp. 52–61.

Alternative Food Production Systems

Mary B. Gregoire and Mary Frances Nettles

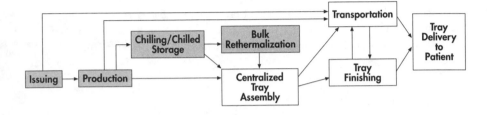

The production of food for patients, employees, and visitors is a major responsibility of health care food and nutrition departments. Various authors have proposed schemes for describing the activities that occur in a food service operation and detailing the positioning of the production process in the flow of food from receiving to delivery to the patient.

Bobeng (1982) developed a model that identifies processes that occur in conventional, cook-chill, and cook-freeze food service systems between the initial procurement of food and supplies and the service of meals to patients. Bobeng's model was the first to illustrate processes common and unique to each system.

Matthews (1982) illustrated product flow in five types of food production systems: cook-serve, cook-chill, cook-freeze, thaw-heat-serve, and heat-serve. Product flow in each starts with procurement and ends with service to the patient. The number of steps varies from four in the heat-serve system to nine in the cook-freeze system.

A second approach to describing how food service systems differ in the processes that occur has been the classification of activities into various stages and the development of unique flow charts depending on the particular activities that occur in a given operation. Escueta, Fiedler, and Reisman (1986) devised the first such classification scheme. They suggested that six components—purchasing, manipulation, processing, preservation, reheating, and distribution—could be combined in various ways to explain the processes of any food service operation. Jones and Heulin (1990) expanded this classification concept in their proposed flow chart, which included 10 stages: storage, preparation, production, holding, transportation, regeneration, service, dining, catering, and dishwashing. They combined these stages in various ways to characterize 10 generic food service systems.

Spears (1995) illustrated the application of systems theory to a food service operation by developing a food service systems model that details input, transformation, and output components specific to a food service operation. This model does not characterize how operations using various production systems differ but rather provides a conceptual framework for components of a food service operation.

Figure 9–1 builds on the work of these authors and illustrates the major processes that can occur in food service operations. The diagram includes all possible processes, and the arrows designate the potential flow between each. Not every process occurs, however, in every food service operation. This diagram is used in this chapter and the next to illustrate the particular flow pattern for each type of operation being discussed. The focus of this chapter is the production, chilling/chilled storage, and bulk rethermalization processes. Chapter 10 discusses the remaining components of the model.

TYPES OF FOOD PRODUCTION SYSTEMS

The food production process was fairly consistent in all health care facilities until research in the 1960s (Bjorkman & Delphin, 1966; MacLennan, 1965, 1969; McGuckian, 1969) introduced ideas that dramatically changed the way production was done. Traditionally, food was prepared and held hot until served. Research of the 1960s led to modifications in this traditional process by introducing ways to chill or freeze foods after preparation and then reheat (or, as it is commonly termed, rethermalize) foods closer to the point of service.

Discussions of the alternatives in food production systems usually group the systems based on definitions first proposed in 1977 by Unklesbay, Maxey, Knickrehm, Stevenson, Cremer, and Matthews. These authors developed a

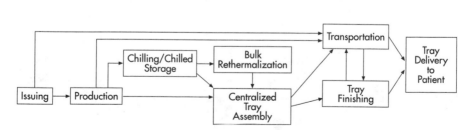

Figure 9–1 Food service operations diagram.

conceptual framework of the food service industry that categorizes food service systems as commissary, conventional, ready food, and assembly-serve.

Commissary systems are defined as those with a centralized food procurement and production function with distribution of prepared menu items to several remote locations for final preparation and service. Most menu items are processed completely in the central facility and then are transported in a heated or chilled state to satellite units (Spears, 1995; Unklesbay et al., 1977).

Conventional systems involve the production and service of food within one food service unit. Menu items are prepared as near to service time as possible to ensure quality. Foods are produced to meet forecasted customer counts and are held hot until time of service (Spears, 1995; Unklesbay et al., 1977). The typical flow pattern for conventional systems as shown in Figure 9–2 would be from production to tray assembly.

A distinct feature of ready food systems, which include cook-chill, cook-freeze, and sous vide (under vacuum), is that menu items are always stored and ready for final assembly and/or heating. Foods are produced in quantities needed to meet inventory levels rather than daily customer counts. In ready food systems, hot food items go through an initial heat processing, are chilled or frozen, and then go through a second heat processing before being served. In cook-chill operations, foods are partially heat processed, chilled either in serving pans in a blast chiller or in bags in a tumble chiller, and then stored in refrigerators for 5 days (panned and blast chilled) to 40 days (bagged and tumble chilled). Sous vide differs somewhat from cook-chill in that raw foods are placed in special bags that are vacuum sealed. Foods are then partially or fully cooked in low-temperature circulating water and rapidly cooled before being held in refrigerated storage. The cook-freeze production system involves partial processing of food items, panning or plating of food items, blast freezing, and storage of frozen items for several weeks (Byers, Shanklin, & Hoover, 1994; Durocher, 1992; Norton, 1991; Spears, 1995; Unklesbay et al., 1977). The typical flow in these systems (see Figure 9–3) would be from production to

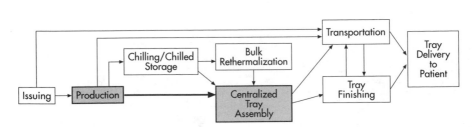

Figure 9–2 Food service operations diagram for conventional food production.

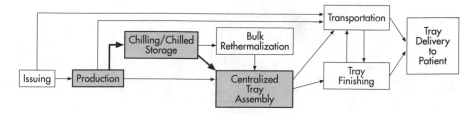

Figure 9–3 Food service operations diagram for cook-chill food production.

chilling/chilled storage to tray assembly. Less common is the flow shown in Figure 9–4, where food is rethermalized in bulk after chilled storage before going to the tray assembly process.

Assembly-serve systems, also referred to as convenience systems, are defined as those in which limited food production occurs. Food products are purchased already prepared and only require heating before service. This rethermalization may occur in the kitchen before food is assembled on trays (which makes it similar to the flow shown in Figure 9–2 for conventional systems), or food may be transported directly to galley kitchens on patient units and be rethermalized there, as shown in Figure 9–5 (Spears, 1995; Unklesbay et al., 1977).

The conventional system has remained the most prevalent system used in hospital food service operations, with 80% or more of hospitals indicating its use (Franzese, 1981; Greathouse & Gregoire, 1988; Matthews, 1982; Nettles & Gregoire, 1993). In 1993, Nettles and Gregoire reported that food service systems in hospitals with more than 100 beds were distributed as 89.2% conventional, 6.9% cook-chill, and 1.5% cook-freeze. Research by Greathouse and Gregoire (1988) and Nettles and Gregoire (1993) suggests that cook-chill and cook-freeze systems are more likely to be found in larger hospitals. Implementation of cook-chill systems appears to be continually increasing (40% of hospi-

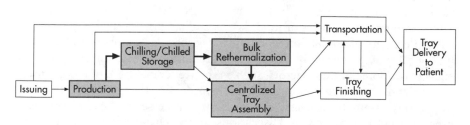

Figure 9–4 Food service operations diagram for cook-chill food production and bulk rethermalization.

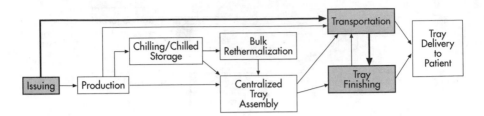

Figure 9–5 Food service operations diagram for convenience food production with delivery direct to floor galleys.

tals with cook-chill systems have implemented them since 1988), whereas implementation of cook-freeze systems appears to be rapidly diminishing (only 4% of current cook-freeze operations were implemented after 1988; Nettles & Gregoire, 1993).

Commissary systems can utilize conventional, cook-chill, or cook-freeze food production. Some hospital administrators have considered relocating food production centers off the premises to utilize potential revenue-generating space within the hospital. With multihospital systems and health care networks increasing, food service directors also are being asked to provide satellite food to smaller sites. Commissary systems are being viewed by many food service directors as an opportunity to expand their services and to become a revenue-generating center (King, 1987a, 1987b, 1989b).

Food service directors are faced with many issues when deciding among the various production options. The production system chosen will affect subsequent processes, as shown in Figure 9–1. For example, the production system will affect whether bulk rethermalization is needed, whether foods will be dished hot or cold on the tray line, what type of temperature support is needed for the meal trays, and so forth.

Often, a first step in the decision process is to gather information about the various production systems. The primary factors discussed related to the system selection appear to be cost of food, labor, and supplies; availability of skilled labor; flexibility of production scheduling; service temperature of food; microbiological quality; sensory quality; nutrient retention; equipment required; and energy use. Some of these factors, such as service temperature of food, sensory quality, and nutrient retention, are actually more directly related to differences in the tray assembly, delivery, and finishing processes and are discussed in greater detail in Chapter 10. Discussions in this chapter focus on the issues related to the food production process itself, chilled storage, and centralized rethermalization processes.

ISSUES RELATED TO THE FOOD PRODUCTION PROCESS

When food service directors evaluate alternative food production systems, many factors must be considered. Although it seems as if labor and food costs are the primary considerations today, other factors are important as well. They include the availability of skilled labor, production scheduling, ingredient control, equipment, energy use, menu, food quality, and food safety.

Food, Labor, and Supply Costs

While one is comparing alternative food production systems, an overall look at cost is recommended. Some systems are inherently labor intensive, but they may save considerable sums in the cost of food and supplies. If a health care facility is located in an area where employees' salaries are relatively low, this type of system may work best. Other systems, such as convenience food systems, are designed to minimize labor costs, but the cost of food is substantially higher. A balance among these costs can be achieved when food service directors are fully aware of the marketplace and how these factors interrelate.

Cost of Food

One of the suggested advantages of ready food systems is reduction in food cost. Corsi (1984), Pizzuto and Winslow (1989), and Durocher (1992), who support this savings, indicate that because an inventory of ready, chilled food is maintained, food is available when needed and less food is wasted because only amounts needed are used. Durocher (1992) also suggests that cooking food products in bags, as is done in some cook-chill operations, reduces the loss in those products. Food service directors should be aware, however, that bagging of food can affect the yield of the product. Dolezal and Brecht (1995) indicated average losses of 10% to 20% in food products that were cooked in large steam-jacketed kettles, pumped into bags, rethermalized in bulk, transferred to steamtable pans, and held hot on steamtable lines. Loss increased as product viscosity increased and could be as much as 25% in extremely viscous products, such as macaroni and cheese.

Food costs in various production systems were predicted by Hysen (1971), Herz and Souder (1979), and Freshwater (1980). Predictive models developed by each suggested that the cook-freeze system would result in the lowest meal cost. Limited research has been done to verify this suggested food cost savings (Department of Veterans Affairs, 1993; Greathouse, Gregoire, Spears, Richards, & Nassar, 1989; Moorshead, 1982), but so far the studies have failed to support a food cost savings for ready food systems.

Cost of Labor

Research by Greathouse et al. (1989) indicated that number of full-time equivalents was the strongest predictor of food service costs. Proponents of ready foods and convenience production systems use reduction in production labor, and thus reduction in labor cost, as a key reason for implementing these systems (Byers et al., 1994; Corsi, 1984; Durocher, 1992; Glew & Armstrong, 1981; Goldberg & Kohligian, 1974; Halling & Frakes, 1981; Pizzuto & Winslow, 1989). Research by the U.S. Department of Agriculture (Freshwater, 1980) and Greathouse et al. (1989) would support this claim. Ready food systems often are able to run production as a Monday-through-Friday, 8-hour-a-day operation because food is being cooked in quantity and chilled or frozen.

Food service directors need to be aware, however, that although ready food and convenience production systems usually require less production labor than conventional systems, they often require more service labor. Many of the hospitals that have ready food or convenience systems include a tray finishing process that involves decentralized rethermalization and often some final tray assembly. This decentralized tray finishing process requires staff to perform these functions. Ready food and convenience systems include an inventory of prepared food items. Monitoring, rotating, and managing this additional inventory also can require additional labor.

Food service directors will find contradictory reports when examining what has been published related to total department labor costs based on the type of food production system being used. Many of the case study reports for individual facilities indicate a labor cost savings. Research comparing data from several hospitals fails to support the cost savings.

Several case studies (Berkman & Schechter, 1991; Kaud, 1972; King, 1987c, 1988, 1989a, 1990) have been published illustrating the labor cost savings that occurred in a given operation when the switch was made from conventional to cook-chill. Food service directors are advised to scrutinize these reported savings carefully by examining the production and service systems that were in place before and after the conversion. Directors should determine how similar the operations being discussed are to their current operation to be sure that the indicated savings could be realized. For example, the conversion at the University of Wisconsin (Kaud, 1972) illustrates an organization that used conventional food production, transportation of food in bulk to decentralized areas, and tray assembly/finishing on individual units. The operation was already labor intensive in service support staff before conversion to a cook-chill system, so that often no additional service employees were needed; a department labor savings was based on the reduction in production labor. The conversion to a cook-chill operation at the University of Iowa Hospitals and Clinics (1994) also included centralization of the tray assembly process, which facilitated a decrease in labor separate from the reduction in production labor. Cedars-Sinai Medical Center (Berkman & Schechter, 1991) converted from a cook-freeze system with rethermalization on decentralized patient galleys to a convenience system where prepackaged convenience foods were delivered directly to patient galleys. Again, because the service labor cost was already in place, a reduction in production labor resulted in an overall labor cost savings.

Rappole (1973) examined the use of convenience products as a means for reducing food service costs and found that hospitals, colleges, and universities using convenience products had not realized the expected labor savings from using these products. Carroll and Montag (1979) compared labor time involved in preparing 59 entree items in cook-freeze and cook-serve food production systems; no significant differences in labor time were found. Hysen (1971), Herz and Souder (1979), and Freshwater (1980), using estimated costs to compare systems, suggested that the ready food systems, specifically the cook-freeze production system, would result in the lowest-cost hospital operation. Moorshead (1982) tried unsuccessfully to validate the Freshwater (1980) model using data from actual food service operations. Moorshead's results indicated that labor costs were not decreased in any of the hospitals surveyed; rather, the hours needed were greater for all functions than those proposed by Freshwater (1980). Greathouse et al. (1989) compared operational data from hospitals with conventional, cook-chill, and cook-freeze systems and were unable to demonstrate a total labor cost savings in hospitals using ready food systems. A recent study by the Department of Veterans Affairs (1993) also indicated that there appears to be no guarantee of labor savings when a cook-chill rather than a conventional production system is used.

Food service labor costs appear to be related to the type of production system used, whether a hot or cold tray line is used, whether decentralized rethermalization is needed, and the amount of tray finishing needed on patient floors. Directors who are considering a change in food service system should evaluate potential labor cost savings carefully. For example, operations currently using a conventional production system with centralized hot tray assembly and have nursing employees delivering trays probably will not realize any overall labor cost savings if a switch is made to a cook-chill production system with cold tray assembly and rethermalization/tray finishing on patient floors because the savings in production labor will be more than offset by the increase in service labor.

Cost of Supplies

Little has been written about the cost of supplies in the various production systems. Supplies that are unique to particular systems include disposable bags/

casing and tipper ties for some forms of cook-chill systems and disposable serving dishes and covers or plastic wrap for individually plated items in cook-chill or cook-freeze systems. Pizzuto and Winslow (1989) suggested that the cost of packaging supplies can be 20% to 25% higher in cook-chill operations compared with conventional production systems.

Skill Level of Labor

Another positive outcome cited for the use of ready food and convenience systems compared with conventional systems is the reduction in the number of skilled employees needed (Byers et al., 1994; Glew & Armstrong, 1981; Maahs, 1993) because food services using these systems typically operate a production unit for fewer hours in a week than conventional operations. Research is limited, however, comparing the actual number of skilled employees needed for each type of production system. A research study conducted in the United Kingdom (Walker, 1988) compared operations that were most successful in implementing and managing a cook-chill operation with those that were least successful. Results indicated that operations that were most successful actually had an increase in skill level of employees because of recipe development and temperature and microbiological controls.

Operating a cook-chill or cook-freeze system usually does not mean that there is no need for skilled employees. Development of recipes that will produce a quality product, monitoring of microbiological issues, and rotation of items in chilled storage are but a few of the specialized skills needed in addition to the traditional preparation skills. The need for skilled production employees is probably least in operations using convenience systems. Such systems require limited preparation, usually only reheating of product. Some operations, such as that at Cedars-Sinai Medical Center (Berkman & Schechter, 1991), have eliminated all production labor by having convenience products delivered directly to galleys on patient floors, where trays are assembled and foods reheated.

Production Scheduling

Production scheduling will differ based on the type of food production system used. These differences often are cited as advantages for the use of ready foods and convenience systems (Byers et al., 1994; Durocher, 1992; Glew & Armstrong, 1981; Halling & Frakes, 1981; Pinkert, 1972).

In conventional systems, all food items needed for a meal are produced that day. Production is geared to having food ready for the tray line three times a day, which creates peak periods of activity. Daily adjustments in recipes and forecast quantities are common based on patient census. Batch cooking techniques are used to help reduce the amount of holding time for each food item for optimal nutrient value and quality.

Production scheduling for ready food systems is quite different. Production is not linked to the tray line process, so that the peaks and valleys of activity are reduced or eliminated. Not all food items on a menu are prepared each day; rather, production is planned to meet inventory levels. Large quantities of fewer items are produced each day. In many cook-chill operations, the food items are dished in a chilled state onto patient trays and are rethermalized after tray assembly. In those operations that rethermalize before the tray line, scheduling of the rethermalization of the food will be needed.

Convenience systems usually require limited production scheduling. If convenience foods are to be heated before being placed on the tray line, then scheduling of this process will be needed. In operations using individual convenience items, usually no production process is needed; rather, these items are placed directly on patient trays and rethermalized as part of the tray finishing process before service.

Ingredient Control

Ingredient control is an issue that is important regardless of the type of food production system used. Effective utilization of a centralized ingredient room has been identified as a cost-effective measure for food service directors to implement (Payne-Palacio, Harger, Shugart, & Theis, 1994; Spears, 1995). Advantages to central assembly of ingredients include increased production control, quality control, and improved security (Payne-Palacio et al., 1994). Less costly employees can be utilized to do simple tasks, such as assembling and measuring ingredients, so that cooks can concentrate their skills on production, garnishing, and portion control (Spears, 1995). Research by Nettles (1993), however, has indicated that the majority (63%) of food service directors are not incorporating ingredient rooms in their facilities. Directors who selected cook-chill systems were more likely to have ingredient rooms in their facilities than directors who had selected conventional food production systems (52% versus 27%).

The primary function of the ingredient room is to coordinate assembly, prepreparation, measuring, and weighing of ingredients (Spears, 1995). The actual tasks that are performed in this area vary from facility to facility. The food service director at Kings County Hospital in Brooklyn, New York, assigns three employees to weigh and measure all ingredients for the kitchen's four cooks (King, 1994). Ingredient room employees at North Mississippi Medical Center in Tupelo, Mississippi, also are weighing ingredients for recipes in addition to preparing fresh vegetables for use (King, 1989b). The ingredient preparation area at St. David's Healthcare System in Austin, Texas, consists of a room where patients' fruit and desserts are preportioned and raw materials to be used in recipes the following day are measured out. The area includes a separate walk-in refrigerator for staging food products (King, 1991).

Food Service Equipment

Food service equipment needs will differ based on the type of food production system used. A food service consultant can guide the food service director in determining the specific equipment requirements for the proposed food production system. Equipment should be selected and sized based on an analysis of the menus to be offered and the number of servings to be prepared in each facility. Several textbooks contain information that can assist food service managers with equipment selection decisions (Byers et al., 1994; Jernigan & Ross, 1989; Kazarian, 1989; Payne-Palacio et al., 1994; Scriven & Stevens, 1989a, 1989b; Spears, 1995).

In conventional kitchens, the equipment should be selected based on the method of preparation and production of food items. Many food service operations are implementing batch cooking concepts, where smaller quantities of food products are prepared closer to the time of service. The quantity of food products to be prepared greatly influences the size of equipment needed in kitchens. Implementation of batch cooking techniques can decrease the size of equipment needed and thus the capital expenditure required. Space requirements for this equipment also may be reduced. The types of equipment needed could include walk-in refrigerators and freezers, ovens (deck, revolving, convection, roll-in, conveyor, combination convection oven/steamer, and/or microwave), steam-jacketed kettles, steamers (pressure, convection, and/or combination convection oven/steamer), tilting fry pans, ranges, griddles/grills, fryers, and food warmers. Innovations in production equipment include the development of hot air impingement/jet sweep ovens, infrared light ovens, combination ovens/steamers, microwave hot-air convection ovens, multi-energy cooking tunnels, and direct steam heating kettles (Kent, 1993; Labre, 1993; Lampi, Pickard, Decareau, & Smith, 1990).

A cook-chill system has many of the same pieces of cooking equipment that are found in conventional kitchens. Because food is not served the same day of preparation, however, specialized chilling equipment is needed. Systems using blast chilling will need to have a large supply of steamtable pans because products are prepared and stored for several days.

Special production equipment is usually found in facilities utilizing the tumble chill type of cook-chill. Steam-jacketed kettles are equipped with automatic temperature controls that ensure uniform cooking of the entire batch of food, and a time–temperature record is maintained for every batch. To further ensure even cooking, the kettle is equipped with a mechanical agitator arm that is activated during cooking yet will not damage delicate items. Kettles are available from 50 to 200 gallons. An air-operated 3-inch draw-off valve is used to empty kettle contents rapidly. A pump-fill station is used to transfer a preset amount of product from the kettle into plastic casings. All cooked items are pumped at aseptic temperatures directly into the casings with no human or utensil contact. Filled casings are immediately loaded into a tumble chiller to allow for rapid chilling of the product.

Water-filled cook tanks often are used to cook meat and poultry products in cook-chill operations. With this technique, pieces of meat are placed in multi-layered bags and vacuum sealed before cooking. Cook tanks use direct steam as a heat source and can be set to cook overnight during off-peak utility hours to effect energy savings. During cooking, the water temperature is maintained between 150° and 175°F. At the end of the cook cycle, the hot water is drained and replaced with chilled water, which stops the cooking process and rapidly drops the temperature of meats before refrigeration.

The cost of equipment and refrigeration for cook-chill operations usually is more than that for a conventional production operation. USECO (1994) indicated that capital costs will be 15% to 20% higher for a cook-chill system compared with a conventional system.

Cook-freeze systems use conventional food preparation equipment to prepare food products. After preparation, food items usually are individually portioned, wrapped, and sent through a shrink tunnel. Food items are labeled and dated. Food products also are frozen in steamtable-size pans for use at a later date.

Convenience systems use preprepared products, so that limited production equipment is needed. Often the only equipment needed are ovens for reheating the products before service.

Energy

One consideration in the selection of a food service system is energy use. Spears (1995) categorized energy use in food service operations into direct and indirect energy expenditures. Direct energy includes the energy used to store, heat, cool, package, reheat, distribute, or serve food. Indirect energy is used to support other functions and includes waste disposal, sanitation, and maintenance of an optimal work environment.

Conserving energy use was recognized as important during the 1970s and early 1980s. Research during that time focused on energy use of cooking and holding equipment. Lampi (1980) reported on the redesign of food service equipment to minimize energy usage. Features being added included solid-state controls to allow for programmed cooking times, reduced equipment size to minimize energy use, and use of multiple energy sources such as hot air jets, microwave, electromagnetic induction, and the like to decrease cooking times and energy use. Studies by McProud (1982) and Oldand and Davis (1982) demonstrated that ovens do not need to be preheated to produce an acceptable product and that eliminating the preheating of ovens could result in a 10% to 15% energy savings for the operation. Hsieh and Matthews (1986) and Tutt, McProud, Belo, Rseng, Ferlin, and Neill (1989) explored the impact on energy consumption of roasting or holding various quantities of product. Their results suggested that energy consumption increased as oven load increased but that use of a fully loaded oven resulted in higher energy savings per serving than use of a partially loaded oven. Energy consumption during hot holding was not affected by the quantity of food being held.

Research also has been conducted to examine energy use of the various food production systems. Barclay and Hitchcock (1984) examined energy consumption for the preparation of food items in conventional production systems and estimated energy use to range from 200 to 3,000 BTU per pound to prepare and hold products. Their results indicated that energy consumption is influenced by the thermostat setting, the quantity of product prepared at one time, the length of the heat processing period, and the type of equipment used. Thomas and Brown (1987) reported that the amount and cost of electricity were minimal for chilling, freezing, holding under refrigeration, and reheating foods in ready food production systems.

Studies to determine whether energy use differs in conventional and ready food systems have produced contradictory findings. McProud and David (1982) compared actual and theoretical energy use in conventional, cook-chill, and cook-freeze systems. Their results indicated that the ready food systems (cook-chill and cook-freeze) required more energy use. More recently, Messersmith, Wheeler, and Rousso (1994b) studied conventional and cook-chill food systems in schools to determine the energy consumption to produce a school meal. Their observations of energy use indicated that the average energy use per meal was 2,690 BTU; the average energy cost per meal was $0.13. The authors reported that there was little consistent difference between cook-chill and conventional facilities and concluded that greater variation occurred within each school system, possibly as a result of menu and production scheduling.

Although energy costs often are considered minor compared with food and labor costs within an organization, conservation of energy is important. Many organizations are installing special equipment to allow monitoring of energy use in food service operations. Several publications exist to help food service directors monitor and conserve energy (Jernigan, 1981; McProud, 1982; Messersmith, Rousso, & Wheeler, 1993; Messersmith, Wheeler, & Rousso,

1994a; National Restaurant Association, 1982, 1986; Thumann, 1992; Unkelsbay & Unkelsbay, 1982).

Menu Considerations

The type of food production system can affect which foods are offered on a menu. Food service directors will need to consider what food products can best be prepared in the system. Many food products that can be prepared and served in a conventional system are not suitable for preparation in ready food systems. Research by Nettles (1993) indicated that hospitals with cook-chill systems (57%) are much more likely than those with conventional systems (22%) to offer a restaurant style menu.

Many facilities are using a combination of cook–tumble chill, cook–blast chill, and conventional preparation. In addition, convenience products also may be used. A food service director should not expect to be able to prepare 100% of menu items using cook-chill technology. Products such as soups, sauces, casseroles, gravies, and meats can be prepared using cook-chill technology, and the majority of food service directors who have cook-chill operations indicate that they use it for these products (Department of Veterans Affairs, 1993; Nettles, 1993). In facilities that use cook–tumble chill technology, menu items must be "pumpable" from the kettle into the plastic casings. This limits the types of food items that can be processed. Foods that usually are not prepared using cook-chill technology include fried foods, vegetables, sandwiches, bakery items, egg dishes such as omelets, and breakfast items such as waffles and French toast.

A test kitchen usually is recommended for facilities utilizing cook-chill or cook-freeze production systems. Food service directors have indicated that considerable time must be spent in recipe modifications to achieve quality food products. Seasoning levels, percentages of liquid versus solid ingredients, ingredient shapes and thicknesses, and product consistency can be affected by the chilling and rethermalization processes. The dietary department of the University of Iowa Hospitals and Clinics (1994) published information about problem solving in cook-chill recipe production and included several recipes that had been developed for its cook-chill operation. Extensive modifications also must be made to the recipes used in cook-freeze systems because frozen foods are subject to structural and texture alterations.

A major concern with convenience systems has been the availability of quality frozen prepared products. Advances in food technology have made this concern less of an issue. The food service staff at Cedars-Sinai Medical Center in Los Angeles found that frozen single-service healthful entrees from local supermarkets equaled or exceeded their quality requirements (Berkman & Schechter,

1991). The major obstacle to placing these items on the patient menu was convincing suppliers to sell retail single-service products to a hospital.

Food Quality

A highly debated issue in comparison of food production systems is the quality of food produced in each system. Pizzuto and Winslow (1989) suggest that cook-chill technology provides the opportunity to serve consistently high-quality food because standardized recipes will be used, food is produced in uniformly controlled batches, and small amounts of food can be rethermalized closer to the point of service, preventing long holding times. Byers et al. (1994) also contend that food quality will be better in cook-chill and cook-freeze systems because of the reduced holding time.

Assessment of food quality is not only a system selection question but a continuous quality improvement issue. Basic to the question of food quality is the issue of the food itself versus the food service system. The quality of food products is affected by the recipes used and the quality of the ingredients. Evaluation of food quality requires standards for each food product served. Spears (1995), Ruf (1989), and Payne-Palacio et al. (1994) have published standards for commonly menued items that can be adapted for use in particular institutions. For example, Spears (1995) provides the following standard for macaroni and cheese:

> Macaroni should be al dente but tender and have a cooked starch flavor. Sauce should have a medium thick consistency with an American or cheddar cheese flavor. Each piece of the macaroni should be completely coated with the light yellow creamy sauce. A portion should spread slightly when spooned on a plate. (p. 741)

The development of such a standard eliminates having food products judged acceptable one day and unacceptable the next based on which employee or manager is evaluating products. The quality food standard helps define an objective measure of what the individual food service team believes is desirable for its clientele. These standards need to reflect what the quality of the food should be when it is served to patients. Use of ready food systems may require two standards for a food product: one for the quality as it leaves the production process, and another reflecting quality after rethermalization. More information about setting quality standards can be found in Chapter 8.

Evaluation of food quality usually is based on several subcomponents: temperature at time of service, retention of nutrients, and sensory attributes. Because quality of the food is affected by the tray assembly, transportation, and finishing processes, a more complete discussion of food quality is provided in Chapter 10.

Food Safety

Food safety is an issue with all types of food production systems. Several authors (Chipley & Cremer, 1980; Klein, Matthews, & Setser, 1984; Snyder & Matthews, 1984) have published review articles summarizing research done on microbiological concerns with various production systems. Each of the studies emphasizes the importance of thoroughly cooking and cooling food and preventing contamination of food in all food production systems.

A Hazard Analysis Critical Control Point (HACCP) program should be established to ensure quality control from food purchasing through food preparation to service. Several authors (Beasley, 1995; Bryan, 1990; Corlett, 1989; Jackson, 1995b) have outlined issues for food service operators to address in implementing HACCP standards in their operations. The 1993 Food Code issued by the U.S. Public Health Service (1993) devotes an entire section to defining HACCP principles and describing how to operationalize these principles. More information about this topic can be found in Chapter 11.

Food safety concerns are particularly important in ready food systems because of the additional critical control points introduced by the chilling and rethermalizing of food items. Jackson (1995b) indicated that conventional food production systems typically have 6 major stages that require risk evaluation; ready food systems may have as many as 11 stages.

Improper cooling has been indicated as the most frequent cause of outbreaks of foodborne diseases (Bryan, 1990; Snyder & Matthews, 1984). The 1993 Food Code requires that cooked, potentially hazardous food be cooled from 140° to 70°F within 2 hours and from 70° to 41°F or below within 4 hours.

Schuster (1993) reported concerns voiced by food service directors related to the time spent cleaning cook-chill equipment. One director indicated that more labor hours are being spent on sanitation activities, such as cleaning additional equipment used in cook-chill production. In another hospital, the food service director indicated that sanitation represented 20% to 25% of the labor hours in the cook-chill area because staff had to pay more attention to the cleanliness of production equipment. The University of Iowa Hospitals and Clinics (1994) provided guidelines for cleaning the kettles, food hoses, and bag filler outlets in its cook-chill operation. These guidelines indicate that cleaning kettles between products can take 5 to 35 minutes, depending on the product, and that cleaning at the end of the day takes at least 2 hours.

Research by Nettles (1993) indicated that most food service directors who selected cook-chill systems are not currently evaluating foods prepared using the cook-chill system for microbiological safety. Several directors indicated that analyses were performed when the system was new but had been discontinued. The cost of having this microbiological testing done could be one reason why testing is not being conducted. A report by the Department of Veterans Affairs (1993) indicated that costs could be $100 or more per sample if testing includes total plate count, anaerobic plate count, and detection of *Clostridium perfringens*, *Escherichia coli*, and *Listeria monocytogenes*.

ISSUES RELATED TO THE CHILLING/CHILLED STORAGE PROCESS

The chilling/chilled storage process occurs only in ready food and convenience systems (Figures 9–3 through 9–5). Special equipment is needed for this process.

Operations using the blast chill form of cook-chill will need blast chill units to chill the cooked food items rapidly. A blast chiller is a quick-chill cabinet that usually holds roll-in racks of food pans. Blast chillers direct frigid air at 1,000 ft/min over the steamtable pans. The smallest blast chiller is capable of dropping the temperature of up to 44 pounds of foods to 37°F within 90 minutes. For large-scale operations, blast chillers capable of chilling 360 pounds or more per batch are common.

A second form of cook-chill involves the bagging of hot food into plastic casings. Filled casings are immediately loaded into a tumble chiller. The chiller is filled with an ice water bath. Depending on product viscosity and casing size, product temperatures are reduced to 40°F in 20 to 60 minutes. Once the food products are chilled, they are transferred to holding crates and stored in refrigerated units until needed.

Water-filled cook tanks are used to cook and then chill meat and poultry products. With this technique, pieces of meat are placed in bags, vacuum sealed, and cooked in the cook tank. At the end of the cook cycle, the hot water is drained and replaced with chilled water, which stops the cooking process and rapidly drops the temperature of meats before refrigeration. For small-scale cook-chill operations, one piece of equipment will serve double-duty as a cook tank and a tumble chiller.

One additional piece of equipment that is needed in operations using tumble chillers and cook tank/chillers is an ice builder, which supplies the ice water for chiller units. The amount of water used in these systems can be of concern, especially in drought areas.

Additional refrigeration space is needed for cook-chill operations for storage of the inventory of chilled food products. The amount of refrigeration will depend on the length of time food products will be stored.

Cook-freeze systems use conventional food preparation equipment to prepare food products. After preparation, food items usually are individually portioned, wrapped, and sent through a shrink tunnel. Food items are labeled and dated. Food products also may be frozen in steamtable pans for use at a later date. Blast freezers are used to reduce the temperature of the food items rapidly. After the food reaches the frozen state, it is moved from the blast freezer to a storage freezer. Sufficient freezer space is needed to store the frozen items. Additional refrigeration space is needed to temper the frozen food before rethermalization. If foods are stored in steamtable pans, additional pans must be inventoried.

Convenience systems also require additional refrigeration and freezer space. Large freezers are required to store the inventory of frozen food products, and refrigeration space is needed to temper the frozen items.

ISSUES RELATED TO THE CENTRALIZED RETHERMALIZATION PROCESS

Centralized rethermalization involves bringing chilled food products to the proper serving temperature. This process involves heating foods in bulk before service on the tray line. For items that were chilled in serving pans, this process may include heating in convection oven or combination convection oven/ steamer. Products that were bagged and chilled can be reheated in the bags, or the bags can be emptied into another pan or piece of equipment. Products that are heated in the bags (e.g., casseroles) often are placed in steam-jacketed kettles of boiling water for heating; the heated product is then transferred to a steamtable serving pan. Sometimes the contents of the bags (e.g., soups and sauces) are emptied directly into steam-jacketed kettles for reheating and then are transferred to steamtable pans, or the contents of the bags are emptied into steamtable pans and then reheated in the pans.

A new concept in bulk rethermalization is the multienergy cooking tunnel (Labre, 1993). The tunnel uses four different forms of energy transfer—microwave, low-pressure steam, forced-air convection, and infrared—separately or in combination, depending on the product being processed. The rationale for each form of energy use is that the microwaves will ensure rapid cooking to the center of the product, low-pressure steam will provide moisture to preserve the color and nutrient content while reducing weight loss, forced-air convection provides crispness and deep browning, and infrared allows rapid surface cooking and browning. The oven can be preprogrammed for a particular food item to ensure the appropriate amount of energy from each source.

SYSTEM SELECTION PROCESS

The food production system decision affects all aspects of a food service operation; therefore, it is vital that professional food service staff be involved in the selection process. Many food service directors begin planning for new food service systems many years before the decision is made to hire an architect or food service consultant. There could be various reasons why a food service director would investigate alternative food production systems. Directors may become aware of new technology and want to determine whether this technology is appropriate for their facility. Other directors may be dissatisfied with their existing production systems and want to investigate other alternatives. The reasons for selecting a food production system should be related to the goals of the individual facility.

Directors should be involved in the planning process from the beginning. They need to be assertive in working with architects and involved in the hiring of a food service consultant. The selection of the appropriate food service consultant can be critical to the success of the project. Directors also should be encouraged to remain an active participant in the selection process after a food service consultant has been hired.

Research has suggested that food service directors are spending different amounts of time in the decision process to select a food service system, varying from 7 to 24 months (Nettles, 1993; Walker, 1988). Some directors have indicated that the length of the decision process is even longer, lasting several years (King & Boss, 1991). Green (1992) indicated that the elapsed time between consideration and implementation of cook-chill systems ranged from 13 months to more than 5 years.

Many food service directors utilize planning committees to assist in the selection process. Most planning committees have a minimum of five members representing food service, administration, finance, maintenance/engineering, and nursing. Food service representatives could be the director, assistant directors, food service supervisors, clinical dietitians, and chef/production representative. Architects, contractors, food service consultants, and manufacturers' representatives also can be members of the planning committee.

The initial period of the selection process involves the gathering of information. The most frequently cited sources of information by food service directors who made the decision to select conventional or cook-chill production systems were other users of the system(s) under consideration, food service equipment manufacturers, and other facilities using the system(s) under consideration (Nettles, 1993). Other sources of information include manufacturers' representatives, food service consultants, seminars and conferences, industry journals, and professional journals (Green, 1992; Nettles, 1993). Nettles (1993) reported that directors who selected cook-chill systems were more likely to consider food service consultants a source of information, to visit other facilities using the system(s) under consideration, and to use seminars/conferences as a source of information than directors who selected conventional food service systems.

Information can be obtained from a variety of sources, but what information is considered the most useful to directors in the food service system decision?

Food service directors have indicated that visits to other facilities using the system(s) under consideration, discussions with manufacturers' representatives, discussions with other users of the system(s) under consideration, and advice from food service consultants provided the most useful information (Nettles, 1993). Walker (1988) indicated that decision makers at successful cook-chill operations utilized many resources during the process of making the decision to select cook-chill. These directors collected information and advice from more than one equipment manufacturer and other cook-chill users. They emphasized visiting a comparable cook-chill facility in terms of size and scope rather than well-known units. Directors of successful operations sent employees to facilities to gain working experience with cook-chill and insight into a working cook-chill operation. These directors also were willing to listen to others with practical experience and knowledge of the applications of cook-chill systems.

There are many issues that food service directors should consider when selecting a food production system. These issues can be categorized into operational, cost, financial, support, informational, construction, and food quality concerns (Nettles & Gregoire, 1993). Specific issues are shown in Exhibit 9–1. These issues can be used to evaluate objectively the present production system and the food service systems under consideration. Research has indicated that the issues food service directors consider most often in the selection of a conventional or cook-chill food service system are patient satisfaction with food quality, manufacturer information, hospital administration support, temperature of food at service, and amount of space available for food production (Nettles, 1993).

The importance of these issues should be determined by the planning committees. Each facility has different goals and expectations that need to be considered in the selection decision. In a study conducted by Nettles (1993), food service directors who selected conventional or cook-chill systems rated additional or new rethermalization equipment, temperature of food at service, payback period, patient satisfaction with food quality, dollars available for the new food service system, and projected total departmental costs as most important.

Food service directors are calculating values for many of the issues before making the system decision. Financial, food, labor, and equipment expenses are calculated most often by directors who select conventional or cook-chill systems (Nettles, 1993). Manufacturers' representatives, food service consultants, financial officers, and maintenance/engineering personnel can assist the food service director with the value or cost calculations. Manufacturers' representatives can be used to calculate the cost of additional or new rethermalization, refrigeration, production, and delivery/transportation equipment. Food service consultants will assist in calculating costs related to construction/renovation or additional equipment. Financial officers can be involved in calculation of dollars available for a new food

Exhibit 9–1 Food Service System Selection Issues

<table>
<tr><td>

Production Operation
Actual and projected food cost
Actual and projected production labor
    cost
Actual and projected service labor cost
Actual and projected total labor cost
Actual and projected total departmental
    cost
Actual and projected meals per labor
    hour
Value of actual and projected raw and
    cooked food inventory
Employee training
Operation of an ingredient room
Payback period
Breakeven point
Return on investment
Net present value
Computerization
Plate waste
Quantity of leftovers
Ability to provide food to other
    facilities
Availability and skill level of labor
Centralization of production

Food Quality
Patient satisfaction with food quality
Cafeteria patron satisfaction with food
    quality
Holding time of prepared foods
Temperature of food at service
Food texture
Standardized recipes
Style of menu

</td><td>

Support and Information
Dollars available for new food service
    system
Viewing of actual operation of other
    facilities
Discussion with other system users
Food service consultant advice
Manufacturer technical assistance and
    training
Journal articles
Seminars and conferences
Administration support
Nursing staff acceptance
Community acceptance
Having food service operation perceived as
    innovative
Staff involvement in decision process
Flexibility in patient meal service

Equipment and Construction
Additional or new production, delivery/
    transportation, refrigeration, and/or
    rethermalization equipment
Installation costs
Production area and/or floor pantry
    construction/renovation
Amount of space available for food
    production and/or floor pantries
Physical relationship between food
    production and service
Energy costs
Overhead costs
Volume of solid waste
Space required for future operations
Routine cleaning and maintenance
    requirements
Employee safety

</td></tr>
</table>

service system and other financial indicators. Food service directors should recognize the importance of calculating financial indicators such as return on investment when considering a change in food production system. They also need to determine whether the costs of the initial investment, maintenance, supplies, energy, and space will be offset by savings in food and labor costs (Jackson, 1995a). Maintenance/engineering personnel can assist in the computation of present utility costs, projected utility costs, and installation costs.

Food service directors should evaluate carefully the food production systems under consideration to be aware of all apparent and hidden costs. Those who are considering cook-chill or cook-freeze will benefit by evaluating the costs that are associated with recipe development in test kitchens and microbiological testing of food products. Directors selecting convenience, cook-chill, or cook-freeze systems should explore the issues of chilled/frozen storage of food products and rethermalization. It is also wise to build in time and money for training and employee job redesign (Schuster, 1993). While making these important decisions, food service directors will benefit by staying aware of the long-range plans for their facilities and by closely aligning their plans with future expectations that are expressed by their administrators.

REFERENCES

Barclay, M.J., & Hitchcock, M.J. (1984). Energy consumption assessment in a conventional foodservice system. *Journal of Foodservice Systems, 3*, 33–47.

Beasley, M.A. (1995). Implementing HACCP standards. *Food Management, 30*, 38, 40.

Berkman, J., & Schechter, M. (1991). Today, I closed my kitchen. *Food Management, 26*, 110–114, 118, 122.

Bjorkman, A., & Delphin, K.A. (1966). Sweden's Nacka hospital food system centralizes preparation and distribution. *Cornell HRA Quarterly, 7*, 84–87.

Bobeng, B.J. (1982). Alternative for menu item flow in hospital patient feeding systems. In *Hospital Patient Feeding Systems* (pp. 113–117). Washington, DC: National Academy Press.

Bryan, F.L. (1990). Application of HACCP to ready-to-eat chilled foods. *Food Technology, 44*, 70–77.

Byers, B.A., Shanklin, C.W., & Hoover, L.C. (1994). *Food service manual for health care institutions.* Chicago: American Hospital Association.

Carroll, G.H., & Montag, G.M. (1979). Labor time comparison of a cook-freeze and cook-serve system of food production. *Journal of the Canadian Dietetic Association, 40*, 39–49.

Chipley, J.R., & Cremer, M.L. (1980). Microbiological problems in the food service industry. *Food Technology, 34*(10), 59–68.

Corlett, D.A. (1989). Refrigerated foods and use of hazard analysis and critical control point principles. *Food Technology, 43*, 91–94.

Corsi, R.M. (1984, Winter). The ready foods system. *Consultant*, pp. 23–25.

Department of Veterans Affairs. (1993). *Advanced food preparation systems. Final report.* Milwaukee: Author.

Durocher, J. (1992). Cook-chill systems. *Restaurant Business, 91*, 154, 156.

Escueta, E.S., Fiedler, K.M., & Reisman, A. (1986). A new hospital foodservice classification system. *Journal of Foodservice Systems, 4*, 107–116.

Franzese, R. (1981). Foodservice systems of 79 hospitals studied. *Hospitals, 55*, 64–66.

Freshwater, J.F. (1980). *Least-cost hospital food service systems.* Washington, DC: Department of Agriculture, Agricultural Marketing Service.

Glew, G., & Armstrong, J.F. (1981). Cost optimization through cook-freeze systems. *Journal of Foodservice Systems, 1*, 235–254.

Goldberg, C.M., & Kohligian, M. (1974). Conventional, convenience, or ready foodservice. *Hospitals, 48*, 80–83.

Greathouse, K.R., & Gregoire, M.B. (1988). Variables related to selection of conventional, cook-chill, and cook-freeze systems. *Journal of the American Dietetic Association, 88*, 476–478.

Greathouse, K.R., Gregoire, M.B., Spears, M.C., Richards, V., & Nassar, R.F. (1989). Comparison of conventional, cook-chill, and cook-freeze systems. *Journal of the American Dietetic Association, 89*, 1606–1611.

Green, G.G. (1992). *Decision making strategy in the selection of cook-chill production in hospital foodservices.* Unpublished doctoral dissertation, Virginia Polytechnic Institute and State University, Blacksburg, VA.

Halling, J.F., & Frakes, B.M. (1981). Product-oriented production in a cook freeze system. *Journal of Foodservice Systems, 4*, 355–361.

Herz, M.L., & Souder, J.J. (1979). Preparation systems have significant effect on costs. *Hospitals, 53*, 89–92.

Hsieh, J., & Matthews, M. (1986). Energy use, time, and product yield of turkey rolls at three oven loads and cooking temperatures in a convection oven. *Journal of Foodservice Systems, 4*, 97–106.

Hysen, P. (1971). Ready foods may provide ready savings. *Modern Hospital, 116*, 95–98, 117.

Jackson, R. (1995a). Equipment can sabotage your budget. *Hospital Food and Nutrition Focus, 11*, 1, 3–5.

Jackson, R. (1995b). Featuring Mildred Cody, PhD, RD. *Hospital Food and Nutrition Focus, 11*, 4–6.

Jernigan, B.S. (1981). Guidelines for energy conservation. *Journal of the American Dietetic Association, 79*, 459–462.

Jernigan, A.K., & Ross, L.N. (1989). *Food service equipment* (3rd ed.). Ames, IA: Iowa State University Press.

Jones, P., & Heulin, A. (1990). Foodservice systems—Generic types, alternative technologies and infinite variation. *Journal of Foodservice Systems, 5*, 299–311.

Kaud, F.A. (1972). Implementing the chilled food concept. *Hospitals, 46*, 97–100.

Kazarian, E.A. (1989). *Foodservice facilities planning* (3rd ed.). New York: Van Nostrand Reinhold.

Kent, R. (1993). Turbo-charged "EasyBake" oven speeds cooking with light. *Hospital Food Service Management, 1*, 73–75.

King, P. (1987a). Expanding a foodservice system. *Food Management, 22*, 64, 68.

King, P. (1987b). Production for profit. *Food Management, 22*, 68, 76.

King, P. (1987c). Solving the space problem. *Food Management, 22*, 54, 60.

King, P. (1988). Changing with the times. *Food Management, 23*, 63, 66.

King, P. (1989a). A gamble pays off. *Food Management, 24*, 80, 86.

King, P. (1989b). A vision comes to life. *Food Management, 24*, 66, 68.

King, P. (1990). From famine to feast at VUMC. *Food Management, 25*, 61, 64.

King, P. (1991). Something old, something new. *Food Management, 26*, 56, 58.

King, P. (1994). The beginning of a dream. *Food Management, 29*, 35.

King, P., & Boss, D. (1991). The politics of a renovation. *Food Management, 26*(7), 104–117, 166.

Klein, B.P., Matthews, M.E., & Setser, C.S. (1984). *Foodservice systems: Time and temperature effects on food quality.* Urbana-Champaign: University of Illinois.

Labre, Y. (1993). The multi-energy cooking tunnel. *Consultant, 26*, 32–33.

Lampi, R.A. (1980). New developments in energy saving equipment. *Journal of Foodservice Systems, 1*, 27–38.

Lampi, R.A., Pickard, D.W., Decareau, R.V., & Smith, D.P. (1990). Perspective and thoughts on foodservice equipment. *Food Technology, 44*, 61–69.

Maahs, J. (1993). Cook/chill—from preparation through service. *Consultant, 26*, 16–18.

MacLennan, H.A. (1965). Ready foods: The application of mass production to a la carte food service using prepared-to-order food. *Cornell HRA Quarterly, 6*, 21–63.

MacLennan, H.A. (1969). Ready foods for hotels. *Cornell HRA Quarterly, 10*, 21–31.

Matthews, M.E. (1982). Foodservice in health care facilities. *Food Technology, 36*, 53–64, 71.

McGuckian, A.T. (1969). The A.G.S. food system—Chilled pasteurized food. *Cornell HRA Quarterly, 10*, 87–92, 99.

McProud, L. (1982). Reducing energy loss in foodservice operations. *Food Technology, 37*, 67–71.

McProud, L., & David, B. (1982). Energy use and management in production of entrees in hospital foodservice systems. *Journal of the American Dietetic Association, 81*, 145–151.

Messersmith, A.M., Rousso, V., & Wheeler, G.M. (1994). Energy management in three easy steps. *School Food Service Journal, 47*, 41, 42, 44.

Messersmith, A.M., Wheeler, G.M., & Rousso, V. (1994a). *Energy conservation manual for school food service managers*. Hattiesburg, MI: National Food Service Management Institute.

Messersmith, A.M., Wheeler, G.M., & Rousso, V. (1994b). Energy used to produce meals in school food service. *School Food Service Research Review, 18*, 29–36.

Moorshead, A.L. (1982). *An empirical investigation of the reliability and validity of the USDA model to determine least-cost hospital food service systems*. Unpublished master's thesis, Virginia Polytechnic Institute and State University, Blacksburg, VA.

National Restaurant Association. (1982). *Energy management system*. Chicago: Author.

National Restaurant Association. (1986). *Facilities operations manual*. Chicago: Author.

Nettles, M.F. (1993). *Analysis of the decision to select a conventional or cook-chill system for hospital foodservice*. Unpublished doctoral dissertation, Kansas State University, Manhattan, KS.

Nettles, M.F., & Gregoire, M.B. (1993). Operational characteristics of hospital foodservice departments with conventional, cook-chill, and cook-freeze systems. *Journal of the American Dietetic Association, 93*, 1161–1163.

Norton, C. (1991). What is cook-chill? *Hospital Food Service*, 24(2), 5–7.

Oldand, D., & Davis, C. (1982). Products cooked in preheated versus non-preheated ovens. *Journal of the American Dietetic Association, 81*, 135–144.

Payne-Palacio, J., Harger, V., Shugart, G., & Theis, M. (1994). *West's and Wood's introduction to foodservice* (7th ed.). New York: Macmillan.

Pinkert, M.S. (1972). Basic planning concepts for ready foods systems. *Canadian Hospital, 49*, 32–34.

Pizzuto, R., & Winslow E. (1989). Why cook/chill systems don't work when they should. *Consultant, 22*, 32–34.

Rappole, C.L. (1973). Institutional use of frozen entrees. *Cornell HRA Quarterly, 14*, 72–89, 99.

Ruf, K. (1989). *Manual for food and nutrition services: Quality control, quality assurance*. Gaithersburg, MD: Aspen.

Schuster, K. (1993). Is your future in cook-chill? *Food Management, 28*, 90, 94, 96, 98, 123–124.

Scriven, C.R., & Stevens, J.W. (1989a). *Equipment facts, revised.* New York: Van Nostrand Reinhold.

Scriven, C.R., & Stevens, J.W. (1989b) *Manual of equipment and design for the foodservice industry.* New York: Van Nostrand Reinhold.

Snyder, P.O., & Matthews, M.E. (1984). Microbiological quality of foodservice menu items produced and stored by cook/chill, cook/freeze, cook/hot-hold and heat/serve methods. *Journal of Food Protection, 47,* 876–885.

Spears, M.C. (1995). *Foodservice organizations: A managerial and systems approach.* Englewood Cliffs, NJ: Merrill.

Thomas, C.J., & Brown, N.E. (1987). Use and cost of electricity for selected processes specific to a hospital cook-chill/freeze food-production system. *Journal of Foodservice Systems, 4,* 159–169.

Thumann, A. (1992). *Handbook of energy audits* (3rd ed.). Lilburn, GA: Fairmont.

Tutt, M., McProud, L., Belo, P., Rseng, R., Ferlin, B., & Neill, C. (1989). Comparison of energy consumption in fully and partially loaded institutional forced-air convection ovens: Preheated and nonpreheated. *School Food Service Research Review, 13,* 146–149.

University of Iowa Hospitals and Clinics. (1994). *Cook chill cookbook.* Iowa City: Author.

Unklesbay, N., Maxey, R., Knickrehm, M., Stevenson, K., Cremer, M., & Matthews, M. (1977). *Foodservice systems: Product flow and microbial quality and safety of foods.* Columbia, MO: University of Missouri–Columbia Agriculture Experiment Station.

Unklesbay, N., & Unklesbay, K. (1982). *Energy management in foodservice.* Westport, CT: AVI.

U.S. Public Health Service. (1993). *Food Code 1993.* Washington, DC: Department of Health and Human Services.

USECO. (1994). *CATR: Chilled food system.* Murfreesboro, TN: Author.

Walker, A.E. (1988). *The transfer of technology: A study of UK cook chill catering operations.* Unpublished doctoral dissertation, Dorset Institute of Higher Education, Dorset, England.

Options in Meal Assembly, Delivery, and Service

Karen R. Greathouse and Mary B. Gregoire

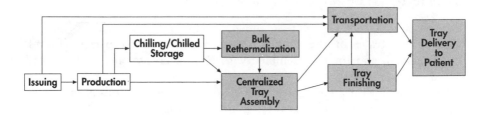

Tray assembly, delivery, and service are important activities that go on for at least three meals per day, 365 days of the year, in all health care facilities. Food service directors are faced with many options when deciding how best to assemble and deliver meals to patients. The possible processes that can occur between the time food is produced and when it is served to patients are indicated in the food service operations diagram (see Figure 10–1). The number of processes in a given operation is affected by the type of production system used, whether foods are dished hot or cold on the tray line, what transportation system is used, and the amount of tray finishing that needs to occur once the carts reach a patient floor.

Figures 10–2 to 10–5 use the food service operations diagram to show some of the variations that exist in operations as food moves from the production process through delivery to patients. Figure 10–2 reflects the most common process flow in a food service operation, one using conventional food production, a hot tray line, transportation of trays to patient floors, and delivery of trays to patients. In this traditional operation, only two processes—tray assembly and transportation—occur between production of the food and delivery to the patient.

The implementation of advanced preparation systems (cook-chill and cook-freeze) has increased the number of processes that occur between food production and service to the patient. Figure 10–3 indicates a system in which food is produced, chilled and held in cold storage, centrally rethermalized, assembled on trays, transported, and served to patients. Another alternative is shown in Figure 10–4, in which food is produced, chilled and held in cold storage, as-

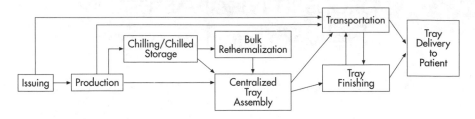

Figure 10–1 Food service operations diagram.

sembled on trays in the chilled state, transported to patient floors, rethermalized, and finally assembled with hot beverages, and so forth and served to patients.

Another major variation in process flow occurs when hot foods or individual convenience products are transported in bulk to patient areas and the centralized tray assembly process is eliminated. Figure 10–5 depicts the processes in the "kitchenless kitchen" concept (Berkman & Schechler, 1991), in which individually prepackaged products are transported to floor galley kitchens, foods are heated, and trays are assembled in these galleys before delivery to patients.

The focus of this chapter is issues and concerns related to the tray assembly, transportation, tray finishing, and patient service processes shown in the food service operations diagram. Quality assessment measures for each process also are included.

CENTRALIZED TRAY ASSEMBLY

The centralized tray assembly process involves placing food items on patient trays in a central location, usually where the food is produced. Centralized tray assembly is used in nearly all hospital food service operations (97% of conventional systems, 96% of cook-chill systems; Nettles & Gregoire, 1993). Advantages commonly cited for centralized tray assembly include elimination of

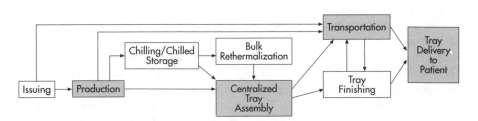

Figure 10–2 Conventional food production with centralized hot tray assembly.

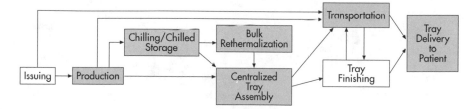

Figure 10–3 Cook-chill or cook-freeze with centralized rethermalization and hot tray assembly.

double handling of food, supervised control of tray assembly in one location, standardized portions and presentation, less staff time for the tray assembly process, and no space requirement for floor kitchens (Byers, Shanklin, & Hoover, 1994). These advantages were responsible for the move toward centralized assembly, which has been in vogue since the early 1950s.

Directors implementing or reevaluating a centralized tray assembly process will make decisions related to the equipment needed for the assembly process as well as the trays and dishes to be used. Assessment of the quality of this process will probably focus on the accuracy and efficiency of the process.

Tray Line Equipment

Centralized tray assembly is accomplished by means of a tray line, which can take several configurations depending on the number of trays to be assembled. The type of equipment selected for the tray line usually differs based on the size of the facility and whether food items are held hot or cold during the tray assembly process.

Small facilities often use a combination cook counter and tray assembly table. Cold food items are placed on a tray, which is pushed down the assembly table to

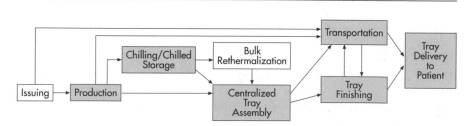

Figure 10–4 Cook-chill or cook-freeze system with centralized chilled tray assembly and rethermalization on patient units.

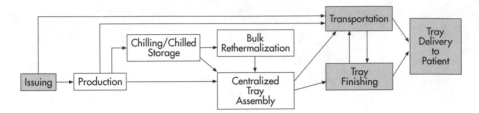

Figure 10–5 Convenience system with rethermalization and tray assembly on patient units.

each station. Hot food is dished from hot wells onto plates, which then are placed on the tray at the end of the assembly process. The hot wells may have fabricated covers to place over them so that the counter may be used as a cook's table. This process would typically require only two employees. The trays may be preset with tray mats, serviceware, and cold food items to expedite tray assembly.

Medium-size facilities may use a roller conveyor that is nonpowered. Mobile hot and cold holding equipment is brought to the tray line and placed so that workers either face the line or work at stations perpendicular to the line. Trays are manually rolled from one station to the next.

Powered conveyors move trays by a mechanized belt, which can be made from different materials and take different shapes. Fabric belts are used for systems that require cut-out trays for specialized rethermalization dishes and is most efficient if the patient menus are placed on the conveyor or in tray stands rather than on the tray. Slat belts are able to negotiate corners so that different configurations can be accomplished. Bandveyor belts consist of four continuous bands that run vertically the length of the tray line. They are the least expensive to purchase and have the lowest maintenance costs.

Circular tray systems are cantilevered over the support equipment and rotate around an oval center. They may be self-contained, with the support equipment built into the base of the unit, or pedestal units, in which mobile support equipment is plugged into the base.

A final tray line configuration is a double line in which the tray moves down one side and then is rotated to the opposite side on the second tray belt so that the starter and checker positions stand next to each other. This allows some distinct advantages not available in other configurations. Hot stations can be positioned directly across from cold stations without the two workers interfering with each other. The checker can easily cycle trays that need corrections to the appropriate station.

In addition to different configurations, tray lines may now be equipped with a programmable microprocessor that automatically turns on and off thermal equipment attached to the tray line. A display panel assures management that proper temperatures have been achieved for both hot and cold equipment, thus reducing the need for personnel to arrive early for the purpose of turning on equipment (Wile, 1985).

The design of the tray line is a function of the number of menu items and the number of trays to be served during the mealtime. As the number of menu items to be offered increases, so does the length of the tray line. To reduce the amount of space needed, a circular or double-sided tray line might be considered.

Tray Line Support Equipment

Operating a tray line usually requires support equipment to help maintain the temperature of the foods being served on the trays. A variety of hot-holding and refrigerated units are available for use with any configuration of tray line. Hot-holding equipment, often termed steamtables, can be units that use dry heat or heated water (steam) to hold pans of food at a proper heated temperature. Fairbrook (1994) stressed that steamtables should not be used to reheat foods that are below recommended serving temperatures. Fairbrook offered several rules for helping ensure that food items held in steamtables remain hot:

- The total amount of food in a steamtable pan should be able to be served within 5 minutes.
- Covers should always be used to help hold heat.
- Adjustable infrared heat lamps should be used above the steamtable.
- Steamtables should have hot water under the pans of hot food.
- Plates should be rewarmed.

Operations using cook-chill production and placing cold food items on patient trays will have refrigerated well units to maintain the chilled temperature of foods. Some ready food operations that have all foods placed on trays in the refrigerated state maintain the tray assembly area at a cooler temperature (e.g., below 60°F) to help keep cold food items at the proper temperature.

Most food service operations also have support equipment for heated or chilled storage of food located close to the line to facilitate replenishing of the line. This equipment may be permanently installed or designed with casters so that it can be loaded in the preparation areas and then moved to the tray line area.

Operations using heated pellets for temperature maintenance of hot food will need equipment for heating these pellets. Equipment may consist of units using radiation or induction heat to heat the wax or metal in the pellets. Transfer of the heated pellet from the warming unit to the tray can require special tools or gloves. The induction heated bases are insulated and can be transferred by hand thus reducing the potential for burns both to employees as well as patients.

The decision about the placement of support equipment on the tray line is as important as the decision about the type of support equipment needed. This equipment can be placed parallel or perpendicular to the tray line and can be positioned at the same height as, lower than, or higher than the tray line. Perpendicular support equipment allows availability of more menu items without adding to the overall length of the tray line.

Linked with the decision of whether to use parallel or perpendicular support equipment is the decision of whether one wants the tray assembly personnel to be able to communicate easily. Having support equipment parallel to the tray line promotes communication; having it perpendicular discourages it. The choice may depend on the internal motivation of employees to communicate only about tray assembly issues as they arise.

The use of parallel versus perpendicular support equipment also can affect the number and type of motions required of personnel. The goal in designing tray line configurations, the layout of the support equipment, and the placement of dishes and supplies should be to minimize the number of turns and reaches that employees will need to make while assembling trays.

An additional consideration for tray line selection involves the ease of cleaning because this task must be performed on a routine basis. The equipment under consideration should be evaluated for considerations such as rounded corners in wells, lack of crevices where food could become lodged, and time required to cool before cleaning can begin.

Trays

Several options are available for patient trays with a wide range of uses and aesthetic appeal. The basic flat tray is available in different materials, including Fiberglas and plastic, and may have reinforced corners and molded separator bottoms for fast drying. The size, color, pattern, and shape options are numerous.

One distinction made between two broad categories of trays is the method of temperature retention. Passive temperature retention refers to insulated trays and components that do not require application of heat or cold. Active heat retention systems, however, require electrical energy for heat maintenance.

Insulated trays are used as an economical method of improving temperature control. They are constructed of plastic with polyurethane foam insulation. A disadvantage often cited is the inflexibility of dish size and menu offerings with a compartmentalized tray.

Split trays are a specialized type that allows the tray to slide into a hot/cold cart for temperature maintenance throughout transportation. The cart is designed to have half the tray held in a heated compartment and the other half in a refrigerated compartment. All cold foods are placed on one side of the tray, and hot foods are placed on the other side of the tray. Service of cold entree items is somewhat difficult with this type of tray because nearly all (if not all) food items need to be placed on one side of the tray.

Finally, specialized trays are required for some conduction rethermalization systems. These trays have special cut-out areas for entree, soup, and vegetable dishes so that, when the trays are loaded onto the rethermalization carts, the dishes make contact with the conduction heat element in the cart.

Dishes

A variety of dishes and styles of dishware are used on patient trays. Insulated component dishes have been designed for holding soups, hot vegetables, cold or hot beverages, and salads. Thermal retention is achieved through the double layer of plastic, which may be filled with air or polyurethane foam.

Regular china is used in many instances, with the shape, size, and glaze dependent upon the particular use and system. Some systems use bases and domes with the entree plate to help achieve greater temperature maintenance. The entree plate is usually the standard 9-inch, round, china plate that rests on a base with a heated wax or metal alloy, commonly called a pellet. When a dome lid is fitted over the casserole base and china plate, the system helps maintain the temperature of hot food during tray delivery. In other systems, a base and dome of double-layer plastic are used to help retain heat.

Dishes for insulated trays are specially sized and shaped to fit inside the tray compartments. In many cases they are square or oblong rather than the traditional round shape. They may be disposable or china.

Special dishes are used in conduction rethermalization systems. The dishes are shaped to fit within cut-out spaces on special trays. Although dishes for these conduction systems often appear similar in shape to regular dishes, the bottom of the conduction system plates and bowls is flat to maximize contact with the heating element within the cart.

The decision of whether to use china or disposable dishes usually involves consideration of several issues:

- the type of dishes that will work with the tray delivery system being considered
- the comparative cost of the dishes
- the comparative costs of energy, detergent, water, labor, waste hauling, and so forth involved in cleaning or removing dishes
- the capital investment in warewashing, pulping, and the like

Limited research has been done to examine this decision in health care food service operations. Several studies, however, have examined variables and costs involved in using permanent versus disposable ware in schools (Davis, 1994;

Mann, 1991; Riley, Shanklin, & Gench, 1991). Pandit (1991) developed a model to assist food service professionals in evaluating the cost of labor, equipment, refuse disposal, and dishes/supplies when comparing disposable and permanent serviceware. Davis (1994) used input from school food service directors to develop an expert computer system to assist with the decision about permanent versus disposable dishes.

Plating

Plating refers to the activity of placing food items on the entree plate during the tray assembly process. The activity becomes especially important when food products are dished in the chilled state for rethermalization after tray assembly. The density of the food product and its location on the plate can affect the quality of the product after rethermalization. Food items that are not plated properly can fail to reach recommended serving temperatures if they are too thick or can be cooked onto the plate if too thin. The placement of food items on the plate is particularly important when microwave ovens are used for rethermalization because the penetration of the microwave is greatly affected by varying product densities.

Quality Assessment

The quality of the tray assembly process is assessed most often based on the accuracy of the trays assembled and the efficiency of the tray assembly process. Documenting results of such assessments can provide important information to help improve the process.

Tray Line Accuracy

Accuracy of the tray assembly process is assessed by observing what has been placed on the patient tray and comparing that with what should be on the tray. Most organizations have someone positioned on the tray line to perform this assessment. This person, usually called a checker, is responsible for ensuring that the food items on the patient tray are what the patient selected and/or are what should be served for that patient's diet. Checking the accuracy of the tray while it is still on the tray line allows corrections to be made easily. The checker position often controls the speed of the tray line.

Organizations differ in their practices of whether the person in the checker position is a manager or an employee. Reasons cited for having a manager in the checker position are that the manager will be more exact in checking trays than an employee and, by being the one checking trays, the manager will be aware of issues related to operating the tray line (e.g., evenness of workload among stations and accuracy of personnel at each station). Having the manager serve as the checker ties that person to the line, however, and makes it impossible for him or her to handle other issues that require management attention while the tray line is running. Some directors feel that well-trained food service employees can be empowered to perform the checking task and that they can handle more responsibility in this role while making sure that trays are accurate and attractive (Jackson, 1995b). Typically no documentation of accuracy is kept of observations from the checker.

A less frequently used but more often documented method of assessing tray accuracy is to check the trays after they have been placed on the cart but before they are delivered to patients. This checking usually is done by a manager, who evaluates actual patient trays or a test tray that is sent to one of the most remote patient units so that temperature retention as well as tray accuracy can be monitored. Assessment of trays at this point does not have the time pressure that exists during the tray line operation, but making corrections on the trays can be more difficult if the trays have been moved from the tray line area.

Dowling and Cotner (1988) suggested a method for studying tray assembly errors. They recommended assessing the number of errors made in tray assembly, the type of error (omission, addition, or substitution), and the severity of the error (whether the error was critical—contradictory—to the patient's diet). The authors indicated that tray accuracy studies are useful diagnostic tools for evaluating the quantity and seriousness of errors in patient tray assembly, evaluating the quality of performance of tray line employees, identifying training needs of individuals assigned to the tray line, and providing feedback for quality improvement projects.

Tray Line Efficiency

Efficiency measures of the tray assembly process reflect the use of resources (staffhours or number of staff) to produce an output (assembled trays). Usually departments will establish a goal for these efficiency measures so that a comparison of actual performance to this goal can be made.

Efficiency most often is measured by calculating a ratio of the amount of time spent assembling the trays to the number of trays assembled. Common calculations include trays per minute or minutes per tray. One concern with these measures is that simply increasing the number of employees will reduce the amount of time spent assembling trays. If the department goal is to assemble trays in the least time possible, then adding personnel to the tray line may be appropriate. A better indicator of efficiency might be one that relates labor time and trays assembled. Calculations such as trays per labor time or labor time per tray better reflect the relationship of input to output. The only way to improve these indicators is by being more efficient in the tray assembly process.

Nichols (1994) suggests targets for tray line efficiency based on the number of tray line positions. The suggested goal for a tray line with five positions is 1.47 labor minutes per meal or 3.4 trays per minute.

An interesting efficiency measure suggested by Nichols (1994) is belt stop minutes. The author states that a tray line is probably running with maximum efficiency as long as tray line stop time stays at or below 4 minutes per hour in an acute care setting. This measure has not been documented in actual operations but may provide an additional indicator for assessing tray line efficiency.

The goal in tray line efficiency is to determine the number of employees/workstations needed on the line and to identify tasks to be performed at each station so that a desired level of output (trays per minute) is achieved (Adam & Ebert, 1989). A technique termed line balancing can be used to assist tray line managers with this task. The line balancing procedure uses six steps as described in Exhibit 10–1.

Lafferty and Dowling (1993) described how line balancing techniques were used to redesign the tray line configuration at Rush–Presbyterian–St. Luke's Medical Center. Changes were made in what items were placed on trays at each station with the goal that each station would have tasks that required approximately the same amount of time. Using this technique, the authors increased the efficiency of the tray assembly process and balanced the workload at each station.

Factors Affecting Tray Line Accuracy and Efficiency

Several factors can affect the accuracy and efficiency of the tray assembly process, such as the speed of the tray line, format of the tray ticket/menu slip, and

---

Exhibit 10–1 Steps for Balancing Labor on the Tray Line

1. Define the elemental tasks being performed on the tray line.
2. Identify the precedent relationships (which tasks must precede which).
3. Calculate the minimum number of workstations needed:

$$\text{Theoretical minimum number of stations} = \frac{(\text{Total labor time per unit}) \times (\text{Desired units/days})}{\text{Total productive time available/day}}$$

4. Specify the work content at each station.
5. Calculate effectiveness (if output goal accomplished) and efficiency (amount of employee productive time versus idle time).
6. Seek further improvement.

number of menu items and modifications offered. The speed of the tray line usually is controlled by the rate at which trays are placed on the line, the availability of food items as needed on the tray line, the evenness of the workload at each station, and, in cases of mechanized belts, the speed of the belt.

The person placing trays on the tray line establishes the pace. When one is evaluating the flow on the tray line, it is important that this station not take significantly more time than other stations because the time between trays will be initiated here. Having food items constantly available as needed on the tray line also is critical to maintaining the flow of trays. Many organizations use a person called a runner to help constantly replenish food items for the line. This is especially important in operations where food items are being cooked in smaller batches to maintain their freshness and thus are constantly being brought to the tray line throughout the entire tray assembly process.

Research by Myers, Konz, and Gregoire (1991), Fankhauser, Vaden, and Konz (1975), and Laurin (1979) suggested that factors related to the readability and complexity of the tray ticket can affect the accuracy of trays assembled. Issues to be considered are the type size and style, the color of the menu ticket/tray slip, the method used to indicate modified diet items, the location of food items on the menu slip, and whether these items are grouped by tray station.

Although there has not been research published examining the impact of the number of items on the speed and accuracy of the tray line, directors have expressed concerns that having more items on the menu can slow the process of reading and determining what a patient is to receive. Some hospitals are going to a spoke-type menu, which allows the patient a choice of entree and then all other items on the menu are linked to that entree; others are implementing nonselect menus for all patients. The goal of each is to reduce the time spent by tray line employees reading the menu slip because the slip often indicates only a number, entree name, or type of diet. Employees at each station know which items are to be given with that menu choice or type of diet.

Recent developments in computer software allow for patient menu selections to be entered and a tray ticket printed with the patient's name, room number, type of diet, and only those items selected by the patient. This reduces the number of items printed on the tray ticket but does require that tray line employees read the ticket. Results of research by Myers et al. (1991) suggested that tray assembly errors were reduced when the tray ticket was individualized with only patient selections, the type of diet was clearly identified, and bold print was used.

TRANSPORTATION

The transportation process involves movement of patient food from the kitchen to the patient floors. This process could involve the movement of food in bulk that will be used to assemble patient trays on the floor or the movement of carts holding trays of food. Carts are the key equipment used in the transportation process. The type of production and tray assembly systems chosen will determine the type of carts needed.

Carts

Carts are designed to transport food trays from the tray line to patient units. The most basic type of cart is for transportation of trays for which no special type of heat or refrigeration maintenance is required from the cart. For example, no temperature support within the cart is required when pellet system and insulated component dishes are used. Similar carts are used for systems that rethermalize hot food on patient units in convection or microwave ovens, with the exception that the carts are built with specific dimensions to fit in refrigeration units in floor galleys. Specialized carts are designed for transportation of insulated trays to accommodate the rather bulky insulated lid that covers the entire tray. These carts also have no temperature support.

Other carts are designed to provide refrigeration and heat maintenance capabilities in the cart. The cart designed for the split tray system houses both refrigeration and heating units for thermal maintenance of cold and hot food items on the tray. Commonly cited advantages are good temperature retention and the fact that no tray finishing is required. The carts themselves, however, are heavy to maneuver, and maintenance cost can be high.

Another specialized cart is used for transportation of the match-a-tray system, which includes separate hot and cold units on the same cart. In this system, the hot food items are removed from the tray and put into heated drawers or slots. The rest of the tray is loaded onto the refrigerated side of the cart. Use of this cart requires tray finishing on the patient floors for reassembly of the tray before delivery to the patient.

Carts for delivery of trays assembled cold on the tray line are available from numerous manufacturers. These carts either contain a refrigeration unit for maintaining the temperature of chilled foods or can be attached to or rolled into refrigeration units. These refrigeration units may be in the central food production area or in galleys or pantries on patient floors. Many of these carts act as the rethermalization equipment also. Some carts contain conduction heating units over which portions of the tray are placed, allowing for rethermalization of hot food items right on the tray. The carts can be programmed for the desired start of rethermalization. Other rethermalization carts have a refrigerated unit on one side of the cart for the cold tray and a convection oven unit on the other. Another option is one that requires two carts for food for each patient area: one for holding the cold trays, which is rolled into a refrigerator, and the other for conduction rethermalization of hot food items. Choosing carts that allow for heat retention or rethermalization to occur on the tray reduces the chance for error when plates are taken off the tray and returned after hot holding or rethermalization.

Delivery carts have numerous options. One of the most basic factors that the food service director should consider is the number of trays to be loaded on carts at one time. To minimize the number of delivery personnel, the inclination is to send as many trays on each cart as possible or as one unit requires. The director, however, should calculate the optimal thermal retention time of the system in use. For example, some carts hold up to 44 trays. Depending on the efficiency of the tray line, the distance that the cart needs to be transported, and the time on the patient unit before delivery, the first tray on the cart could well be beyond the recommended thermal retention time if it sits on the cart waiting for 43 more trays to be dished and loaded before it is delivered to the patient.

The director should talk to other users of the product before final selection. Some critical questions to ask are as follows:

- How difficult is the cart to push and maneuver when loaded? (Maneuverability will affect how many carts can be delivered at one time and the chances of damage to walls, railings, etc.)
- How well does the inside molding on seams hold up? (Water inside moldings can promote vermin breeding inside carts.)
- How well do the casters, brakes, and wheels hold up?
- Does the cart have tray slides designed to anchor the tray in place, and, if so, how much space on the tray is lost when the trays are loaded onto the carts?
- Are locking wheels needed?
- Which wheels should be swivel type?
- How easy is the cart to clean?
- Will it easily pass through all doors along the route?

In addition to food transportation within a unit, advanced preparation systems have popularized the commissary or food factory system. This food production unit prepares food items for shipment to a number of medical centers in food service locations. Palmer (1984) stated that savings result from economies of mass production, lower inventory and purchases cost, and improved monitoring of employee productivity. The author believes that a successful commissary operation is total cost analysis, which minimizes the sum of the costs of transportation, warehousing, inventory, order processing, and production lot quantity costs while achieving a desired customer service level.

Quality Assessment

A key indicator of quality of the transportation process is the timeliness with which the trays are delivered to the unit. Observing the transportation process and documenting the time it takes and possible reasons for delays will provide data to help improve the process. Another indicator of quality is the appearance of the trays after the transportation process, particularly whether the transportation process has resulted in items that have shifted or spilled on the tray and if food temperatures have been successfully maintained.

TRAY FINISHING

The tray finishing process includes any required activities on the patient unit before final presentation of the tray to the patient. The range of activities may be as simple as adding hot beverages or may be quite complex and involve rethermalization of food products. Operations with a decentralized tray assembly system require complete tray assembly on the floor, which often requires additional space and rethermalization or holding equipment.

Limited Finishing

Many systems require limited final tray finishing, such as placement of hot beverages, frozen desserts, or cold beverages. Because not all foods undergo rethermalization equally well by conduction or convection, tray finishing may be carried out on patient floors for products such as toast or poached eggs. Increased efficiency of the tray finishing process can normally be achieved after the patient menu is evaluated to identify the foods that require more labor-intensive finishing tasks. These menu selections can be replaced with others that are equally acceptable to patients but require less handling time.

Rethermalization

There are three methods for heating or rethermalizing foods: conduction, convection, and microwave.

Conduction Rethermalization

Part of the tray finishing process may be accomplished within the transportation cart itself, as mentioned earlier. Conduction rethermalization often occurs in the refrigerated carts that were used in the transportation process. In these carts, heating occurs on special plates that are designed to make contact with heating elements located under portions of the shelves holding the trays. Another version of conduction heating involves having separate carts with heated shelves for holding plates and bowls to be rethermalized. These carts have numbered shelves to correspond with numbered shelves in a refrigerated unit where the cold trays are stored. Trays are reassembled after rethermalization.

The conduction heating units are activated in a number of ways. They may be activated by the stainless steel rim of the plate cover making contact with the conduction element. Food items that are not to be heated are covered with a plastic dome, which will not activate the conduction unit. In other carts, the conduction units are activated by the tray cover coming in contact with a switch that controls the conduction element for that tray. Trays containing an entree that is not to be heated are turned around before being placed in the cart so that the conduction heating switch is not activated by the tray cover. In some carts, personnel can program whether a dish is heated or kept cold. Conduction heating equipment differs in whether the temperature of the heating elements can be changed, whether the heating time can be modified, and whether heat maintenance options are available. Having the option of heating or not heating each tray allows service of popular entrees such as shrimp salad or chicken caesar salad. Food service directors should consider the number of decisions that must be made by employees related to rethermalization; increasing the number of decisions made can result in the need for more training.

Other options now available with conduction heating carts are bun warmer drawers, security locks for safe storage during chilling and rethermalization, numbered tray shelves, and special clips to hold trays in place on the cart and reduce the chances of improper rethermalization because of tray shifting during transport.

Convection Rethermalization

Convection rethermalization requires special carts or ovens that are available from several manufacturers. In all cases, the hot food items are heated in a convection unit separate from the cold tray.

One variation of conduction rethermalization involves the assembly of all food items onto patient trays, transportation of these trays in refrigerated carts to patient units, and transfer of the hot food item dishes to a special convection oven unit for rethermalization. A newer form of this concept involves a specialized cart with an oven insert rack for the hot food items. Dishes are placed on this rack during the tray assembly process and transported in an unrefrigerated section of the cart to the patient floor, and the rack of dishes is loaded into the convection oven. This eliminates moving individual dishes during rethermalization. The oven insert is pulled back into the delivery cart after rethermalization, and hot dishes and cold trays are on the same level in the cart to ease matching of entrees with trays (Nichols, 1994). A third version of convection rethermalization involves carts that contain a refrigerated compartment for the cold trays and a separate compartment in which convected heat actually flows throughout the cart to reheat food. Hot food items are placed on shelves during tray assembly. These have separate cold compartments to prevent the transfer of heat during the rethermalization process.

Microwave Rethermalization

Rethermalization by microwaves was reported by 22% of cook-chill systems and 59% of cook-freeze systems in a study by Nettles and Gregoire (1993). Improvements in convection and conduction systems have probably decreased the decision to use microwave rethermalization. Commonly cited disadvantages include overheating and scorching of foods, uneven heating due to differing densities, and low productivity because only one tray is heated at a time. Typically, rethermalization using microwave ovens occurs in galleys on patient floors.

A modified version of microwave rethermalization was introduced in the 1980s as a means of centralized rethermalization (Smith, 1981). Termed a food finisher, this piece of equipment was designed to move food products on a mechanized conveyor through a tunnel that consisted of numerous sections for microwave heating; some sections also included steam jets to circulate moist warm air. This food finisher, or microwave tunnel, could be programmed for the number of microwave applications to be used on a given food product. Use of the food finisher has been limited, however, to a few installations in the early 1980s.

Decentralized Tray Assembly

Decentralized assembly involves menu items being produced in one location and transported in bulk, either hot or cold, to various locations for assembly in areas near patients (Spears, 1995). Options for rethermalization in bulk include convection ovens, steamers or convection steamers, hot water baths, or steam-jacketed kettles. Up to 75 meals can be rethermalized simultaneously within one or two convection ovens (Fasano, 1993).

Even though centralized tray assembly has several distinct advantages, food service directors may be using decentralized assembly for some or all of their patient units because there is less time lapse between assembly and service of food trays, and the quality of some products may be improved. Additionally, last-minute changes in patient selections are facilitated by a system where the tray is assembled on the patient floor immediately before service. Implementation of advanced preparation systems (cook-chill, cook-freeze, and convenience) has in some instances resulted in a variation of decentralized systems in which food may be placed on trays in a central location but is rethermalized in patient floor galleys, and hot beverages and other temperature-sensitive items are placed on trays before delivery to the patient. Use of decentralized tray assembly usually requires additional labor for the tray finishing process. Supervision of the final tray assembly process also becomes more difficult because this tray assembly is occurring in several different floor galley kitchens simultaneously.

Some of the issues that should be addressed when one is considering whether to implement a centralized or decentralized tray assembly process are outlined below; this selection decision is closely linked with the type of production system used and whether rethermalization of food will be needed before delivery to patients:

- What questions might be considered to find the optimal place to use such a system?
- How many different menu items and variations on each would need to be transported in bulk to patient areas?
- Could patient service times be staggered sufficiently so that personnel and equipment could receive maximum use?
- Could sufficient training and empowerment of employees be achieved so that centralized supervision would be unnecessary?

Quality Assessment

Assessment of quality of the tray finishing process should focus on issues such as the appearance and temperature of food on the tray as well as the efficiency of the personnel assembling the tray. When rethermalization occurs during the tray finishing process, it can affect the appearance and aroma of the food items being served.

DELIVERY TO PATIENTS

The process of delivering trays to patients involves personnel taking trays from the food cart and delivering them to the patients. This process is the service portion of the food service operation. This activity has received much attention in recent years as patient-focused care concepts have increasingly been implemented in facilities across the nation.

Personnel Delivering Meal Trays

Hospitals differ on which department's personnel are responsible for the delivery of patient trays. In some hospitals the food and nutrition department has this responsibility, in others nursing personnel deliver trays, and in some the responsibility is shared. Research by Nettles and Gregoire (1993) indicated that the responsibility for tray delivery appeared to be related to the type of food production system in place at the hospital. In hospitals with conventional food production systems, hospitals were split in about half on whether nursing or dietary employees delivered trays. Hospitals with cook-chill systems were much more likely, however, to have trays delivered by food service employees.

Recent innovations in tray delivery include the use of host/hostess or patient service associate programs. Hospitals with host/hostess programs have designated employees for each floor who are responsible not only for delivery of meal trays but also for serving beverages and snacks between meals.

The concept of patient service associate developed concurrent with the trend toward patient-focused care in hospitals. The concept involves service personnel who are assigned to specific patient rooms and who have multiple responsibilities for a given patient. The position often combines the roles of housekeeper, nurse aide, and tray passer into one position, thus reducing the number of different personnel entering a patient's room in a day's time. (See Chapter 3 for a discussion of the impact of restructuring on employees' responsibilities and an example of how tasks can be reassigned to members of the direct patient care team.)

Results of a study by Gregoire (1994) suggest that patient satisfaction with meal service may be related to personnel who deliver meal trays. Patients in hospitals where dietary employees delivered trays gave higher ratings for food quality issues than patients in hospitals where nursing personnel delivered meals. Conversely, patients in hospitals where nursing personnel delivered meals were more positive about the care and concern given by the personnel passing trays.

Quality Assessment

Assessment of the quality of the tray delivery process should be done by both the food and nutrition department staff and the patients themselves. Food and nutrition staff need to be concerned about the efficiency of the tray delivery process as well as the quality of the food served to patients. Patients can provide valuable information about their satisfaction with the food and service provided at mealtimes. Several researchers (Dubé, Trudeau, & Belanger, 1994; Gregoire, 1994; Oldford, 1989) have suggested that patient satisfaction with meal service is multidimensional and that assessments of patient satisfaction should focus on all dimensions. Results of their research suggest that assessment of patient satisfaction should focus on issues related to the food, the personnel serving the food, and the environment in which the food is served. Quality of the food typically is assessed as part of the production process, but quality of the food as it is served to the patients also needs to be assessed. Factors to be considered include taste, appearance, and temperature. In addition, accuracy of the tray from the patient's perspective is important.

Having patients evaluate the food and service while they are still in the hospital allows food and nutrition staff to correct issues identified by the patients. Results of several research projects suggest that patient satisfaction with meal service is related to variables such as age (Carey & Posavac, 1982; DeLuco & Cremer, 1990; Dubé et al., 1994; Maller, Dubose, & Cardello, 1980), gender (Carey & Posavac, 1982; DeLuco & Cremer, 1990; Dubé et al., 1994), level of education (DeLuco & Cremer, 1990; Dubé et al., 1994), and appetite (DeLuco & Cremer, 1990; Dubé et al., 1994; Maller et al., 1980). Research has failed to show a relationship between satisfaction and factors such as medical diagnosis (DeLuco & Cremer, 1990; Maller et al., 1980) and type of diet (Carey & Posavac, 1982; Dubé et al., 1994; Maller et al., 1980).

Although some nutrient loss is inevitable in any process applied to foods, generally the advantages of improved palatability, texture, and eating properties as well as production of new products, elimination of microorganisms, and destruction of toxins are considered to outweigh nutrient losses. Food service directors will, however, want to develop standard procedures that minimize cooking losses during holding, assembly, rethermalization, transportation, tray finishing, and delivery to patients.

A number of studies have evaluated the relationship between nutrient destruction and time food is held. Williams and Miller (1993) summarized results of 66 studies that examined nutrient retention in cook-chill and conventional cook–hot hold food service systems and concluded that under normal operating conditions, with less than 90 minutes of hot holding, less nutrient loss occurred in conventional compared to cook-chill systems. Kahn and Livingston (1970) compared thiamine retention in stew, chicken, shrimp, and peas held 1, 2, and 3 hours. They found retention rates of 78%, 74%, and 76%, respectively. Ang, Chang, Frey, and Livingston (1975) studied the ascorbic acid retention of mashed potatoes held hot for 0.5 and 3.0 hours and found 66% and 30% retention rates, respectively. They also found that a cook-freeze system did not offer improvement if the product was held any longer than 0.5 hour. In general, prolonged hot holding at high temperatures has a direct effect on nutrient retention.

The distribution process has not been studied widely, but Wagner (1971) compared the ascorbic acid content of food held hot in insulated containers and foods held in refrigeration for various periods of time. Significantly greater amounts of vitamin C were lost in vegetables held for 3 hours in an insulated container than in vegetables held in refrigerators and reheated.

In advanced preparation systems, food service directors should be aware of potential nutrient loss during prolonged storage. Augustin (1975) found that vitamin losses after 6 hours in potatoes held in refrigeration were not changed significantly by storing the potatoes up to 24 hours. Charles and Van Duyne (1958) studied several vegetables and found that they all lost significant vitamin C with refrigerated holding for 24 hours.

Williams (1996) recommended the following practices to reduce nutrient losses:

If using a cook-chill system

- chill foods quickly
- maintain chilled foods below 10°C during storage, plating, and delivery
- minimize the amount of time food is above 50°C, preferably no more than 1 hour
- reheat food after plating rather than in bulk
- avoid long storage times

If using conventional cook–hot hold system:

- batch cook vegetables
- minimize the amount of hot holding time

Varying conclusions have been reached about nutrient retention and different methods of reheating food. Engler and Bowers (1976) and Bowers and Fryer (1972) concluded that different methods of reheating, such as microwave ovens compared with convection ovens, did not significantly affect nutrient retention.

DECISION ISSUES IN TRAY ASSEMBLY, TRANSPORTATION, AND FINISHING

The innovations in tray assembly, transportation, and finishing available in recent years have given the food service director a wide assortment of choices for system selection. A comprehensive comparison of the various systems by manufacturer name or detailed descriptions of systems are available in different sources (Goldberg & Kohligian, 1974; Hysen & Harrison, 1982; Norton, 1991; Pinkert & Hysen, 1973). Sources compare the advantages, disadvantages, and distinguishing characteristics of different systems. Norton (1991) offers other helpful comparative data such as cart dimensions, warranty information, voltage, training, cycle duration, and manufacturers' years of experience in food delivery systems. In addition, manufacturers have developed extensive product brochures that outline their systems and their benefits.

Also of use to the food service director is a background reading of case studies of different hospitals' experiences with implementation of new systems. The benefits of reviewing such cases include consideration of the use of different combinations of systems available as well as acquaintance with problems to be avoided by preplanning (Exhibit 10–2).

Integral to the selection process is the question of food quality. The food service director will want an objective measurement of food quality. A number of food quality studies have been carried out using reproducible methodology to document the sensory quality of food from various systems. A summary of those studies is provided in Exhibit 10–3. Assessment of food quality is not only a system selection question but a continuous quality improvement issue. Basic to the question of food quality is the issue of the food itself versus the food service system. The quality of the food itself has to do with the food, the recipes used, the quality of the ingredients, and the desired product for the target clientele. These issues can best be addressed by developing quality food standards for the products served as referenced in Chapter 9.

The food service director must assess the ongoing quality of the food service system itself. That is, how well does the chosen system protect the microbiological, nutrient, and sensory quality of the products? The microbiological quality of the products is best evaluated by the time–temperature relation of the products as they move through the phases of tray assembly, storage, transportation, and finishing. This responsibility translates into the use of the hazard analysis critical control point (HACCP) methodology, in which a thorough analysis of each step in production and distribution is conducted to determine the points of potential microbiological danger. Safety procedures and processes are then established at these points. Bobeng and David (1978) first defined critical control points for HACCP models for food service systems as ingredient control and storage, equipment sanitation, personnel sanitation, and time and temperature. There are numerous reports on HACCP implementation (Beasley, 1995; Bryan, 1990; Corlett, 1989; Jackson, 1995a). The Food Code 1995 issued by the U.S. Public Health Service devotes an entire section to defining HACCP principles and describing how to operationalize these principles.

A list of studies examining microbiological issues in various food service systems is given in Exhibit 10–4. Some of the studies were carried out in actual operations; others were simulated. Klein, Matthews, and Setser (1984), in their summary of microbial studies, indicated that microbial concerns exist for all types of food service systems. The microbial quality appears to be dependent on issues such as type of food, quality of raw ingredients, batch size, type of equipment used for cooking, and position of food item in cooking equipment. Management of time–temperature relationships throughout all processes is critical.

Research on the maintenance of appropriate temperatures in cook-chill systems indicates that safe temperatures are not always maintained. Ridley and Matthews (1983) tracked internal temperatures of 93 food items at meal assembly, after distribution to patient galleys, after cold holding in the galleys, and

Exhibit 10–2 References for Case Studies of Alternative Food Service Systems

Berkman, J., & Schechler, M. (1991). Today I closed my kitchen. *Food Management, 26,* 110–114, 118, 122.

Bjorkman, A., & Delphin, K.A. (1966). Sweden's Nacka hospital food system centralizes preparation and distribution. *Cornell HRA Quarterly, 7,* 84–87.

Bryan, L., & Fritz, M. (1976). Increase employee productivity and patient satisfaction. *Hospitals, 50,* 125–128.

Corsi, R.M. (1984). The ready food system. *Consultant, 17,* 23–25.

Glew, G. (1973). The technology for improved service. *Hospitals, 47,* 51–52.

Glew, G., & Armstrong, J.F. (1981). Cost optimization through cook-freeze systems. *Journal of Foodservice Systems, 1,* 235–254.

Goldberg, C.M., & Kohligian, M. (1974). Conventional, convenience, or ready food service? *Hospitals, 48,* 80–83.

King, P. (1987). Expanding a foodservice system. *Food Management, 22,* 64, 68.

King, P. (1987). "First class" food production. *Food Management, 22,* 70, 75.

King, P. (1987). Production for profit. *Food Management, 22,* 68, 76.

King, P. (1987). Solving the space problem. *Food Management, 22,* 54, 60.

King, P. (1987). The final step. *Food Management, 22,* 73, 78.

King, P. (1988). A system with room to grow. *Food Management, 23,* 61, 64.

King, P. (1988). Changing with the times. *Food Management, 23,* 63, 66.

King, P. (1988). Cook/freeze succeeds in Hawaii. *Food Management, 23,* 55–56.

King, P. (1988). "Plate-ready" debuts at Texas A&M. *Food Management, 23,* 61–64.

King, P. (1989). A gamble pays off. *Food Management, 24,* 80, 86.

King, P. (1989). A vision comes to life. *Food Management, 24,* 66–68.

King, P. (1989). The future of central production. *Food Management, 24,* 52, 57, 71.

King, P. (1990). At St. Francis, time's on their side. *Food Management, 25,* 76–77.

King, P. (1990). Best of both worlds. *Food Management, 25,* 68, 76.

King, P. (1990). From famine to feast at VUMC. *Food Management, 25,* 61, 64.

King, P. (1990). Michigan DOC: Food production in a state of flux. *Food Management, 25,* 64, 68.

King, P. (1994). Overcoming the age barrier. *Food Management, 29,* 42.

King, P. (1994). Support components make the system at the New York Hospital. *Food Management, 29,* 41.

King, P. (1994). The only constant is change. *Food Management, 29,* 54.

Millross, J., & Glew, G. (1974). Staff, equipment, and wastage. *Hospitals, 48,* 72–74.

Millross, J., Hill, M.A., & Glew, G. (1974). Consequences of a switch to cook-freeze. *Hospitals, 48,* 118–126.

Ricklin, A.H., McCoy, G., & Kotimsky, S.R. (1975). Microwave system reduces costs, improves meals. *Hospitals, 49,* 47–49.

Ross, V. (1974). Virginia hospital triples meal service without adding cooks through FF. *Quick Frozen Foods, 37,* 40–41.

Stephenson, S. (1992). New cook-chill system earns high grades. *Restaurants and Institutions, 112,* 114.

Exhibit 10–3 Research Studies Comparing Sensory Attributes of Meal Systems by Means of Objective Methods

Dahl & Matthews (1980):	Reheating precooked foods results in loss of moisture.
Bobeng & David (1978):	Sensory scores for color of meat and uniformity of color were significantly lower for beef loaves prepared in cook-chill or cook-freeze systems.
Zallen, Hitchcock, & Goertz (1975):	Sensory scores of beef loaves served without prior storage were significantly higher than for similar products stored and re-heated.
Allen, Noble, & Schilmore (1991):	Comparison of conventionally and cook-chill prepared egg and cheese product showed significantly higher scores for conventionally prepared.
Glew (1973):	Precooked frozen food reheated was as acceptable to patients as conventionally prepared foods.
Cardello, Maller, & Kluter (1984):	Results of a survey of patient acceptance of food products before and after implementation of cook-freeze showed lower ratings for flavor and texture and higher ratings for temperature after implementation.
Sawyer & Naidu (1984):	Under full meal reheating conditions, conduction reheated meals were significantly superior in sensory evaluation compared with those reheated in convection or microwave systems.

after microwave reheating. Few of the food items were found to be in the recommended temperature range (i.e., $\leq 7°C$ or $\geq 74°C$). At meal assembly, only 20 of 93 items were at 7°C or lower; after distribution to the patient galley, only 11 of 93 were at 7°C or lower; after cold holding, 26 of 93 were at 7°C or lower; and after microwave reheating, 25 of 40 were at 74°C or higher. In a more recent study, Williams and Miller (1993) examined hold time and temperature of vegetables prepared in conventional and cook-chill operations and reported similar concerns. They found that vegetables prepared in conventional systems were held hot (above 50°C) for significantly longer periods of time (72 versus 49 minutes) than vegetables prepared in cook-chill operations; vegetables in cook-chill operations, however, were held in the 10° to 50°C temperature range for extended periods of time (mean, 157 versus 16 minutes).

Lacey (1994) discussed issues related to food safety, particularly to *Listeria monocytogenes*. Because of the thermotolerance nature of this bacterium, it is expected to flourish in cook-chill prepared foods at the expense of other relatively harmless bacteria. The author expressed concern that regular consumption of food prepared using cook-chill technology could alter the intestinal mi-

Exhibit 10–4 Research Studies Comparing Microbiological Concerns for Meal Systems by Means of Objective Methods

Chipley & Cremer (1980):	The authors reviewed 20 research projects that focused on accessing microbiological concerns in food service operations. They concluded that thorough cooking, cooling, and reheating of food and prevention of recontamination are the most important factors in maintaining a safe food supply.
Dahl, Matthews, & Marth (1980):	The fate of *Staphylococcus aureus* in cook-chill systems before and after microwave heating was determined. The number of *S. aureus* decreased as time of microwave heating increased.
Klein, Matthews, & Setser (1984):	The authors summarized 23 studies that have examined the microbiological quality of foods prepared in conventional, ready food, and commissary food service systems. The authors concluded that all types of food service systems need to protect against microbiological contamination of the foods served.
Ridley & Matthews (1983):	Temperatures of nearly 100 food items were monitored during meal assembly, distribution, and service in a hospital using a cook-chill system. The temperatures of many of the food items often were greater than 45°F and less than 165°F.
Snyder & Matthews (1984):	The authors reviewed 40 studies of the microbiological quality of menu items produced and stored in cook-chill, cook-freeze, cook–hot hold, and heat-serve systems. They concluded that steps requiring thermal processing may have a greater effect on all aspects of food quality than any other food handling procedure.
Williams & Miller (1993):	This study compared time and temperature of vegetables prepared in conventional and cook-chill operations. Vegetables prepared in conventional systems were held hot for extended periods of time; vegetables prepared in cook-chill systems often were between 10° and 50°C.

crobial flora from that resulting from the ingestion of conventionally prepared foods.

The sensory quality of the products in systems that rethermalize is considered a function of several issues. Plate selection and reheating influence the sensory quality of the meal and should be considered. The dome or covering in reheat systems may also have a detrimental effect on sensory quality of the meal. Condensate from hot food will collect on the top of the dome and drip onto the food. In the case of sandwiches, for example, producing an acceptable, nonsoggy product becomes a challenge. Innovations by at least one manufacturer diminish the condensate under the dome. In addition to the condensate, a dome covering plates that contain several food items the odors of which are combined may produce an undesirable sensory effect. Plating in reheat systems should therefore avoid combining foods with strong odors with other foods on the same plate.

Gravies, sauces, and glazes enhance the sensory quality of products for cook-chill systems. In general, most meats should have at least a thin glaze to protect them from drying during conduction or convection rethermalization.

DECISION AND EVALUATION TOOLS

Several of the total quality management tools lend themselves well to both the system decision and assessment processes. The tree diagram tool is best used when a complex process such as implementation of a project is to be initiated. In the tree diagram, completion team members first brainstorm all the tasks needed to accomplish a goal. After the initial brainstorming, those tasks considered most important are placed on the major tree headings. The next level of detail tasks can then be assigned under the major tree headings as detailed steps. As the tree diagram is reviewed for logical sequence of steps, team members may also break down the detailed steps into subtasks. The tree diagram then lends itself to further work as individual tasks are assigned and deadlines are set.

Figure 10–6 shows a first attempt at building a logical sequence of necessary steps to implement a new tray delivery system. Team members build the diagram such that the accomplishment of each detailed task on the right leads to the completion of the broader level goal on the left. The tree diagram works particularly well for complex tasks in keeping the team focused on the major goal and not missing an important intermediate step. As the process of tray delivery system implementation continues, team members may further refine the plan.

The sequence flow chart is used to analyze the flow of work in a process and to identify opportunities for improvement. Figure 10–7 shows a sample of a sequence flow chart developed to analyze the steps between trays loaded on carts in the tray assembly area and trays delivered to patients in a convection rethermalization system. In preparing the chart, members write out tasks as they actually occur rather than how they should occur. At each step in the process, the people involved are identified and listed along the top of the chart. Each task in the process should take a certain amount of time and is recorded on the right. Team members can use the chart to direct their efforts in further study to determine how to reduce the time within the cycle. Several other tools, such as cause and effect diagrams, force field analyses, and affinity diagrams,

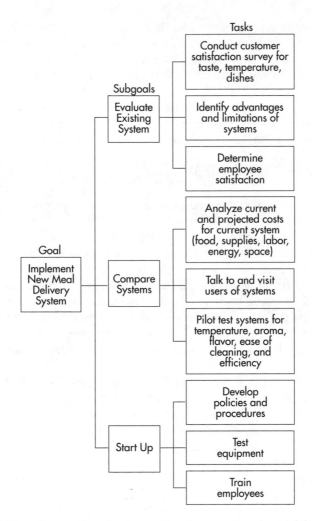

Figure 10–6 Tree diagram for selection and implementation of meal delivery systems.

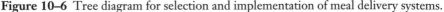

may help with this process. Chapter 14 provides more information about total quality management/quality improvement methods.

CONCLUSION

Rapid advancements in technology are reshaping the way that food service directors are delivering their products and services. The combination of tech-

TASK \ WHO	Tray Assembly				Hostess				Nursing Service			Time Per Task	Elapsed Time
Load Trays												8	15
Deliver to Floor												12	15
Remove Entree												7	7
Place in Oven													
Place in Refrigerator												.10	.10
Start Retherm												3	15
Check Diet for Changes												11	12
Prepare Beverages												8	10
Place on Trays													
Remove Entree from Oven												10	15
Unwrap													
Place on Trays													
Notify Nursing Service												2	2
Roll Cart to Nursing Unit												2	2
Deliver to Patient												10	30
TOTAL												73.1	123.1

Figure 10–7 Sequence flow chart for meal assembly and service.

nological advances makes possible a wide array of system combinations. This environment, coupled with the pressure for increased client satisfaction and decreased use of resources, makes it imperative that the food service director use the collective energy of the food team as well as the many tools available to create the best possible system combination for a given food service operation.

REFERENCES

Adam, E.E., & Ebert, R.J. (1989). *Production and operations management* (4th ed.). Englewood Cliffs, NJ: Prentice-Hall.

Allen, A., Noble, J., & Schilmore, D. (1991). Sensory and objective evaluation of conventionally prepared versus cook-chill prepared egg and cheese products in a hospital foodservice operation. *Journal of Foodservice Systems, 6,* 1–14.

Ang, C.Y.W., Chang, A.M., Frey, A.E., & Livingston, G.E. (1975). Effects of heating methods on vitamin retention in six fresh or frozen prepared food products. *Journal of Food Science, 40,* 997–1003.

Augustin, J. (1975). Variations in the nutritional composition of fresh potatoes. *Journal of Food Science, 40,* 1295–1299.

Beasley, M.A. (1995). Implementing HACCP standards. *Food Management, 30,* 38, 40.

Berkman, J., & Schechler, M. (1991). Today I closed my kitchen. *Food Management, 26,* 110–114, 118, 122.

Bobeng, B.J., & David, B.D. (1978). HACCP models for quality control of entree production in hospital foodservice systems. Quality assessment of beef loaves utilizing HACCP models. *Journal of the American Dietetic Association, 73,* 531–551.

Bowers, J.A., & Fryer, B.A. (1972). Thiamin and riboflavin in cooked and frozen reheated turkey (gas vs. microwave ovens). *Journal of the American Dietetic Association, 60,* 399.

Bryan, F.L. (1990). Application of HACCP to ready-to-eat chilled foods. *Food Technology, 44,* 70–77.

Byers, B.A., Shanklin, C.W., & Hoover, L.C. (1994). *Food service manual for health care institutions.* Chicago: American Hospital Publishing.

Cardello, A.V., Maller, O., & Kluter, R. (1984). Multi-user assessment of a hospital cook-freeze foodservice system. *Journal of Foodservice Systems, 3,* 153–169.

Carey, R.G., & Posavac, E.J. (1982). Using patient information to identify areas for service improvement. *Health Care Management Review, 7,* 43–48.

Charles, V.R., & Van Duyne, F.O. (1958). Effects of holding and reheating on the ascorbic acid content of cooked vegetables. *Journal of Home Economics, 50,* 159–162.

Chipley, J.R., & Cremer, M.L. (1980). Microbiological problems in the food service industry. *Food Technology, 34,* 59–68.

Corlett, D.A. (1989). Refrigerated foods and use of hazard analysis and critical control point principles. *Food Technology, 43,* 91–94.

Dahl, C.A., & Matthews, M.E. (1980). Cook/chill foodservice system with a microwave oven: Thiamin content in portions of beef loaf after microwave heating. *Journal of Food Science, 45,* 608–612.

Dahl, C.A., Matthews, M.E., & Marth, E.H. (1980). Fate of *Staphylococcus aureus* in beef loaf, potatoes and frozen and canned green beans after microwave-heating in a simulated cook/chill hospital foodservice system. *Journal of Food Protection, 43,* 916–923.

Davis, C.L. (1994). *An expert computer system developed for serviceware selection in school foodservice.* Unpublished doctoral dissertation, Kansas State University, Manhattan, KS.

DeLuco, D., & Cremer, M. (1990). Consumers' perceptions of hospital food and dietary services. *Journal of the American Dietetic Association, 90,* 1711–1715.

Dowling, R., & Cotner, C. (1988). Monitor of tray error rates for quality control. *Journal of the American Dietetic Association, 88,* 450–453.

Dubé, L., Trudeau, E., & Belanger, M. (1994). Determining the complexity of patient satisfaction with foodservices. *Journal of the American Dietetic Association, 94*, 394–398.

Engler, P.P., & Bowers, J.A. (1976). B-vitamin retention in meat during storage and preparation. *Journal of the American Dietetic Association, 69*, 253–257.

Fairbrook, P. (1994). The trouble with steamtables. *Food Management, 29*, 48.

Fankhauser, W., Vaden, A.G., & Konz, S.A. (1975). Applying concepts of visual perception to formats of hospital menus. *Journal of the American Dietetic Association, 67*, 464–469.

Fasano, J. (1993). Cook-chill question and answer corner. *Consultant, 26*, 32–33.

Glew, G. (1973). The technology for improved service. *Hospitals, 47*, 51–52.

Goldberg, C.M., & Kohligian, M. (1974). Conventional, convenience, or ready food service? *Hospitals, 48*, 80–83.

Gregoire, M. (1994). Quality of patient meal service in hospitals: Delivery of meals by dietary employees vs. delivery by nursing employees. *Journal of the American Dietetic Association, 94*, 1129–1134.

Hysen, P., & Harrison, J. (1982). *State-of-the-art review of healthcare patient feeding system equipment. Hospital feeding systems*. Washington, DC: National Academy Press.

Jackson, R. (1995a). Featuring Mildred Cody, PhD, RD. *Hospital Food and Nutrition Focus, 11*, 4–6.

Jackson, R. (1995b). What's new in labor-saving equipment. *Hospital Food and Nutrition Focus, 11*, 7–8.

Kahn, L.N., & Livingston, G.E. (1970). Effect of heating methods on thiamin retention in fresh and frozen prepared foods. *Journal of Food Science, 35*, 349–351.

Klein, B.P., Matthews, M.E., & Setser, C.S. (1984). *Foodservice systems: Time and temperature effects on food quality*. Urbana-Champaign, IL: University of Illinois.

Lacey, R.W. (1994). *Listeria*, implications for food safety. *British Food Journal, 94*, 26–32.

Lafferty, L.J., & Dowling, R.A. (1993, October). Reengineering foodservice processes through quantitative analysis. Presentation at the American Dietetic Association annual meeting, Anaheim, CA.

Laurin, J.P. (1979). *Comparison of two menu designs on error rate and assembly time in a centralized patient tray assembly system*. Unpublished master's thesis, University of Missouri, Columbia, MO.

Maller, O., Dubose, C.N., & Cardello, A.V. (1980). Consumer opinions of hospital food and foodservice. *Journal of the American Dietetic Association, 76*, 236–242.

Mann, N.L. (1991). *A decision model for solid waste management in school food service*. Unpublished doctoral dissertation, Texas Woman's University, Denton, TX.

Myers, E., Konz, S.A., & Gregoire, M.B. (1991). Individualized menu slips improve the accuracy of patient food trays. *Journal of the American Dietetic Association, 91*, 1425–1428.

Nettles, M.F., & Gregoire, M.B. (1993). Operational characteristics of hospital foodservice departments with conventional, cook-chill, and cook-freeze systems. *Journal of the American Dietetic Association, 93*, 1161–1163.

Nichols, J. (1994). *Trayline doctor* (4th ed.). Kansas City, MO: Crimsco, Inc.

Norton, L.C. (1991). *Keep it hot?? Keep it cold!!* Missouri City, TX: Norton Group.

Oldford, C.L. (1989). *Patient hospital foodservice satisfaction: An exploratory framework and analysis*. Unpublished doctoral dissertation, New York University, New York, NY.

Palmer, J.D. (1984). The logic and logistics of commissaries. *Cornell HRA Quarterly, 25*(1), 104–109.

Pandit, R. (1991). *Disposable versus reusable ware: Cost evaluation model development*. Unpublished master's thesis, Rochester Institute of Technology, Rochester, NY.

Pinkert, M.S., & Hysen, P. (1973). Pros and cons of three food systems. *Canadian Hospital, 50*(3), 13–15.

Ridley, S.J., & Matthews, M.E. (1983). Temperature histories of menu items during meal assembly, distribution and service in a hospital foodservice. *Journal of Food Protection, 46,* 100–104.

Riley, L.K., Shanklin, C.W., & Gench, B. (1991). Comparison of volume of waste generated by and cost of two types of serviceware systems. *School Food Service Research Review, 15,* 32–36.

Sawyer, C.A., & Naidu, Y.M. (1984). Sensory evaluation of cook/chilled products reheated by conduction, convection and microwave radiation. *Journal of Foodservice Systems, 3,* 89–106.

Smith, D. (1981). Food finishing of frozen food. In proceedings of the 37th Conference of the Society for the Advancement of Food Service Research (pp. 161–166). Washington, DC.

Snyder, P.O., & Matthews, M.E. (1984). Microbiological quality of foodservice menu items produced and stored by cook/chill, cook/freeze, cook/hot-hold and heat/serve methods. *Journal of Food Protection, 47,* 876–885.

Spears, M.C. (1995). *Foodservice organizations: A managerial and systems approach.* Englewood Cliffs, NJ: Prentice-Hall.

U.S. Public Health Service. (1995). *Food Code 1995.* Washington, DC: Department of Health and Human Services.

Wagner, K.H. (1971). *On the question of vitamin preservation in food which has been treated according to the multimet-multiserve procedure as compared to the preservation in orthodox containers.* Cleveland, OH: Crown X.

Wile, B. (1985). Innovations in tray handling/make up. *Consultant, 18,* 44–45.

Williams, P.G., & Miller, J.C.B. (1993). Warm-holding of vegetables in hospitals: Cook/chill versus cook/hot-hold foodservice systems. *Journal of Foodservice Systems, 7*(2), 117–128.

Zallen, E.M., Hitchcock, M.J., & Goertz, G.E. (1975). Chilled food systems: Effects of chilled holding on quality of beef loaves. *Journal of the American Dietetic Association, 67,* 552–557.

Current Issues in Food Safety

Mildred M. Cody

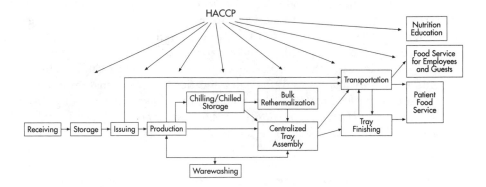

Recent authoritative estimates place the number of individual cases of foodborne illness at 6.5 million to 33 million annually. Although many of these cases result in simple gastrointestinal upset, more than 500 per year result in death. Additionally, 2% to 3% may result in long-term consequences, such as birth defects in offspring, arthritis, hemolytic uremic syndrome and Guillain-Barré syndrome (Cody & Keith, 1991; Council for Agricultural Science and Technology, 1994; Knabel, 1995).

GENERAL TRENDS

Three general trends are important to institutional food safety. First, the populations served within institutions are more fragile now than in the past. More limited hospital stays, greater proportions of immunosuppressed patients, and larger numbers of elderly are the current trends. These patients are more susceptible to foodborne disease. Foodborne disease may exhibit more severe outcomes for these populations, too. Second, as identified in Chapters 9 and 10, more types of food service systems are now available. Institutions are purchasing more value-added foods requiring less on-site preparation. In some instances, foods are prepared days before they are consumed. Many of these foods require special handling to keep them safe. Third, fewer food preparation skills are taught in schools and homes than in the past; new workers are unlikely to have even basic food preparation skills or food safety knowledge.

THE ROLE OF FOOD SERVICE MANAGERS AND DIETITIANS

Managers and dietitians who work in food service and nutrition departments can best serve their employees, patients, and other customers by being well versed in the principles of food safety. To do this, it is important for them to understand fully how food can become contaminated and how they can recognize potentially hazardous conditions. Effective systems for monitoring food service activities can be established, and employees can be trained to apply the principles they learn on the job. Patients and other customers can benefit by learning these principles as well through education programs that are offered by health care professionals. In this manner, the objectives regarding food safety identified in *Healthy People 2000* (U.S. Department of Health and Human Services, 1992) are more likely to be achieved.

Outbreaks

The Centers for Disease Control and Prevention (CDC) compile data from state and local health departments to produce national reports of confirmed outbreaks of foodborne illness. A case is a single episode of illness. An outbreak is an incident involving two or more cases of illness caused by the consumption of food from the same source (but a single case of botulism or chemical poisoning is classified as an outbreak). Outbreaks are confirmed by analytically matching the suspected food with the disease in several cases (or a single case for botulism or chemical poisoning). These data are not inclusive of all foodborne disease. Rather, they identify and track problems that threaten public health.

Surveillance

The CDC also maintains surveillance data on several foodborne diseases: botulism, campylobacteriosis, cholera, hepatitis A, listeriosis, salmonellosis, shigellosis, trichinosis, and typhoid fever. Surveillance data differ from outbreak data in several important ways. First, surveillance data report individual cases, not just cases associated with outbreaks. For example, about 10,000 campylobacteriosis cases are reported annually to the CDC, and only 145 of these cases are from outbreaks (Bean & Griffin, 1990). Second, unlike confirmed foodborne outbreak cases, not all surveillance cases are foodborne. Many bacteria are transmitted through water, person-to-person contact, or other routes. Additionally, outbreak data report food vehicles (carriers) and factors that contribute to food toxicity.

Confirmed Reports of Foodborne Disease

In all reporting periods, bacterial pathogens have been responsible for most of the foodborne disease outbreaks in the United States. During the latest reporting period, bacterial agents were responsible for 66% of the outbreaks,

92% of the cases, and 96% of the deaths from confirmed foodborne illness. Table 11–1 shows data for bacterial and other toxic agents, including parasites, viruses, and toxic chemicals.

Underreported Foodborne Disease

Experts agree that foodborne disease is underreported (Bean & Griffin, 1990; Cody & Keith, 1991; Council for Agricultural Science and Technology,

Table 11–1 Confirmed Outbreaks of Foodborne Illness in the United States, 1983–1987

Category	Toxic Agent	Outbreaks	Cases	Deaths
Bacterial	*Bacillus cereus*	16	261	0
	Brucella spp	2	38	1
	Campylobacter spp	28	727	1
	Clostridium botulinum	74	140	10
	Clostridium perfringens	24	2,743	2
	Escherichia coli	7	640	4
	Listeria monocytogenes	3	259	70
	Salmonella spp	342	21,245	30
	Shigella spp	44	9,971	2
	Staphylococcus aureus	47	3,181	0
	Streptococcus, group A	7	1,001	0
	Streptococcus, other	2	85	3
	Vibrio cholerae	1	2	0
	Vibrio parahaemolyticus	3	11	0
	Total bacterial	**600**	**50,304**	**132**
Chemical	Ciguatoxim	87	332	0
	Heavy metals	13	176	0
	Monosodium glutamate	2	7	0
	Mushrooms	14	49	2
	Scombrotoxin	83	306	0
	Shellfish	2	3	0
	Other chemical	31	371	1
	Total chemical	**232**	**1,244**	**3**
Parasitic	*Giardia* spp	3	41	0
	Trichinella spiralis	33	162	1
	Total parasitic	**36**	**203**	**1**
Viral	Hepatitis A	29	1,067	1
	Norwalk virus	10	1,164	0
	Other viral	2	558	0
	Total viral	**41**	**2,789**	**1**
	Combined total	**909**	**54,540**	**137**

Source: Data from N.H. Bean and P.M. Griffin, Foodborne Disease Outbreaks in the United States, 1983–1987: Pathogens, Vehicles, and Trends, *Journal of Food Protection,* Vol. 53, 1990.

1994; Knabel, 1995). There are many reasons for this. First, most cases result in mild symptoms that are not diagnosed or treated. Second, state staffs are not equipped to monitor foodborne disease effectively. Almost a quarter of the states have no staff specifically assigned to monitor foodborne or waterborne pathogens (disease-causing organisms), and no states have enough staff to investigate all potential cases of foodborne illness. Third, medical data based on hospital discharges and causes of death are incomplete. Also, some diseases are more likely to be diagnosed than others. Physicians are more likely to diagnose and report diseases that have life-threatening potential, distinctive symptoms, or familiar names. Large outbreaks, especially those involving pathogens that produce symptoms quickly, are more likely be diagnosed and reported. For newer bacterial pathogens and viruses, lack of efficient, effective diagnostic tests hampers diagnosis.

OVERVIEW OF FOODBORNE ILLNESS

To cause foodborne illness, pathogens or chemicals must be present in food in toxic (disease-causing) amounts. Factors that affect the amounts of pathogens and toxic chemicals in food include level of original contamination (occurrence), time held under compromising conditions, and use of processes that inactivate or remove toxins or pathogens. Although the toxic level of pathogens and chemicals does vary for individuals based on age and physiological condition, food that contains these pathogens or toxic chemicals in potentially toxic amounts is called contaminated.

Contamination

The presence of pathogens or toxic chemicals on food or articles that contact food is called contamination. Pathogens and toxic chemicals can contaminate foods during agricultural production, transport, preparation, and service. For most chemicals and some pathogens, the levels that originally contaminate (occur in) foods do not increase over time. Bacteria, however, can grow and produce toxins in foods. Because most foodborne illnesses are caused by bacteria, their growth and toxin production must be controlled to reduce the risk of foodborne illness. Additionally, some toxic chemicals can leach from inappropriate containers or surfaces over time.

During growth, plants are exposed to naturally occurring soilborne and waterborne pathogens, pathogens from sewage and raw manure, and pesticides. Risks from these contaminants can be minimized by thoroughly washing or scrubbing produce in cool, clean water. Peeling after washing, if desired, can further reduce risk, but it also reduces the fiber content of produce. Soaps and detergents are not used for washing fresh produce; they are not approved for food use and will leave residues on foods. Because severely immunosuppressed individuals are susceptible to parasitic infections from contaminated produce, raw fruits and vegetables are typically eliminated from their food plans unless they can be peeled effectively. For example, a banana peel would protect the fruit inside against contamination, but lettuce has no protective "package." A traditional tossed green salad would not be an appropriate food for this population, but a whole, washed banana could be safely presented.

Foods can be contaminated during transport, preparation, or service by fomites, inanimate objects that carry pathogens. It is common for fomites to be contaminated by contact with naturally contaminated raw foods. Examples of fomites are knives that have been used to cut raw meats, surfaces contaminated by pathogens from raw foods or shipping cartons, unsanitized sinks, and used gloves. Even dust particles in the air may contain bacterial spores, making it important to keep food covered during holding and transport.

When fomites come into contact with foods, some of the contaminates will be transferred to the food. This is called cross-contamination because inanimate objects must touch each other for it to occur. Cross-contamination contributes to foodborne disease in almost half of bacterial outbreaks. Common examples of cross-contamination include using the same knife and/or cutting surface to prepare raw and cooked foods, using a contaminated sink for thawing, and pooling fresh shell eggs instead of using pasteurized egg products. Other examples from health care facilities include putting patient meals onto contaminated carts for service or putting contaminated waste, such as tongue depressors, near or on patient trays. Use of sanitary, packaged, single-service utensils, napkins, and condiments may reduce cross-contamination from handling; these items are discarded after one use.

Because food handlers frequently carry bacteria on their hands and in nasal passages, they can contaminate unprotected food by touching it or by sneezing or coughing on it. Food handlers include kitchen staff, service staff, caregivers who feed clients, and the clients themselves. Contamination of food by kitchen staff can easily occur when individuals prepare foods without washing their hands and changing gloves between products, sneeze or cough over food, touch food after touching themselves or fomites, or fail to wash their hands before unloading the dishwasher between cycles. Of particular concern is contamination of hands by feces from handlers who do not wash their hands thoroughly after toileting or working with client body fluids, contamination of patient food by a single caregiver feeding two or more people at the same time, and contamination of patient food by handlers who "sample" food from patient trays. Food can be protected from handler-transmitted pathogens by single-use gloves (used for a single task and discarded when they are damaged or soiled or when a task is interrupted); by plate covers; by masks that cover the nose, mouth, and beard areas; and by hair nets.

Animals can also contaminate foods. Flies can bring pathogens from garbage or sewage areas into the kitchen or service area. Rodents can transmit pathogens from fecal contamination and from orally carried pathogens. Even asymptomatic pets used in pet therapy can carry organisms that are pathogenic for humans. For these reasons, pest controls are important and include appropriate use of approved pesticides, barriers to food storage and preparation areas, and handwashing for everyone who handles pets, including clients and caregivers. Additionally, no animals, including pets, are permitted in food preparation service areas except patrol dogs accompanying security officers and support animals such as guide dogs. These dogs are not permitted on chairs, tables, or other surfaces, only the floor.

Enhanced safety precautions are important in some clinical food service areas (Schiller & Ctakis, 1992). Patients in isolation areas require enhanced protection against infection because their immune systems are suppressed. In these areas, all food handlers adhere to rigorous sanitation procedures, all foods are cooked or processed to minimize pathogen loads, and no outside food is permitted. In cases where nutrient is supplied by enteral or parenteral formula, cautions include keeping all tubes and peripheral areas as clean as possible to reduce infection risk. Additionally, foods should be consumed as soon after service as possible to reduce risk of contamination and bacterial growth during holding. When patient food is kept on floors, it should not share space with food from outside sources, including staff lunches, or with medications.

Because food served in health care settings can be contaminated by patient contact, airborne pathogens, or inappropriately discarded medical waste, leftovers from patient meals should never be taken from patient areas in "doggy bags" or consumed by facility staff. Additionally, food service waste should be inspected carefully for contaminated waste inappropriately discarded on trays.

Holding Times

In general, food should not be held at room temperatures for longer than 2 hours. This has relevance for patients who may be asleep or undergoing tests during meal service. Simply reheating their food may not destroy pathogens if they are present. Reheating chilled foods on service floors requires sanitary handling of the patient tray and frequent cleaning of microwave ovens to reduce the risk of cross-contamination. Meals left uneaten should be discarded appropriately.

Food service managers can monitor foods from the point of receipt at the loading dock to the time of actual consumption by patients and other customers to ensure that this recommendation is followed. There is no opportunity to destroy foodborne pathogens in menu items that do not undergo cooking on-site, so that it is wise to be aware of the cumulative effect of holding at room temperature in the receiving area and during the processes of issuing, food preparation, tray assembly, transport to patient units, and service.

Toxic Agents

Table 11–2 identifies the major pathogens in foods and some of the factors that are important to their ability to cause disease. It also describes symptoms and time to onset of the symptoms. The listing of foods associated with each pathogen can be used as a guide for incorporating precautions in recipes and other guidelines followed by food service personnel.

Control of Foodborne Illness

Prevention and control of foodborne illness are important at each point in the food production and delivery chain. Internal quality assurance programs and external oversight help ensure that food sold or served to clients is safe. Internal quality assurance programs include adherence to good manufacturing practices (GMPs), implementation of hazard analysis critical control point (HACCP) systems, and delivery of educational programs to all personnel.

External Oversight

Government agencies provide external oversight for food safety (see Table 11–3). Their regulatory activities include:

- development of regulations designed to protect the public
- inspection of products and processes to ensure that regulations are followed
- removal of unsafe products and closure of unsafe facilities
- legal action against individuals and facilities that do not follow regulations

At the federal level, most regulatory oversight is by the Food and Drug Administration (FDA) and the U.S. Department of Agriculture. At the state and local levels, regulatory oversight is typically through state departments of agriculture and health, which develop regulations and monitor compliance for food produced and consumed within their jurisdictions.

Additionally, many health care institutions are accredited by the Joint Commission on Accreditation of Healthcare Organizations (Joint Commission),

Table 11-2 Major Characteristics of Pathogens

Pathogen	Symptoms [Complications]	Time to Onset [Duration]	Source	Associated Foods	Prevention
Bacteria					
Bacillus cereus Emetic	Nausea, vomiting	0.5–6 hours [24 hours]	Soil (airborne)	Rice dishes and pasta products	Hold at 140°F, cool rapidly
Diarrheal	Watery diarrhea, abdominal cramps	6–15 hours [24 hours]	Soil (airborne)	Meat products, soups, puddings, sauces	Hold at 140°F, cool rapidly
Campylobacter spp	Diarrhea (sometimes bloody), fever, headache, nausea, abdominal pain [arthritis, carditis, cholecystitis, colitis, endocarditis, erythema nodosum, Guillain-Barré syndrome, hemolytic-uremia syndrome, meningitis; pancreatitis, septicemia]	2–5 days [7–10 days]	Animals, flies, raw poultry	Poultry, unpasteurized milk, raw vegetables	Thorough cooking, pasteurization, washing raw produce
Clostridium botulinum	Fatigue, weakness, double vision, vertigo followed by severe nervous system damage, respiratory paralysis	18–36 hours [death can occur if not immediately treated]	Soil and water	Home-canned foods, smoked and salted fish, cooked root vegetables held at warm temperatures too long	Appropriate heat treatments, acidulation, refrigeration (some strains)
Clostridium perfringens	Intense abdominal cramps, diarrhea	8–22 hours [24 hours]	Soil, dust, sewage, manure, water	Meats, soups, gravies, stews, casseroles	Hold at 140°F, cool rapidly, reheat to 165°F
Escherichia coli Enterohemorrhagic	Severe cramping, bloody diarrhea [hemolytic uremia syndrome, erythema nodosum, seronegative arthropathy, thrombotic thrombocytopenic purpura]	12 hours–3 days [2–9 days]	Animal and human feces, untreated water	Raw or undercooked ground beef, unpasteurized milk	Thorough cooking to 155°F, pasteurization

continues

Table 11-2 Continued

Pathogen	Symptoms [Complications]	Time to Onset [Duration]	Source	Associated Foods	Prevention
Enteropatho-genic (EPEC)	Fever, diarrhea (watery, profuse)	12 hours–several days	Human feces	Raw foods	Sanitation, thorough cooking to 155°F
Enterotoxigenic (ETEC)	Diarrhea (watery, profuse), cramps, vomiting	10 hours–3 days [3–5 days]	Human feces	Raw foods	Sanitation, thorough cooking to 155°F
Enteroinvasive (ETEC)	Fever, cramps, diarrhea (sometimes dysentery)	At least 18 hours [uncertain]	Human feces	Raw foods	Sanitation. thorough cooking to 155°F
Listeria monocyto-genes	Flulike symptoms, septicemia, meningitis, spontaneous abortion, perinatal septicemia	12+ hours for gastrointestinal symptoms; 4 days–3 weeks for other symptoms [2–3 days for gastrointestinal symptoms; duration longer for other symptoms]	Soil, plants, water, animal feces, refrigeration condensate	Milk, soft cheese, raw produce, deli items	Sanitation, thorough cooking and reheating to 165°F, pasteuriza-tion
Salmonella spp	Abdominal cramps, diarrhea, fever, chills, headache [aortitis, cholecysti-tis, colitis, endocarditis, epididymoorchitis, meningitis, myocarditis, osteomyelitis, pancre-atitis, Reiter's disease, rheumatoid syndromes, septicemia, splenic abscesses, thyroiditis, septic arthritis (persons with sickle-cell anemia)]	0–48 hours [2–7 days]	Raw meat and poultry, human and animal feces	Eggs, poultry products, meat, fish, shellfish	Thorough cooking, sanitation, pasteurization, hygiene

continues

Table 11–2 Continued

Pathogen	Symptoms [Complications]	Time to Onset [Duration]	Source	Associated Foods	Prevention
Shigella spp	Abdominal cramps, diarrhea (stools may contain blood or mucus), fever, vomiting [erythema nodosum, hemolytic uremia syndrome, peripheral neuropathy, pneumonia, Reiter's disease, septicemia, splenic abscesses, synovitis]	12–50 hours [several days]	Human feces	Salads, raw vegetables, poultry	Hygiene, sewage control, cooking
Staphylococcus aureus	Nausea, vomiting, abdominal cramping	1–7 hours [2 days]	Skin, nasal passages, hair, sores	Protein salads, meat, poultry, milk and egg products	Thorough cooking, refrigeration, hygiene
Vibrio cholera	Diarrhea (profuse, watery), variable fever	9–72 hours [several days]	Polluted water	Seafood	Sewage control, cooking
Vibrio parahaemolyticus	Diarrhea (explosive, watery), abdominal cramps, vomiting, headache, fever [septicemia]	4–96 hours [2–3 days]	Warm marine waters	Raw or undercooked shellfish	Thorough cooking, refrigeration
Vibrio vulnificus	Chills, fever, prostration, often death	1 day (persons with high serum iron, liver damage)	Warm marine waters	Raw or undercooked clams and oysters	Thorough cooking
Yersinia enterocolitica	Severe abdominal pain mimicking appendicitis, fever, diarrhea, vomiting [arthritis, cholangitis, erythema nodosum, liver and splenic abscesses, lymphadenitis, pneumonia, pyomyositis, Reiter's disease, septicemia, spondylitis, Stills's disease]	24–48 hours [1–3 days]	Intestinal tracts of animals	Chocolate milk, reconstituted dry milk, tofu, pork chitterlings, meat	Sanitation, hygiene, cooking

continues

Table 11-2 Continued

Pathogen	Symptoms [Complications]	Time to Onset [Duration]	Source	Associated Foods	Prevention
Parasites					
Anisakiasis spp	Abdominal pain, nausea, vomiting	Hours to weeks	Occur naturally in seafoods	Raw or undercooked marine fish, squid, or octopus	Thorough cooking, freezing at −4°F for 30 days
Ascaris lumbricoides	Bowel obstructions, reduced nutrient absorption, damage to lung capillaries predisposing to pneumonia	10 days–8 weeks or longer	Human feces	Raw fruits or vegetables that contact soil	Sanitation, cooking
Cryptosporidium parvum	Severe diarrhea, sometimes fever, nausea and vomiting	1–12 days or longer	Human feces	Mishandled foods	Sanitation, thorough cooking
Diphyllobothrium latum	Reduced vitamin B_{12} absorption	3–6 weeks or longer	Naturally occurring in fish muscle	Raw or undercooked freshwater fish	Cooking or freezing 24 hours at 0°F
Entamoeba histolytica	Severe diarrhea, fever, chills, cirrhosis	2–4 weeks	Human feces	Raw or mishandled foods	General sanitation, thorough cooking
Giardia lamblia	Severe diarrhea [cholangitis, dystrophy, joint symptoms, lymphoidal hyperplasia]	5–25 days	Human and animal feces	Mishandled foods	General sanitation, thorough cooking
Taenia saginata	Worm segments in feces, nausea, abdominal pain, aberrant appetite, sometimes digestive disturbances [arthritis]	10–14 weeks or longer	Beef muscle	Raw or undercooked beef	Thorough cooking or freezing below 23°F for 4 days
Taenia solium	Worm segments in feces, nausea, abdominal pain, aberrant appetite [cysticercosis of muscles, heart, brain or other organs, arthritis]	8 weeks–10 years or longer	Pork muscle, human feces	Raw or undercooked pork; food mishandled by T. solium carrier	Thorough cooking or freezing below 23°F for 4 days

continues

Table 11-2 Continued

Pathogen	Symptoms [Complications]	Time to Onset [Duration]	Source	Associated Foods	Prevention
Toxoplasma gondii	Severe fatigue, abortion or stillbirth [encephalitis and other central nervous system diseases, pancarditis, polymyositis]	10–23 days	Pork or mutton muscle, cat feces	Raw or undercooked meats, raw milk, mishandled foods	Thorough cooking, pasteurization of milk, general sanitation
Trichinella spiralis	Muscle pain, fever [cardiac dysfunction, neurologic sequelae]	8–15 days or longer	Animal muscle	Raw or undercooked pork or meat of carnivorous animals (bears, etc.)	Thorough cooking, freezing pork at 5°F for 30 days, irradiation
Viruses					
Hepatitis A virus	Fever and nausea; can be followed by acute hepatitis	2–6 weeks	Human feces	Raw or undercooked shellfish, mishandled foods	Thorough cooking, general sanitation
Norwalk and Norwalk-like viruses (astrovirus, calicivirus, small round structured viruses)	Nausea, vomiting, diarrhea, headache, fever	12–60 hours for Norwalk, longer for some others [24–48 hours for Norwalk, may be longer for others]	Human feces and vomit	Raw or undercooked shellfish, mishandled foods	Thorough cooking, general sanitation
Rotavirus	Vomiting, fever, diarrhea, respiratory illness, temporary lactose intolerance	1–3 days [virus shed for 5–7 days, symptoms may be longer]	Human feces	Raw or mishandled foods	General sanitation

Source: Data from the Council for Agricultural Science and Technology, Foodborne Pathogens: Risks and Consequences, 1994; S.J. Knabel, Foodborne Illness: Role of Home Food Handling Practices. Food Technology, Vol. 49, p. 119, © 1995; M. Cody and M. Keith, Food Safety for Professionals: A Reference and Study Guide; American Dietetic Association, 1991, and Y.H. Hui; J.R. Gorham, K.D. Murrell, and D.O. Cliver (Eds.), Foodborne Disease Handbook, Vol. 1 and 2 © 1994, Marcel Dekker, Inc.; with assistance from Dr. Virginia S. O'Leary.

Table 11–3 Food Safety Regulators and Laws

Agency	Major Laws or Objectives
U. S. Food and Drug Administration	Federal Food, Drug, and Cosmetic Act of 1938 Food Additives Amendment of 1958 Pesticide Amendment Act of 1960 Color Additive Amendments of 1960 Saccharin Study and Labeling Act of 1977 Public Health Service Act of 1944 Tea Importation Act of 1897 Fair Packaging and Labeling Act of 1966
U.S. Department of Agriculture	Federal Meat Inspection Act of 1907 Filled Milk Act Wholesome Meat Act of 1967 Wholesome Poultry Products Act of 1968 Egg Products Inspection Act of 1970 Swine Health Protection Act of 1980
U.S. Department of Transportation	Sanitary Food Transportation Act of 1990
State departments of agriculture and state health departments	These agencies typically have jurisdiction over processing, warehousing, transport, and retailing of food produced and marketed within their borders. Responsibilities and regulations vary.
Joint Commission on Accreditation of Healthcare Organizations or other accrediting agencies	Accreditation is not a requirement for a facility to have a license to operate, but it is important to illustrate "superior" quality.

which seeks to optimize health care delivery through documented continuous improvements in infection control, patient care, and other components of health care delivery. Because food service is linked to infection control and to delivery of medical nutritional therapy, its activities are reviewed in Joint Commission site visits.

Another important government activity is establishment of food safety standards to guide both internal quality assurance programs and external oversight. The *Food Code 1995* describes the FDA's recommendations to state agencies that inspect retail food establishments in the United States. Sometimes called the unicode, it was developed to unify practices across the wide range of food retailing establishments. One of the health objectives for the year 2000 is to extend to at least 70% the proportion of states and territories that have implemented model food codes for institutional food operations and to at least 70% the proportion that have adopted the new uniform food protection code that sets recommended standards for regulation of all food operations.

Exhibit 11–1 gives an example of a unicode recommendation for receiving food products. The term *food* is defined in the Food Code 1995 as "a raw, cooked, or processed edible substance, ice, beverage, or ingredient used or intended for use or for sale in whole or in part for human consumption, or chewing gum" (FDA, 1995, p. 6). A potentially hazardous food is defined as "a food that is natural or synthetic and is in a form capable of supporting: (i) the rapid growth and progressive growth of infectious or toxigenic microorganisms; (ii) the growth and toxin production of *Clostridium botulinum;* or (iii) in shell eggs, the growth of *Salmonella enteritidis*" (FDA, 1995, p. 11). Potentially hazardous foods are defined in the code as shown in Exhibit 11–2. Additional information regarding the Food Code 1995 is provided in Chapter 1.

Internal Programs

GMPs are standards for universal practices. Examples of GMPs are appropriately cleaning and sanitizing food contact surfaces and equipment, maintaining appropriate temperature settings for storage areas, and using equipment properly. GMPs are monitored routinely, and deviations from standards are corrected immediately.

Exhibit 11–1 Example of a Standard from the FDA's Food Code 1995: Specifications for Food Receiving Temperatures

---

3-202.11 Temperature.*

(A) Except as specified in paragraph (B) of this section, refrigerated, potentially hazardous food shall be at a temperature of 5°C (41°F) or below when received.

(B) A FOOD may be received at the temperature specified in LAWS governing its distribution.

(C) Except as specified under paragraph (D) of this section, potentially hazardous food that is cooked to a temperature and for a time specified under XXX3-401.11 - 3-401.15 and received hot shall be at a temperature of 60°C (140°F) or above.

(D) Upon receipt, POTENTIALLY HAZARDOUS FOODS shall be free of evidence of previous temperature abuse.

---

*An asterisk (*) after a title indicates that all of the provisions within that section are critical unless otherwise indicated.

Source: Reprinted from FDA *Food Code 1995*, U.S. Government Printing Office, the U.S. Food and Drug Administration.

Exhibit 11–2 Definition of Potentially Hazardous Foods from the FDA's Food Code 1995

---

(60) Potentially Hazardous Food.

(a) **"Potentially hazardous food"** means a FOOD that is natural or synthetic and is in a form capable of supporting:

(i) The rapid and progressive growth of infectious or toxigenic microorganisms;
(ii) The growth and toxin production of *Clostridium botulinum*; or
(iii) In shell eggs, the growth of *Salmonella enteritidis*.

(b) **"Potentially hazardous food"** includes an animal FOOD (a FOOD of animal origin) that is raw or heat-treated; a FOOD of plant origin that is heat treated or consists of raw seed sprouts; cut melons; and garlic and oil mixtures.

(c) **"Potentially hazardous food"** does not include:

(i) An air-cooled hard-boiled egg with shell intact;
(ii) A FOOD with a WATER ACTIVITY (AW(a_w)) value of 0.85 or less;
(iii) A FOOD with a hydrogen ion concentration (PH(pH)) level of 4.6 or below when measured at 24°C (75°F);
(iv) A FOOD in an unopened HERMETICALLY SEALED CONTAINER, that is commercially processed to achieve and maintain commercial sterility under conditions of nonrefrigerated storage and distribution; and
(v) A FOOD for which a variance granted by the REGULATORY AUTHORITY is based upon laboratory evidence demonstrating that rapid and progressive growth of infectious and toxigenic microorganisms or the slower growth of *C. botulinum* cannot occur.

Source: Reprinted from FDA *Food Code 1995*, U.S. Government Printing Office, the U.S. Food and Drug Administration.

HACCP programs are quality assurance programs that specifically target food safety (Cody & Keith, 1991; FDA, 1995; International Association of Milk, Food, and Environmental Sanitarians, 1991; International Life Sciences Institute, 1993). The purpose of HACCP programs is to prevent food safety problems. Pillsbury, the National Aeronautics and Space Administration, and the U.S. Army–Natick Laboratories developed the first HACCP programs to eradicate pathogens from foods used by astronauts during space exploration. The FDA already requires HACCP analysis for the low-acid canned food industry. In 1994, HACCP analysis was proposed for most of the remaining food industry inspections. The FDA has also incorporated HACCP programs into its Food Code 1995, and many local regulators require HACCP programs for restaurants and other retail food establishments.

There are several advantages to using HACCP systems for safety assurance. HACCP analysis is scientifically sound because it focuses on reducing known risks. The process is practical because it is tailored to the ingredients and processes actually being used. HACCP analysis permits effective collaboration between facilities and regulators. The facility is responsible for developing and implementing an HACCP plan; government oversight can be more effective over time as regulators begin to audit HACCP records. When regulator oversight is tied to HACCP analysis, it will be easier to designate common problem areas for research and training.

APPLICATION OF HACCP PROGRAMS

There are seven steps in an HACCP program. These steps are followed by the HACCP team. Ideally, the HACCP team includes experts in food safety and facility experts who know how food is prepared and served in the facility. External experts, by themselves, may not be effective at tailoring an HACCP plan to a given facility. Internal experts may need help in identifying hazards and critical control points (CCPs), establishing critical limits and a verification system, and developing effective reporting procedures and documents.

Step 1: Identify Hazards

Hazard analysis is the identification of ingredient and process factors that increase the risk of foodborne illness. In food service, this activity requires review of recipes to identify potentially hazardous ingredients and review of processes to identify potential points of contamination and/or bacterial growth. Any time the specifications for a food ingredient are changed or a recipe is modified, hazard analysis must be repeated.

Step 2: Identify CCPs

After hazards are identified, points at which these hazards can be prevented, controlled, or eliminated are established. All phases of food procurement, receiving, storage, thawing, preparation, cooking, holding, cooling, reheating, and serving are considered to establish the most appropriate CCPs. Table 11–4 highlights some processes to review for different types of food service systems. Figure 11–1, the Food Code 1995 CCP decision tree, is a guide to determining essential CCPs for food preparation steps. Although each CCP gives an additional barrier to foodborne illness, tracking redundant CCPs is expensive. If there is no way to prevent, control, or eliminate a hazard (no CCP and no process or ingredient modification), the potential food is not appropriate for use in health care settings.

Table 11–4 Potential Processes for CCPs

Operation	Conventional Cook and Serve	Assemble and Serve	Ready Prepared (Cook-Chill or Cook-Freeze)	Commissary Operations
Procurement	X	XX	X	X
Storage	X	XX	X	X
Preprocessing	X	N/A	X	X
Cooking	XX	N/A	XX	XX
Chilling/freezing after cooking	N/A	N/A	XX	XX
Storage after cooking	N/A	N/A	XX	XX
Thawing after storage	N/A	N/A	X	X
Meal assembly	X	X	X	X
Serving	X	X	X	X
Holding	XX	XX	XX	XX
Transporting	N/A	N/A	N/A	XX
Reheating	N/A	XX	XX	XX

N/A, not applicable to the type of food service.
X, requires some monitoring; may be a standardized GMP.
XX, appropriate CCP required.

CCPs typically include a description of what, how, and how much. Most CCPs can be written using the Food Code 1995 as a guide. For example, based on item 3-202.11 from the unicode (see Exhibit 11–1), an appropriate CCP is "Temperature of ground beef must register 41°F or below when received." What is the temperature of the ground beef? How is measurement by thermometer (register)? How much is 41°F or below? CCPs can be included in forms and recipes, posted near the appropriate task, and used as the basis for training.

Step 3: Establish Critical Limits

Once CCPs are established, their critical limits are determined. These limits are food safety boundaries. Most critical limits in food service will include time/temperature limits or barrier assurance. The goal is to inactivate pathogens during cooking, to hold prepared food in the danger zone (between 40°F and 140°F) for no longer than 2 hours, and to reduce contamination/recontamination. That means that food should be cooked to appropriate internal temperatures, held at appropriate temperatures during service, chilled rapidly during storage, and reheated thoroughly before serving. Whenever possible, food should be covered or packaged to prevent contamination from environmental dust or other foods or by food handlers.

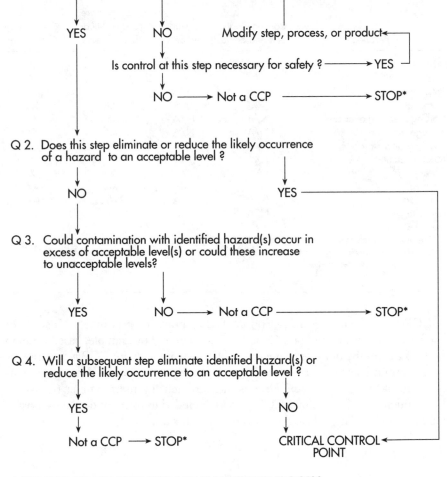

Figure 11–1 CCP decision tree (apply at each step in food preparation that has an identified hazard). *Source:* Reprinted from FDA *Food Code 1995*, U.S. Government Printing Office, the U.S. Food and Drug Administration.

Step 4: Establish Procedures

Next, procedures to monitor CCPs are established. Monitoring is a planned sequence of observations and/or measurements. It tracks the process so that loss of control can be corrected before deviations occur, indicates when deviations requiring corrective action have occurred, and provides a written record for verification. Monitoring of procedures includes determining who monitors, what is observed or measured, and how often the observation or measurement is made. Monitoring must be done rapidly to be effective because the time between production and consumption is usually short.

Step 5: Establish Corrective Actions

If critical limits are not met, corrective actions must be established. Corrective actions include determining what to do with food produced when the deviation occurred, correcting the cause of the deviation, and recording the corrective actions for the HACCP record. Common actions for handling potentially hazardous foods are reprocessing a product (sensory quality may suffer) or discarding a product (expensive). Correcting a deviation cause may include changing temperatures of storage equipment or requiring a food handler to wash his or her hands.

Corrective actions are established in advance of a problem occurring because concerns for product quality or cost may overwhelm appropriate safety considerations during an event. Also, establishing written procedures in advance ensures that employees will know what to do even when supervisors are not available. HACCP is designed to be a standard, objective system with the sole purpose of maintaining product safety.

Step 6: Establish Effective Recordkeeping

The HACCP plan and records must be on file at the food establishment. The Food Code 1995 lists the following examples of HACCP documents:

- a listing of the HACCP team members and their assigned responsibilities
- a description of the product and its intended use
- a flow diagram of food preparation indicating CCPs
- hazards associated with each CCP and preventive measures
- critical limits
- monitoring system
- corrective action plans for deviations from critical limits
- recordkeeping procedures
- procedures for verification of the HACCP system

In addition to a list of the HACCP team members with their responsibilities, the product description and uses, and a flow diagram, other information can be tabulated for easy reference (see Figure 11–2). These records are important because they are the basis for problem solving and future decision making.

Process Step	CCP	Chemical Physical Biological Hazards	Critical Limit	Monitoring Procedures Frequency Person(s) Responsible	Corrective Action(s) Person(s) Responsible	HACCP Records	Verification Procedures/ Person(s) Responsible

Figure 11–2 Sample Food Code 1995 HACCP record table. *Source:* Reprinted from FDA *Food Code 1995*, U.S. Government Printing Office, the U.S. Food and Drug Administration.

Step 7: Establish Procedures To Verify That the System Is Appropriate and Is Working Satisfactorily

The first stage of verification is a review of critical limits to verify that they are adequate to control hazards that are likely to occur. The second stage is frequent internal review of the HACCP plan and records to verify that the plan is appropriate and that it is being followed. The third stage is audit by the HACCP team or an external auditor to confirm that the HACCP plan is working satisfactorily or to make modifications to the HACCP plan. The fourth phase is review by regulatory agencies.

Food service HACCP plans are developed specifically for the facility that will prepare/serve the food. Several HACCP guides are available that give examples that can be modified to meet facility needs (La Vella Food Specialists, 1994; National Restaurant Association, 1993; Norton Group, 1994; Olin E. Teague Veterans Center, 1991).

INTEGRATING HACCP ANALYSIS IN THE FOOD SERVICE SYSTEM

As one example, consider an original recipe for vegetable beef soup that uses fresh vegetables and raw meat delivered in the frozen state (see Table 11–5). This traditional recipe does not highlight CCPs that can prevent product contamination and reduce pathogen growth. No instructions are provided for storing the ingredients, cleaning the vegetables, thawing the meat, and other critical processes. These activities have been traditionally left up to the judgment of employees, who may or may not be trained to follow proper procedures.

Examples of potential CCPs for the soup recipe are shown in Table 11–6. Specific control limits are identified along with corrective actions that can be taken when conditions are found to be unsafe.

If the recipe is rewritten, it can reflect CCPs. The revised recipe in Exhibit 11–3 shows not only the conventional processes but alternative procedures that can be followed for systems that hold food products hot after preparation and those that use the cook-chill food service system. Note that the more complex the food service system, the more CCPs. In this way, employees can have clear and complete instructions so that they can produce the food from start to finish in a safe manner.

Figure 11–3 is a flow chart that outlines potential processes for preparation and service of the soup as well as many other menu items. Although the systems are outlined individually, they can be linked. A commissary system may include an on-site conventional cook-and-serve system with some food transported to another site. The secondary site then becomes an assemble-and-serve system.

Depending on the system used by the facility, some of the CCPs in Table 11–6 may be GMPs, that is, standard processes that focus on total facility safety instead of safety for the individual product. CCP₂ and CCP₃ are examples of potential GMPs; they are standard processes that depend on proper maintenance of equipment.

Figure 11–4 shows how the HACCP record table for the vegetable beef soup would be started. This documentation makes review and modification more efficient and effective. It ties directly into recipe standardization, job descriptions, and employee training, evaluation, and remediation.

Table 11–5 Traditional Recipe for Vegetable Beef Soup

Ingredients	Amount for 50 6-oz servings	Procedures
Vegetable oil	0.5 cup	In a large stock pot, saute onions, celery, and carrots in oil until tender.
Onions, chopped	2 cups	
Celery, chopped	2 cups	
Carrots, sliced	2 cups	
Beef broth	1.5 gallons	Add broth and beef. Bring to the boiling point then simmer for 1 hour.
Cooked roast beef, diced	4 pounds	
Noodles	1 pound	Add noodles. Return to a boil and simmer for 15 minutes or until noodles are tender but still firm. Serve.

Table 11–6 Potential CCPs for Vegetable Beef Soup*

Operation		CCP	Control Limit(s)	Corrective Action(s)
Procurement	CCP₁	Upon receipt from an approved vendor (3-201.11), roast beef will be frozen with no indications of previous temperature abuse (3-202.11) or damage to packaging (3-202.16).	Observation: Labeling information Intact packaging Meat frozen Measurement: Package temperatures not above 41°F	Do not accept food in receiving unless it meets the standard. If accepted at receiving, it must be discarded. Contact vendor. Rewrite specifications to reflect safety considerations.
Storage	CCP₂	Roast beef will be maintained frozen (3-501.11).	Observation, measurement: 0°F or below, maximum 1 week	If freezer temperature rises to 32°F, check for thawing. If thawed, move to refrigerator (41°F or below, maximum 1 day). If freezer temperature rises to 41°F, use product immediately or discard. If product temperature rises above 41°F, discard. Have equipment serviced, if necessary.
	CCP₃	Oil, onions, celery, carrots, broth, and noodles will be stored in a clean, dry location; not exposed to splash, dust, or other contamination; and at least 6 inches above the floor (3-305.11); and separated from potentially hazardous foods (3-302.11).	Observation: Appropriate storage	Discard potentially contaminated food. Retrain/counsel staff.
Preprocessing (preparing)	CCP₄	Equipment food contact surfaces shall be cleaned and sanitized after roast beef is diced (4-602.11, 4-703.11).	Observation: Appropriate cleaning and sanitizing	Discard products that come in contact with unsanitized equipment food contact surfaces. Retrain/counsel staff.

continues

Table 11-6 Continued

Operation	CCP	Control Limit(s)	Corrective Action(s)
	CCP5 Clean and rinse the onions, celery, and carrots with cool running water. Cut as directed (3-302.15). Cover and refrigerate until needed for preparation.	Observation: Appropriate labeling and dating	Discard unused vegetables at maximum storage or if undated (assume maximum storage). Retrain/counsel staff.
	CCP6 Clean can before opening (3-302.11).	Observation, measurement: 41°F, maximum 1 day	Retrain/counsel staff.
		Observation: Routine cleaning	
Cooking	CCP7 Soup will be cooked to heat all parts to a temperature of at least 165°F for 15 seconds (3-403.11).	Measurement: Internal temperature at 165°F, 15 seconds	Continue cooking until appropriate temperature is met.
Chilling/freezing	CCP8 Soup will be cooled to 41°F or below within 4 hours of preparation (3-501.14, 3-501.15).	Measurement: Internal temperature 41°F or below within 4 hours of preparation	If product is not cooling quickly, cool in ice bath while stirring or place food in more shallow pans.
	CCP9 Soup to be frozen will be chilled to an internal temperature of 41°F within 4 hours of preparation and held in the freezer at 0°F until use.		
Storage	CCP10 Soup shall be stored in the refrigerator (3-501.15, 3-501.16).	Measurement: Internal temperature at 41°F or below, 10 days	If product temperature exceeds 41°F for less than 2 hours, reheat to 165°F and serve immediately. If product temperature exceeds 41°F for longer than 2 hours or is past date, discard.
Thawing	CCP11 Thaw frozen roast beef under refrigeration (3-501.13).	Observation, measurement: Refrigerator temperature of 41°F or below, 1 day	If refrigerator temperature drops below 41°F, check temperature of beef. If temperature of beef is above 41°F, discard. Have equipment serviced, if necessary.

continues

Table 11-6 Continued

Operation	CCP	Control Limit(s)	Corrective Action(s)
Meal assembly	CCP$_{12}$ Meals will be assembled by food handlers who meet standards of personal cleanliness (2-3), using appropriate serviceware (4-1, 4-7, 4-9). CCP$_{13}$ Meal components meet dietary prescriptions.	Observation: Food handler hygiene Serviceware selection, cleaning, sanitizing, storage Observation: Compare tray to order	If meal assembly is inappropriate, discard food. Retrain/counsel staff. If assembled meal does not meet standard, re-assemble. Retrain/counsel staff.
Serving	CCP$_{14}$ Meals will be served by food handlers who meet standards of personal cleanliness (2-3), using appropriate serviceware (4-1, 4-7, 4-9).	Observation: Food handler hygiene Serviceware selection, cleaning, sanitizing, storage	If service is not appropriate, discard potentially contaminated food, remediate, and resume service. Retrain/counsel staff.
	CCP$_{15}$ For self-service, food must be presented to reduce cross-contamination (3-304.15, 3-306.11, 4-302.12, 4-904.11).	Observation: Consumer practices Protection of displayed food Appropriate serving and eating utensils available	
Holding	CCP$_{16}$ Hold cooked soup at 140°F or above for no longer than 4 hours (3-501.16).	Measurement: Internal temperature of 140°F or above, taken every thirty minutes	If temperature drops below 140°F, reheat to 165°F and hold at a minimum of 140°F for the remainder of the holding period. If temperature drops below 140°F again, discard.

continues

Table 11-6 Continued

Operation	CCP	Control Limit(s)	Corrective Action(s)
Distribution	CCP17 During distribution food will be maintained at appropriate temperature (3-202.11) and protected from cross-contamination (3-302.16).	Measurement: Internal temperature of 41°F or below or 140°F or above taken at receipt Observation: Packaging is intact	For chilled food, if distribution and service times exceed 4 hours, discard. For hot food, if temperature drops below 140°F, reheat to 165°F and hold at a minimum of 140°F for the remainder of the holding period; if temperature drops below 140°F again, discard. Discard potentially contaminated food.
Reheating	CCP18 Soup that is cooked, cooled, and reheated for hot holding shall be reheated within 2 hours so that all parts of the food reach at least 165°F for 15 seconds (3-403.11).	Measurement: Internal temperature of 165°F or higher at end of heating	If food is not reheating quickly enough, increase heat, with stirring, if possible. Divide food into smaller units for reheating, if necessary.

*CCPs are developed from the FDA's Food Code 1995. These CCPs are examples; they are not the only CCPs that might be written by a specific facility.
Source: Reprinted from the FDA.

Exhibit 11–3 Revised Recipe for Vegetable Beef Soup Incorporating HACCP Analysis Results

Ingredients	Amount for 50 6-oz servings	Procedures for conventional cook-and-serve systems
Raw beef roast, chuck, frozen	5.5 pounds	1. Thaw beef in refrigerator (41°F maximum) and dice into 1/2" squares. If not used immediately, cover, label, date, and return to refrigerator until needed (41°F maximum, 1 day maximum). **CCP**$_{11}$
Onions, whole Celery stalks Carrots, whole	1 pound 0.5 pound 0.7 pound	2. Clean and rinse the onions, celery, and carrots with cool running water. Chop and if not used immediately, cover, label, date, and return to refrigerator until needed (41°F maximum, 1 day maximum). **CCP**$_5$
Vegetable oil	0.5 cup	3. Saute onions, celery, and carrots in oil until tender for approximately 10 minutes.
Beef broth	1.5 gallons 4 pounds	4. Add broth and beef. Bring to the boiling point then simmer for 1 hour. **CCP**$_7$
Noodles	1 pound	5. Add noodles. Return to a boil and simmer for 15 minutes or until noodles are tender but still firm. Assemble meal and serve immediately. **CCP**$_{12,14}$

Modifications for Other Food Service Systems

Conventional cook-and-serve systems with hot holding
    Procedure #5—Instead of serving immediately, product is transferred to service containers, covered, and held for service (**CCP**$_{16}$). Then it is served.

Cook-chill systems with hot holding
    Procedure #5—Instead of serving immediately, product is cooled to 41°F or below within 4 hours of preparation (**CCP**$_8$).
    Procedure #6 is added for storage in the refrigerator (41°F maximum, 10 day maximum; **CCP**$_{10}$).
    Procedure #7 is added for reheating (**CCP**$_{18}$).
    Procedure #8 is then added for assembling and serving immediately (**CCP**$_{12,14}$).

HACCP implementation improves recordkeeping for food production. To complete food safety recordkeeping in health care institutions, recordkeeping in dietary departments is linked to food service. Careful documentation of food served to and consumed by patients is important. From a dietary standpoint, this

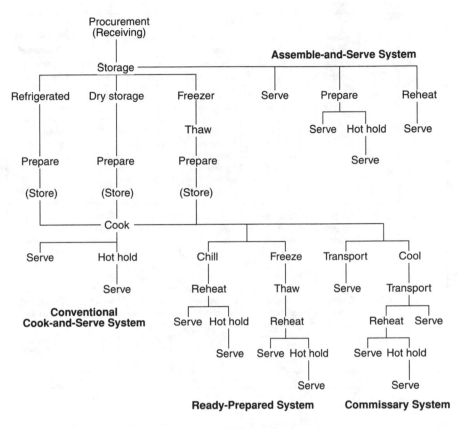

Figure 11–3 Flow chart of process using different food service systems.

documentation is useful for assessment of nutritional health. Also, should an outbreak of foodborne illness occur, this documentation will help track the potential food vehicle. Without careful documentation of patient consumption, outbreak data in health care settings are difficult to compile. First, many infections in health care settings may be foodborne or transmitted by person-to-person contact or by an environmental contaminant. Second, printed cycle menu items may be inaccurate, especially if item substitution is necessary for some patients.

REPORTING INCIDENTS OF FOODBORNE ILLNESS

When an outbreak of foodborne illness is suspected, internal procedures include notification of public health authorities. Public health authorities will try

Process Step	CCP	Chemical Physical Biological Hazards	Critical Limit	Monitoring Procedures Frequency Person(s) Responsible	Corrective Action(s) Person(s) Responsible	HACCP Records	Verification Procedures/ Person(s) Responsible
Thawing	CCP₁₁	Enteric pathogens	Thaw frozen roast beef under refrigeration (41°F, 1 day).	Department personnel transfer roast beef from freezer to refrigerator the day before it is needed.	Discard/ have equipment checked (Person A)	Food preparation log	Monitoring of process and review of log by supervisor
Cleaning	CCP₅	Residues, dirt, rocks, enteric pathogens	Clean and rinse vegetables with cool, running water.	Department personnel wash vegetables.	Rewash (Person B)	Food preparation log	Monitoring of process and review of log by supervisor
Cooking	CCP₇	Enteric pathogens	Cook all parts to a temperature of at least 165°F for 15 seconds.	Department personnel cook soup.	Continue heating until appropriate temperature is reached (Person C)	Food preparation log	Monitoring of process and review of log by supervisor

Figure 11–4 Sample HACCP record table for vegetable beef soup.

to confirm the outbreak by identifying a causative organism and linking it with suspect food(s). When the cause of the outbreak and its contributing factors are confirmed, internal procedures are reexamined, and changes in food preparation, handling, and service are made where appropriate (HACCP step 7).

EMPLOYEE TRAINING

The person in charge of a food service facility has the dual role of training and monitoring. According to the Food Code 1995, the person in charge of a facility shall be able to describe the relationship between prevention of foodborne illness and the management and control of the following:

- cross-contamination
- hand contact with ready-to-eat foods
- handwashing
- maintenance of the food establishment in a clean condition and in good repair

Furthermore, the person in charge is responsible for ensuring that employees are effectively cleaning their hands (see Exhibit 11–4), appropriately checking foods at receiving, properly cooking potentially hazardous foods, using appropriate methods of cooling foods, and properly sanitizing cleaned multiuse equipment and utensils before they are reused.

Providing effective, continuous, applicable training is a critical component of establishing a quality food safety program. New hires may bring their home habits to the institution, where poor food handling is more likely to cause an outbreak of foodborne illness. To protect compromised clients from foodborne illness, good food handlers know and practice appropriate handling practices. Effective training teaches the whys and hows of food safety and monitors participants to determine when remediation is necessary. The strongest food service staff members learn to monitor each other for inappropriate behaviors and take a role in group training. On-site, current reference materials can help in preparation of training materials and in answering questions that surface after training. Reference materials may be print or electronic, but they should be reliable and represent appropriate standards of practice.

PATIENT EDUCATION

Food safety is a critical component of education for all immunocompromised patients and for many other patients with compromised health status, including renal, diabetic, geriatric, pediatric, and postsurgical patients. Patient education includes working with the patient and with the family food preparers. Because many people do not routinely follow good food preparation practices at home, patient food safety instruction is a time for reeducation. Food safety is an important topic even for institutionalized patients because well-meaning visitors may bring in favorite foods that do not meet food safety standards. Only the patient can protect himself or herself against potentially hazardous food gifts.

Although many patients will remember "always doing it that way and never getting sick," they are more fragile as a result of being sick and will need to follow their food safety "prescriptions." Caregivers should involve the patient and family food preparers in the training by assessing their current practices and consumption patterns and addressing the whys and hows of appropriate choices and food handling. For example, consumption of tossed green salads is

Exhibit 11-4 Sample Handwashing Lesson for New Employees

Topic:	Handwashing	Audience:	New employees
Purpose:	To teach employees why, how, and when to wash their hands	**Level:**	Entry and remediation
		Time:	20–30 minutes
Equipment:	Sink, soap, paper towels	**Reference:**	*Food Code 1995* (2-301.13)

Objectives for Evaluation	Content	Activities
The employee will demonstrate knowledge of the relationship between the prevention of foodborne disease and the personal hygiene of food service workers.	There are many different causes of foodborne illness, but most foodborne illness is caused by bacteria. Some of these bacteria are on our hands, on the things we touch, and in our mouths and noses.	Demonstrate some of the ways that hands can become contaminated. Ask for examples of things that the workers have touched in the last 5 minutes.
The employee will demonstrate appropriate handwashing technique.	Washing hands appropriately takes at least a full minute. To wash hands (and exposed portions of your arms), thoroughly wet your hands. Using our cleaning compound, vigorously rub the surfaces of your lathered hands and arms for at least 20 seconds. Then rinse with water. Dry hands with a clean paper towel, and turn off water.	Demonstrate handwashing while you are talking. Be sure to count out the 20 seconds. Remind audience that the spigot is dirty and that the paper towel is a barrier between their hands and the spigot. The paper towel keeps them from recontaminating their hands.
	Sometimes you may have dirt under your fingernails. This can happen when you work with food, especially doughs.	Have employees demonstrate handwashing.
	Then you need to use a nailbrush to clean your fingertips, under your fingernails, and between your fingers.	Demonstrate using a nailbrush while you are talking.
	After defecating, contacting body fluids and discharges, or handling waste, you need to wash your hands twice. The first time, use a nailbrush. The second time you do not need to use a nailbrush.	Have employees demonstrate using a nailbrush.

Demonstrate double handwashing. |

continues

Exhibit 11–4 Continued

Objectives for Evaluation	Content	Activities
The employee will demonstrate knowledge of when to wash his/her hands.	When do you need to wash your hands? • After touching bare human body parts other than clean hands and clean, exposed portions of arms. • After using the toilet room. • After caring for or handling support animals. • After coughing, sneezing, using a handkerchief or disposable tissue, using tobacco, eating, or drinking. • After handling soiled equipment or utensils. • Immediately before engaging in food preparation. • During food preparation as often as necessary to remove soil and contamination and to prevent cross-contamination when changing tasks. • When switching between working with raw foods and working with ready-to-eat foods. • After engaging in other activities that contaminate hands.	Ask the question. Answers that do not come from participants should be listed and discussed when relevant to the facility.
Employees will know and follow institutional policies.	You must wash your hands before putting on gloves and before changing gloves. You may use lotion after handwashing if your hands will not come into contact with food.	Discuss why hands must be clean, even when gloves are worn. Lotion can leave a residue on food. That's why people who will be working with food shouldn't use lotion, even if they will be wearing gloves.

Evaluation: Supervisor will monitor handwashing practices of employees. Each time an employee does not wash hands appropriately, he or she will be required to complete the training.

Courtesy of Anna Iglesisa.

much riskier for a patient with acquired immunodeficiency syndrome than for a healthy adult. To be effective, dietary advice to eliminate this menu item would include the why (to reduce risk of infection by common pathogens) and the how (substitute canned fruit salads, pickled beets, or bean salads).

Because many patients eat out frequently (or bring in prepared foods), defensive eating is a useful topic to consider. Patients need to know which foods are potentially hazardous and how to handle food deliveries. For example, patients may have accepted "doggy bags" from favorite restaurants. This is a risky practice for compromised patients because typically this food has been in the danger zone for too long.

As discussed in Chapter 5, all patient education materials should meet the needs of the patient. They must consider reading level (and appropriate language), content, and availability. Materials are available through the American Dietetic Association, the FDA, the U.S. Cooperative Extension Service, and hospitals. Some locally produced materials are excellent. In all cases, the content of all materials should be evaluated before they are used. If one needs to update written materials, this can be done in writing, preferably with an overlay sticker that has correct information. The patient should not be simply told to make the changes. Later, the patient or a care provider may not remember the change. Professionals are responsible for the materials they distribute or recommend.

REFERENCES

Bean, N.H., & Griffin, P.M. (1990). Foodborne disease outbreaks in the United States, 1973–1987: Pathogens, vehicles, and trends. *Journal of Food Protection, 53*, 804.

Cody, M., & Keith, M. (1991). *Food safety for professionals: A reference and study guide.* Chicago: American Dietetic Association.

Council for Agricultural Science and Technology. (1994). *Foodborne pathogens: Risks and consequences.* Ames, IA: Author.

International Association of Milk, Food, and Environmental Sanitarians, Inc. (1991). *Procedures to implement the HACCP system.* Des Moines, IA: Author.

International Life Sciences Institute. (1993). *A simple guide to understanding and applying the HACCP concept.* Washington, DC: Author.

Knabel, S.J. (1995). Foodborne illness: Role of home food handling practices. *Food Technology, 49*, 119–131.

La Vella Food Specialists. (1994). *HACCP for food service: Recipe manual and guide.* St. Louis, MO: Author.

National Restaurant Association. (1993). *HACCP reference book.* Chicago: Author.

Norton Group. (1994). *HACCP: The future challenge: Practical application for the food service administrator.* Missouri City, TX: Author.

Olin E. Teague Veterans Center. (1991). *Food quality and hazard control plan: Keep your turkey out of jeopardy with HACCP.* Temple, TX: Author.

Schiller, M.R., & Ctakis, A. (1992). Hazard analysis critical control points: Implications for clinical nutrition service delivery. *Topics in Clinical Chemistry,* 7, 52–59.

U.S. Department of Health and Human Services, Public Health Service. (1992). *Healthy people 2000: National health promotion and disease prevention objectives.* Washington, DC: Government Printing Office.

U.S. Food and Drug Administration. (1995). *Food Code 1995.* Washington, DC: Government Printing Office.

Revenue-Generating Opportunities

Jimmy R. Lloyd

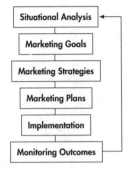

Institutional food service has slowly altered its patient-anchored identity to a more commercially flexible one. Profit is replacing subsidy, marketing supplants complacency, productivity is measured rather than excused, and growth opportunity is welcomed. The accompanying challenges are formidable: tougher competition, increased accountability, declining margins, and environmental pressures. Internal and external influences must be balanced for operational and personal success. These varied influences and the expectations they give rise to may seem contradictory, but they must be incorporated into sound operating plans to produce the synergy required for positive results.

MARKETING FOOD SERVICES

Marketing entails individual and organizational processes that occur to facilitate and expedite satisfying exchange relationships through the creation, distribution, promotion, and pricing of goods, services, and ideas (Pride & Ferrell, 1993). To meet the current and future challenges, directors of food and nutrition services and managers of their commercial operations will benefit by taking a thoughtful, well-organized approach to marketing the organization's food services. The first question that needs to be asked is: Where are we now? An objective view of current programs to determine their level of success from many points of view is needed before one can set future plans. Sometimes called a situational analysis, this process entails an internal assessment of the strengths and weaknesses of current programs as well as an external assessment of environmental influences and how well the expressed needs of customers are being met.

The second question is: Where should we be going? An integrated approach is also required for the identification of goals. Input from customers, administrators, staff members, and the community at large is necessary for a realistic view of the future role of the commercial food service operation. In the dynamic and ever-changing health care environment, there are many exciting opportunities available, and professionals in the field can certainly enjoy using their creative talents as they take a leadership role in developing new markets for their services.

After goals are identified, a marketing strategy is designed in answer to the next question: How should we get there? This is where the planning team members rigorously identify creative ways to achieve the desired goals. Their efforts yield a carefully thought through marketing plan, which is implemented over time while results are closely monitored to determine whether the goals are actually being met.

The food service marketing model shown in Figure 12–1 was especially designed to reflect the needs of leaders who wish to continuously improve their commercial food services. This model includes six major activities: situational analysis, identifying marketing goals, designing the marketing strategy, developing a marketing plan, implementing the marketing plan, and evaluating outcomes. It can be used as a guide for professionals as they strive to adapt their services to the needs of their customers. As stressed in previous chapters, customers are forever changing, and the marketing process therefore must be dynamic and ongoing. As results of the marketing plan are evaluated, even more opportunities for improvement can be identified, and this, of course, brings the manager back to the situational analysis stage again.

SITUATIONAL ANALYSIS AND IDENTIFICATION OF GOALS

Situational analysis is the identification of marketing opportunities and potential problems confronting an organization (Spears, 1995). This process works well when the expectations of customers and administrators are studied. Some common expectations are evident for managers involved in institutional food service. Consumer expectations typically produce administrative goals. Food service managers must interpret and incorporate these expectations into responsive operational plans. Table 12–1 demonstrates the collateral effect of these relationships. These expectations must be reflected in departmental goal statements for successful operations.

In addition to the expectations of customers and administrators, environmental factors play a major role in the establishment of realistic goals. Situational analysis should also entail review of the external influences that affect customer behavior and administrative priorities. These factors include the

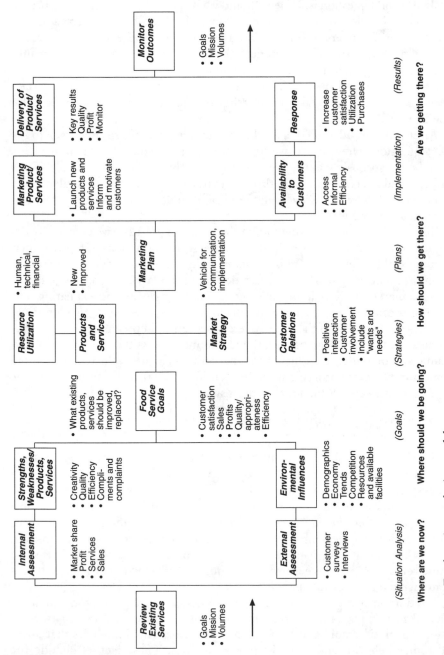

Figure 12–1 Food service marketing model.

Table 12-1 Collateral Effect of Consumer and Administrative Expectations

Consumers	Administration	Food Service Management
Fast service	Responsive service	Increased customer satisfaction
Self-service	Upscale dining	Innovative services
Value	Subsidy versus profit	Increased productivity
Quality	Consistency	Increased choices/variety
Menu variety	Current market trends	Effective marketing
Brand names	Fiscal accountability	In-house or contracted branding
Healthy selections	Innovation	Appropriate product mix

changing demographics of the population, the economy, industry trends, and competition. Readers are referred to Chapters 1 and 8 for detailed descriptions of these considerations.

The organization's systems, processes, and functions must be evaluated to track for the presence of appropriate goals. The model for hospital or institutional food service depicts the primary components and corresponding goals. All systems, components, and functions must be affected to produce satisfied customers (see Table 12-2).

Successful marketing plans must be developed to respond to the wants and needs of customers. Customers are the impetus, and systems are the method of providing responsive service. Strategic plans should reflect all available input, such as administrative philosophy, financial conditions, survey results, trends, standards of service, market conditions, and management creativity. The fusion of progressive management concepts with desirable service plans can yield customer-pleasing, profit-generating operations.

Evaluating Alternatives

The pressure to introduce new and creative services must be evaluated in the context of the financial environment of each facility. Total quality management methods can be used for the evaluation of cost-effective, creative services to provide a quick analysis useful in prioritizing possible service options. Services can be considered and selected based on the application of simple criteria. Projected customer satisfaction, profit or revenue, operating expenses, and capital investment are the essential components that guide the decision-making process. By factoring in these components, one can measure the potential impact of new services. Table 12-3 provides an example of this analytical model as applied to the actual commercial food services offered at Shands Hospital at the University of Florida.

High-volume, high-revenue, low-expense ideas are usually a "quick sell" to administration. Some services may be offered even though they are not profit-

Table 12–2 Food Service Components and Goals

Systems	Components	Functions	Goals
Materials management	Purchasing	Specifications, bids, requisitions, vendor relations	Optimal quality and value
	Receiving	Product storage, rotation, handling	Meet hazard analysis critical control point (HACCP) guidelines
	Issuing	Inventory distribution	Supply on demand
Food production	Ingredient control [Cook-chill/freeze]	Recipe ingredient assembly [Bulk preparation of food inventory]	Optimal quality
			Adequate and timely supply
	Hot production	Conventional preparation or retherm	Meet HACCP guidelines
	Cold production	Assembly of salads, sandwiches, etc.	
Food service	Patient tray line	Meal assembly and delivery	Satisfy patients with Joint Commission–approved standards of service
	Catering	Special services and presentation	Provide enhanced service, revenue
	Cafeteria	Plating and service	Provide a variety of services, revenue
	Food court	Light preparation, assembly, service	⌐ Expedite service and enhance revenue ⌐
	Vending	Assembly and stocking	
	Satellites	Assembly, transport, service	
Management	Financial	Budgeting, cash receipts, deposits, reports	Fiscal accountability
	Quality control	Monitor, intervene, document	Meet and exceed quality standards, correct deficiencies
	Human resources	Payroll, time and attendance, education, inservice training, counseling	Provide environment for well-trained, productive, motivated staff
	Clerical	Office operations	Process information and reports
	Committees	Planning, quality, directors, staff, safety, infection control, special events, others	Comply with regulatory standards, enhance departmental operations, communicate with staff/institution

continues

Table 12-2 Continued

Systems	Components	Functions	Goals
	Customer service	Focus groups, advisory groups, marketing	Interact with customers, promote department services
	Other	Planning, interdepartmental, community services, professional affiliations, productivity	Contribute to profession and community, enhance services
	Accreditations	Joint Commission, state/local regulations, American Dietetic Association	Demonstrate competencies

able because they are expected services of the institution (e.g., off-hours service and faculty and administrative dining). It is necessary to understand the customers of the food service to provide appropriate service and meet their needs. Table 12–3 can be useful in determining the impact of decisions about new services and how to prioritize their implementation.

A strong marketing plan provides the instrument to enhance customer satisfaction and ensure operational success. The marketing plan is critical for the creation of a positive image, effective communication with customers, development of sound strategies, collection and utilization of essential data, and design and promotion of attractive services. Some of the goals of the marketing plan are as follows:

- Identify who you are and what you do.
- Describe services.
- Enhance customer satisfaction.
- Sell additional products and services.
- Develop a market profile.
- Expand the market base.
- Solicit customer feedback.
- Design suitable services.

Market Surveys

An effective market survey will supply the information necessary to develop a sound marketing strategy and obtain favorable results. Identification of customers, buying patterns, and market potential is a vital management objective. This infor-

Table 12-3 Analytical Model Applied to Commercial Food Service Operations, Shands Hospital, University of Florida*

Services	Volumes (Utilization and Measurement of Customer Acceptance)	Profit/Revenue (Return on Investment)	Operating Expense (Labor, Food, and Supplies)	Investment Capital (Initial Capital Purchases)
Deli	H	H	L	L
Espresso cart	M	M	M	L
Branding	H	L	L	L
Vending	H	H	L	M
Catering	H	H	L	L
Bake shop	H	H	L	L
Conference facilities	H	H	L	M
Pizza outlet	H	H	L	L
"Make your own" bars	H	H	L	L
Faculty services	L	L	H	H
Healthy selections	M	L	M	M
Satellite services	H	H	L	L
Grab and go	H	H	L	L
Off hours	L	L	H	M
Storefront	H	M	L	L

*H, high impact; M, medium impact; L, low impact.

mation forms the basis for an effective operating strategy. Daily operations are affected as important decisions are enabled. Some of the results might include:

- addition of new products or services
- assurance of quality for repeat customers
- identification of untapped markets for growth
- provision of items or services for which customers go to competitors
- elimination of items that do not sell
- increased use of the most popular menu items

With regard to the competition in the community, Sneed and Henderson Kresse (1988) state "Astute foodservice managers always know their competitors, the products they offer, and the prices they charge. Just like the restauranteur, the manager in institutional foodservice operations should conduct market research to identify and describe the competition" (p. 110).

Although many managers do not view themselves as being in direct competition with local restaurants, grocery stores, and fast food operations, it is wise to learn about other sources of food that potential customers have in the immediate area. This type of research is also helpful in identifying market trends, and one can learn about the various types of foods and services that succeed in a given community. Sneed and Henderson Kresse (1988) suggest that the following information be used as a basis for tracking competitors:

- location
- size (number of seats and business volume)
- products (product mix, service mix, distinguishing features, image, quality, consistency, special advantages, benefits)
- pricing (objectives, methods, product prices, sensitivity to customers and competitors' pricing)
- promotions

The market survey presents an image of the food service and communicates the desire to be responsive to customers. The survey should be designed so that it is easy to complete and simple in general appearance. The customer should find it easy to handle the survey in pick-up, completion, and return. An incentive may be offered to increase participation in the survey. The form can provide information about the department's services and products as well as request information. One should focus on the objective of the survey and make certain that the format is frequently reviewed and revised. For maximum results, the collected data should be used on a timely basis.

Market research and surveys are useful for collection of basic information, but they are often not scientific as a result of distribution methods, levels of participation, and other variables. According to Spears (1995), marketing research should be systematic, not haphazard or disjointed. It involves a series of steps that include the collection of data from many sources, accurate recording, and careful analysis. It helps managers identify the most appropriate marketing goals, strategies, and plans.

MARKETING STRATEGIES AND PLANS

According to Pride and Ferrell (1993), marketing strategies include selecting and analyzing a target market and creating and maintaining an appropriate marketing mix that will satisfy this market. Marketing strategies and plans should have concrete objectives that are measurable. These objectives most often relate to customer satisfaction and financial benefit. Quite often, marketing tactics are developed to target specific market segments, such as the following:

- medical staff
- administrators

- clerical staff
- students and interns
- patients' families
- visitors
- community groups

Target populations can also be categorized in other ways. According to Sneed and Henderson Kresse (1988), "Foodservice operators in other settings identify the market segments that they wish to serve. Examples of market segments are young families, double income no kids (DINKS), well-off older people, children, working people, or any number of potential segments" (p. 109). The profit motive can be clearly seen in this type of scheme.

Marketing plans can be simple or complex, but they cannot be neglected. Some common examples of food service marketing techniques include the following:

- *Signage:* Designed to get customer attention with the greatest visibility and impact
- *Point of sale:* Concise, informative notices providing customer prompts
- *Printed announcements:* Menu distribution or special, informative communications
- *Employee newsletter:* Communication of service news through wide circulation
- *Giveaways:* Customer-pleasing promotions to attract new customers and reward regulars
- *Premiums:* Including discounts, combination deals, and frequent customer rewards
- *Ads:* Fliers, mailers, bulletins used to inform customers and promote services
- *Phone-in service:* Daily menu recording and order placement
- *List of service:* Phone numbers for primary services
- *Interdepartmental:*
  1. Guest speaking to external groups to promote services
  2. E-mail to announce and promote services
  3. External communications to market to specific groups
  4. Meal or snack tickets for requesting departments, groups, or individuals

Branded Products and Services

It is difficult to justify price increases with customers for generic, institutional products. Customers are willing to pay more for a branded product that they associate with quality. The concept of branding is currently generating great interest in the institutional marketplace. Products must be enjoyed and valued, or meal patronage will decrease. Selected brands that offer name recognition, quality, and reliability can enhance or supplement existing services. Institutional managers have been slow to tap into this new resource, but branding can be an advisable and attractive option. Although operators may fear this as a competitive threat to their independent survival, branding is actually a cooperative enterprise that can benefit both the supplier and the operator. Branding can be tastefully introduced with dedicated carts, kiosks, counters, and other presentations. Companies also contract to provide fully operated franchises to sell their branded products in the nontraditional, institutional markets. It is necessary to evaluate the market potential for this concept. The product quality and taste must be sampled before a brand is designated. Besides determining what will work best at each facility, it is important to assess the financial impact as well.

Many operational problems can be addressed with branding. The reasons for offering branding can vary, but branded products seem to correct some of the deficiencies often noted in subsidized operations. It is possible to increase customer satisfaction with the provision of brands found desirable by patrons. Products of recognized quality are the best received and most popular. Customer traffic increases as innovative, professionally marketed products are introduced. This also increases revenue for the department. The department's image can be boosted as branded marketing is shared with the food service department. All these factors, as well as the responsiveness they denote, produce greater credibility. As margins shrink and financial objectives become more challenging to obtain, the low operating costs of this arrangement offer further inducement.

Other operational deficiencies may be corrected and significant advantage realized. Most independent operators face some criticism from captive customers, who want to see more than superficial menu changes. It is challenging to develop new programs with all the vital components for success: consistency, effective marketing, supportive systems, and profitability. The pressure to create new services, along with the need to design and monitor their delivery, does not account for the high incidence of management frustration resulting from limited resources such as time, merchandising, systems, and quality control. Few restaurant concepts or branded items can even be duplicated by the independent operator because of the inherent difficulty in ensuring products of consistent quality, accurate portioning, and recognizable name. Brands provide a premium of profit potential, market share, consumer confidence, and hands-on assistance.

Branding can significantly reduce the labor and food costs that accrue to the department because these are allocated to the branding company. This produces significant savings for subsidized departments. It is also difficult to adapt to current market trends when capital funding is unavailable within the institution. The expense for the design, installation, and operation of the branded service is avoided by the department while revenues are generated. One of the most significant justifications is that generic selections will be replaced with customer-preferred branded items.

Food service operators must consider a variety of financial factors to determine the most favorable branding alliance. When evaluating a possible brand, one should critique the branded service as a stand-alone business, and develop a profit and loss schedule to determine potential success. This is best accomplished by applying the profit and loss calculation on a square footage basis. One can then compare the results with the performance of other department services and consider the return on investment as a final determination.

There are some apparent cautions to consider as well. It is critical to make certain that the brand image and the institution are compatible. One should know the facts about franchise fees and be able to track the terms of the agreement. Franchise fees may exceed 10%. Multiple contract options can be confusing and difficult to analyze. One should avoid duplication of existing department products or services and not create unfavorable comparisons between these and brand selections. If operators are unable to provide service as a result of excessive volume or desire a specialized product and menu, then branding can be a prudent alternative.

Determining Price Structure

The process of price assignment has become an important management function. Appropriate pricing is the formula for planned recovery of expenses and generation of profit as dictated by institutional philosophy. Many factors influence the price assignment practice: financial objectives of the institution and department, customer perception about food and service, and competition. The process begins with knowledge of the costs associated with providing products and service. Expenses for food and labor, cost/benefits, production costs, shrinkage, sales cost, and equipment depreciation must be detailed. The most common method for pricing has been 2.5 times food cost, which produces a 40% food cost. Subsidized food service typically utilizes this formula (see Table 12–4).

Product costs are affected by the degree of purchased convenience. Highly processed and ready-to-serve products are the most costly to purchase, but the use of raw ingredients is more labor intensive, and the resulting expense may reduce the advantage of the low food cost. An effective selling price will accommodate these variables. An informed mark-up should be applied to the raw food cost that recovers the full range of expense for labor-intensive and convenience-

Table 12-4 Application of the Standard Mark-up Formula

Food	Cost per Serving	Price (2.5 × raw food cost)
Frozen French fries	12¢	30¢
Instant "mashed" potatoes	5¢	13¢
Au gratin potatoes	34¢	85¢
Fresh potatoes	17¢	43¢

oriented production. Labor costs must be allocated to menu items so that the correct value is assigned that will decrease the inappropriate spread in selling price between convenience and "from scratch" products. Failure to include this in the mark-up formula will limit sales because convenience products will always be higher priced and labor costs will not be recovered for other products. Two of the largest components of profit and loss are controlled in the pricing function.

Pricing is a volatile subject in most operations because institutional customers are accustomed to generous subsidies that enable low food prices. It is possible to introduce price increases sensitively in a gradual manner. It may be best to identify the items that are lowest in price and thus recover the lowest expenses as immediate targets for increase. It is also advisable to look at the competition and its pricing. By pricing just below the competition, the increase is usually defensible for quality products.

Discounting is a popular pricing strategy that offers a bargain to customers and generates increased sales volumes. It is an artful method of marketing. Discounting has not been popular with institutional operators because of historically low prices and limited mark-ups. As pricing strategy has become more advanced, the opportunity has arisen to provide premiums such as discounting. Discounting encourages increased customer participation by adding value. There are three common methods for discounting:

- straight discounting (e.g., two-for-one specials or percentage discounts),
- meal bundling (e.g., value meals and combination deals), and
- frequent diner (i.e., loyalty incentives).

Discounting can be of equal benefit to customers and the food service. Discounting is not just to give something away but rather to increase the customer count so that it will offset the loss of profit margin. The customer perceives the value, and the operator receives the volume. Incremental sales increases must be produced or the impact will be an erosion of core business. The discount must be significant and meaningful to the customer. The promotion should be simple, expeditious, and attractively priced. Discounting requires operational flexibility, but with defined objectives it can provide market growth, customer incentives, and added value.

Team Planning

The food service director and manager of commercial food services can tap the creative abilities of many resourceful individuals inside and outside the institution to assist in developing marketing strategies and plans. Point-of-service employees are frequently good at identifying customers' needs and identifying the most effective marketing methods. Implementation of the marketing plan is facilitated when staff members are involved in planning because they perceive themselves as an integral part of the project. Readers are referred to Chapters 2 and 3, where team involvement is stressed. Chapter 2 also fully discusses the functions of planning, directing, and coordinating services. In addition, it shows how policies, procedures, and methods are developed from the goals and objectives of the organization and department.

IMPLEMENTATION AND MONITORING

When plans are carefully developed, implementation becomes easier. All the equipment, supplies, and methods that employees need to get a project underway must be at their fingertips. Although the philosophy of "learning as we go" may provide much needed flexibility, it also sometimes results in chaos, which can lead to defeat. Expectations need to be clearly understood by all staff members involved, and adequate training should occur so that they have the knowledge and skills to launch the marketing plan.

Existing and potential customers can be made aware of new services that are being offered through the marketing techniques described above. They will want to know how and when they can gain access to the new goods or services, how much it will cost, and whether it will suit their needs and desires. Customers' initial reactions are important. Managers will be able to learn if they are on the right track, or if any unforeseen factors are causing the need for adjustments in the program, by being physically present in service areas and having informal conversations with customers. This can be followed up with more formalized methods, such as surveys, to determine whether consumer needs have been met.

The success of a new marketing plan should be evaluated with respect to the goals that were initially set forth. The case study shown in Exhibit 12–1 shows how many objectives were achieved in one hospital. These objectives included use of employees' downtime, increased variety, improved morale of the hospital staff, customer satisfaction, and increased revenues.

Exhibit 12–1 Case Study in Creative Marketing

Silsby Doctors' Hospital is a small facility in Silsby, Texas. At about 2:30 pm one can hear an announcement over the intercom that says "a batch of gourmet cookies has just come out of the oven."

"They come down like cattle!" says Larry Dalo, the director of dietary services. Cookies quickly disappear as employees and guests of the hospital share a welcome break from their busy schedules. During an otherwise tranquil mid-afternoon, Dalo cleverly uses food service employees and space to increase profits. His customers are excited about the fact that he keeps them wondering what surprises he has in store for them next!

Dalo learned that small things make a big difference to people, and tries to promote a fun atmosphere for each and every customer. "Every Tuesday morning," he says, "we have a trivia question and the person who answers it correctly wins a free muffin and a beverage." This stimulates business and, more importantly, it makes the cafeteria a fun place to be.

The lessons Dalo learned from working in the restaurant industry have applied well in the hospital setting and keep his customers coming back for more. As the newly appointed director at Silsby, he has already remodeled the kitchen and cafeteria, and improved the morale of employees of the hospital while increasing revenue. In 1995, Dalo showed his appreciation by treating everyone to free frozen yogurt every Friday. This may cut into his profits a little, but customers receive a very special message from this—that the cafeteria is not there only to make a profit, but the hospital really cares for its employees!

Source: Reprinted from R. Jackson, Increasing Cafeteria and Vending Profits, *Hospital Food & Nutrition Focus,* Vol. 11, No. 6, pp. 7–8, © 1995, Aspen Publishers, Inc.

Specific methods for the routine monitoring of quality are covered in detail in Chapter 14. Cash operations have a definite advantage over patient food services because immediate feedback is received by simply reviewing cash sales.

Financial Reporting

Numerous reporting methods are available to ensure appropriate controls and document performance. Cost center allocation is a practical method to isolate revenue and expenses within a functional area. These functional units are treated as independent businesses with all subsequent revenue and expenses reported there. This functional separation promotes more effective decision making and fiscal accountability. Cost centers are based on product, service, or operational distinction. Some department units that easily accommodate cost center designation are cafeteria, catering, vending, faculty dining, ingredient control, patient food service, clinical services, and administrative.

Budgetary performance can be measured at any interval to account for the success of operations. A simple profit and loss statement can document the food service department's processing of revenues and expenses. The profit and loss formula is:

Sales (revenue) – Cost of food = Gross profit
Gross profit – Labor and operating costs = Net profit/loss

Cost Center Allocation

Although some managers still practice "shoebox accounting," it is probably not wise to toss all revenues in one category and compare them against total expenses. This is not to say that the bottom line is not important, but wise and successful managers have learned that appropriate cost and revenue allocations help them complete financial analyses that enable them to identify trends and learn the outcomes of their decisions. The advantages of cost center allocation are that it:

- provides a focused report for an individual service unit to determine success in budget management and performance
- identifies budget variances (i.e., where the budget exceeds or fails to meet objectives)
- contrasts actual performance with expected performance
- divides total budget into usable components

Some disadvantages of cost center allocation are that it often:

- segments operations and imposes boundaries
- effects strict allocation of expenses even though the mechanism is sometimes limited (e.g., it can be difficult to assign an expense category for food supplied by central production to all recipients, such as cafeteria, patients, and catering)
- causes managers to miss the "big picture" because attention is given to many small operating units

Therefore, while one is identifying cost centers, it is important to establish the most realistic and achievable method for a given institution. One must also keep in mind that some programs may elicit a lower profit margin than others, but this does not necessarily mean that they should be discontinued. For example, the case study given at the end of Chapter 7 describes community programs offered at Gundersen Lutheran Medical Center in La Crosse, Wisconsin. Some of the programs at this medical center have higher profit margins than others. The *One-Minute Morsel*, which is a nutrition education spot on the local television station, brings no profit whatsoever but reaps many other rewards for the medical center from a marketing perspective. Again, one is brought back to the initial goals of the marketing plan, which are not always based in financial success. In the overall financial scheme, other programs should act to subsidize the programs that are less profitable but should still be maintained because they also fulfill the mission of the institution.

Figure 12–2 provides a sample format for summarizing and analyzing revenues and expenses for one cost center. It also provides data on productivity, which is discussed below.

Productivity

As the economic environment has changed, the effects have rippled through the food service industry. Diagnosis-related groups, managed care, government regulation, and health care reform have produced drastic reductions in re-

	Actual	Budgeted	YTD Variance
Revenue:			
Cash Sales	$_____	$_____	$_____
Units of Service: Meal Equivalents	_____	_____	_____
Customers	_____	_____	_____
Direct Expenses:			
Labor Dollars (regular, overtime, benefits)	_____	_____	_____
Food Expense	_____	_____	_____
Supply Expense	_____	_____	_____
Other Direct Expenses	_____	_____	_____
Total Direct Expenses	$_____	$_____	$_____
Labor Hours (productive + nonproductive)	_____	_____	_____
Net Gain/Loss (total revenue – total expenses)	$_____	$_____	$_____
Productivity			
Meal Equivalents per Labor Hour	_____	_____	_____
Cost per Meal Equivalent:			
Labor Cost per Meal Equivalent	$_____	$_____	$_____
Food Cost per Meal Equivalent	_____	_____	_____
Supply Cost per Meal Equivalent	_____	_____	_____
Other Cost per Meal Equivalent	_____	_____	_____
Total Cost per Meal Equivalent	$_____	$_____	$_____

Figure 12–2 Monthly summary of cafeteria income and expenses.

sources and financial support for labor-intensive service departments. With computerized technology advancements in equipment and systems and more educated staffs, operational efficiency and productivity have increased. Because operational success remains the paramount goal of food service managers, productivity indicators are utilized to measure and document performance. Measurement of productivity remains an industry goal because it has not been standardized for practical use.

Numerous measures are currently used: meal equivalents per labor hour, cost per meal equivalent, return on investment, and benchmarking. Each measure is useful for its intended application. Meal equivalents per labor hour is the most common formula used to measure productivity:

$$\text{Meals per labor hour} = \frac{\text{Total meal equivalents}}{\text{Total labor hours}}$$

This formula can be used for comparison of reporting periods (meal to meal, day to day, or month to month) and even for comparison with other facilities when the same formula is used. Since the composition of a meal is not yet standardized in the industry because it is calculated internally, external comparisons are not always valid.

The cost per meal equivalent can also be an effective tool in expense management. This formula focuses on department costs and enables the evaluation of expenses. Because meals are the department's ultimate product, the examination of all input is critical for cost-effective management:

$$\text{Cost per meal equivalent} = \frac{\text{Total direct expenses}}{\text{Total meal equivalents}}$$

Return on investment is a bottom line approach that assesses profitability. Net profit is related to equity and total assets, or to sales as shown below:

$$\text{Profit margin} = \frac{\text{Net income}}{\text{Revenues}} - 100$$

Benchmarking has become an effective industry tool for comparative measurement of productivity. This process involves the standardized reporting of operational data for effective comparison. Competitors and peers provide base data in essential service categories relating to meal equivalents and procedures, labor hours, and operational methods. This establishes a base standard for comparison. These standards form the benchmark for departmental operational reports. Because administrators desire independent confirmation of productivity and the Joint Commission on Accreditation of Healthcare Organizations requires comparisons with other facilities, participation in benchmarking has become more critical.

CONTINUOUS IMPROVEMENT

Exciting new technologies and disciplines are evolving to effectively measure food service productivity and determine appropriate resource allocation. This section presents case studies and ideas for managers who wish to expand and improve their commercial food service operations.

The Shands Hospital Experience

The Department of Food and Nutrition Services at Shands Hospital at the University of Florida has partnered with the Department of Management Systems Engineering to study, measure, and document food service staff task performance. Management engineering methods are utilized to evaluate staff positions, establish critical tasks, evaluate time and motion performance, and develop standards. These compiled data are used as a measure of productivity. They form the basis for future operating plans and staffing requests. Although such evaluation can generate some staff and department anxiety, it actually serves to credit appropriately the most productive units and individuals. This also enables additional training and development to address documented deficiencies.

Vending

To increase profits, all existing and potential services should be examined for their profit potential. Vending is an excellent subject to examine. Self-operated versus contracted vending is a beneficial case study. Contracted services involve negotiation of a commission submitted as a fee for provision of vending at a facility. Self-operation of vending provides a revenue-producing service with minimal labor expense, a modest capital investment, and an excellent return on investment. In 1991, Shands Hospital converted to predominantly self-operating vending in high-volume locations and contracted low-volume locations for an attractive commission. The subsequent results are shown in Table 12–5. Vending volumes increased with the introduction of self-operation. Negotiations with vending contractors have yielded higher annual commissions. Vending is now the most profitable department cost center.

"Grab and Go" Packaged Sandwiches

Many staff members need to return to work promptly. Because lines form at peak hours, alternative services that reduce customer wait time are essential. One option that accomplished this was the creation of a daily menu of six sandwich selections that are prepared and packaged the morning of service. This

Table 12–5 Results of Vending Decision, Shands Hospital at the University of Florida

Year	Vending Commission	Vending Revenue	Total
1991	$56,006	$330,499	$386,505
1992	49,071	425,504	474,575
1993	84,151	448,305	532,456
1994	90,109	449,712	539,821

quick service option provides the most popular customer selections without service delay. The result has been an annual revenue increase of $40,000.

Deli Service

Fresh, made-to-order deli sandwiches are available two shifts per day to customers. Top-quality ingredients are specified, including breads supplied fresh from a local specialty bakery. Although long lines form for this quality product service, they are acceptable. Staff average assembling a sandwich in approximately 40 seconds. Deli sales now exceed $300,000 annually. Customer satisfaction is extremely high.

Food Court or Mini Mall

A series of specialty food outlets was constructed to provide a variety of freshly prepared food selections and to diffuse patronage by offering an attractive alternative to the cafeteria. Four shops provide additional food selections: pizza, bake shop, burgers, and ice cream. A variety of fast food selections are offered. More than 90% of the products are prepared in the shops. A bright, common dining area contains 120 seats. Results have exceeded expectations. Customer volume is shown in Table 12–6. This increased variety of services and food outlets provided an opportunity for staff development and promotion. New services and skills were gained. Customer response has been positive, and prices are market competitive. Revenue exceeds $1 million annually.

Other Marketing Experiences

The Department of Food and Nutrition Services at the University of Alabama at Birmingham has planned for the opening of an innovative retail bakery in a main corridor location adjacent to the cafeteria. The bakery will be supplied with products from the main bakery and will be supplemented with point-of-sale finishing. Skilled cake decorators will showcase their talents and products in a highly publicized demonstration. Cookies, tarts, pies, cakes, French

Table 12–6 Annual Customer Volume for Mini Mall, Shands Hospital at the University of Florida

Outlet	Annual Customer Volume
Pizza	185,674
Baked Goods	256,264
Burgers	168,294
Ice Cream	104,779

pastries, bar cookies, and whole grain and specialty breads are featured. Sales projections are $150,000 for the first year (J.M. Van Zutphen & B. Bagley, personal communication, 1995). Future marketing will focus on a cook-to-order station and more specialty carts featuring nachos and other high-profit items.

The University of Iowa Hospitals and Clinics has experienced great success with marketing of patient education material. The director of food and nutrition services reports that outside sales of education materials exceeded $10,000 in 1995 (J. Gilmore, personal communication, 1995). A systematic approach was applied to the production and sale of these materials:

1. registered dietitian review and revision
2. formal review before publication
3. new covers and format
4. use of *Paradox* database for tracking inventory, cost, and usage
5. development of video presentations
6. bulk mailing of catalogs

The department has been successful with marketing ventures featuring popular menu items. A pasta bar special received great reviews from the 591 cafeteria customers who paid $2.98 for it. The cafeteria was also specially decorated with coordinated theme tablecloths. Revenue of more than $1,700 was generated, and customers were pleased.

The director of food and nutrition services at the University of Utah Health Science Center reports success with a variety of unique marketing concepts (L. Rackly, personal communication, 1995). Patronage has increased, as evidenced by the long customer lines. Customer favorites include the following:

- ethnic specials: Southwestern, Thai, and salad entrees
- pasta bar: three pastas with various sauces
- "Slice-to-order" station, featuring prime rib, roast turkey, or roast pork
- display cooking, featuring stir frys
- stuffed potato bar

North Carolina Baptist Hospital features several notable services. Customers have expressed appreciation for the delivery service provided by the hospitals' pizzeria. Heart-healthy meals are packaged for take-out ease. The food service department also provides meals to a local high school.

According to Bishop, the director of food service at Primary Childrens' Hospital, in Salt Lake City, Utah, "My administration believes that the best thing we can do for our employees is to get them away from the work place for a while" (Jackson, 1995, p. 7). She initiated outdoor summer barbecues whereby grills are set up under a canopy once a week. Sales volume often exceeds $1,400 in just two hours. Bishop also focused on other customers' needs to realize a profit. Because their main cafeteria, the "Rainbow Cafe," is located at one end of the facility, box lunches, soups, and beverages on carts were made available for employees that were too busy to travel to it. The program soon generated $4.00 per minute (Jackson, 1995).

More, the director of food services at Stormont-Vail Regional Medical Center, a 500-bed facility in Topeka, Kansas, says "employees get a kick out of performing" as they provide visual stimulation to increase profits by giving Asian stir fry and other demonstrations in the cafeteria once a week. A table is set up in the seating area; food is prepared in batches, and customers pay the cashier. Daily revenues exceed $250 from this service. The cafeteria is also used in the evening to provide meals for the "Healthwise–55" senior program. This not only fills the cafeteria during off-peak hours, but it provides a community service as well. Costs total $2.00 per meal and $3.50 is generated for each (Jackson, 1995, p. 7).

All of these directors have one thing in common: Their enthusiasm and willingness to please customers is contagious. From them, staff members learn what service is all about, and customers return because the food tastes good, prices are reasonable, and they feel welcomed and appreciated by the employees who serve them. As food service operators strive to control costs and generate greater revenue, their success will be affected by quality marketing, introduction of innovative services, effective pricing strategies, and beneficial networking.

REFERENCES

Jackson, R. (1995). Increasing cafeteria and vending profits. *Hospital Food and Nutrition Focus, 11*, 6, 7-8.

Pride, W.M., & Ferrell, O.C. (1993). *Marketing: Concepts and strategies* (8th ed.). Boston: Houghton Mifflin.

Sneed, J., & Henderson Kresse, K. (1988). *Understanding foodservice financial management.* Gaithersburg, MD: Aspen.

Spears, M.C. (1995). *Foodservice organizations: A managerial and systems approach.* Englewood Cliffs, NJ: Prentice-Hall.

Preparing for Future Challenges

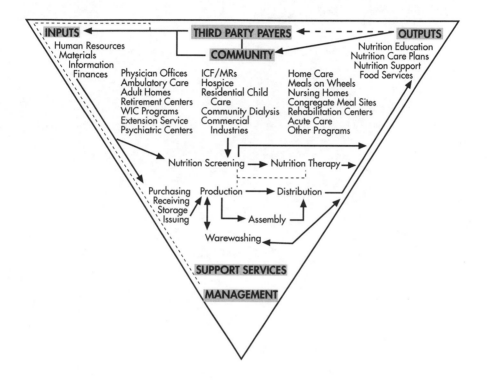

INPUTS ← THIRD PARTY PAYERS ← ← ← ← ← ← OUTPUTS

Human Resources | COMMUNITY | Nutrition Education
Materials | | Nutrition Care Plans
Information | | Nutrition Support
Finances | | Food Services

Physician Offices | ICF/MRs | Home Care
Ambulatory Care | Hospice | Meals on Wheels
Adult Homes | Residential Child | Nursing Homes
Retirement Centers | Care | Congregate Meal Sites
WIC Programs | Community Dialysis | Rehabilitation Centers
Extension Service | Commercial | Acute Care
Psychiatric Centers | Industries | Other Programs

Nutrition Screening → Nutrition Therapy

Purchasing Production → Distribution
Receiving
Storage
Issuing → Assembly

Warewashing

SUPPORT SERVICES

MANAGEMENT

A Systems Approach to Productivity

Ruby P. Puckett and Rita Jackson

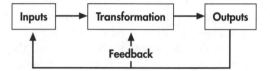

Health care and its delivery of services continue to undergo a metamorphosis. There is little doubt that major changes will continue to take place throughout the remaining century and into the next decade. Downsizing, rightsizing, reengineering, and restructuring are common occurrences in the health care environment. Managers and employees are confronted with longer work hours, fears, hostilities, stress, and anxiety. The mottos vary: "Do more with less," "Meet customers' needs," "Do it right the first time," and "Quality performance is the most important thing." Managers and workers are to do these things while continuing to be highly productive and providing quality service to their customers. They continually seek new and improved ways to do their jobs more efficiently and effectively, to provide the same or more customer services while containing or reducing the cost of operation.

This chapter presents methods that are commonly used to measure and improve the productivity of clinical nutrition and food services. To understand better how managers and workers will meet these ongoing challenges while dealing with complex, ever-changing issues, it is important to understand the past and how it affects the future.

EARLY PRODUCTIVITY STUDIES

Frederick Taylor (1865–1915) is commonly accepted as the father of scientific management. Taylor started his career as a day laborer in the Bethlehem steel mills and progressed to a position in middle management. While in this position, his major concern was: What is a fair day's work? Taylor's research emphasized developing the best method to perform the job, selecting and training workers at all levels of the organization, utilizing proper methods, and achieving close cooperation between managers and workers.

Carl G.L. Barth (1860–1939) and Henry L. Gantt (1861–1919) scientifically studied workers, the machines they used, and the environment where work was accomplished. Gantt developed the Gantt chart, which is used to measure actual versus planned performance, as well as the process chart and flow diagram. He also developed a task and bonus plan that rewarded workers for production levels above the standard. These pioneers originated the practice of standardization of parts, work methods, and assembly line production. They were more interested in the work being produced than the workers who performed the tasks.

Other pioneers, such as Frank Gilbreth (1868–1924) and Lilian Gilbreth (1869–1924), a psychologist and his wife, were behavioralists who focused their studies on the worker. They developed a class of fundamental motions called therbligs (*gilbreth* spelled backward with the *th* transposed) as the most elemental motions. Elton Mayo and F.J. Roethlisberger, between 1927 and 1932, at the Western Electric Hawthorne Works, conducted behavioral science studies of workers' productivity and interaction while stressing group dynamics and psychological needs. Douglas MacGregory, Rensis Likert, and Charles Argyris used behavioral science and human relations approaches to link the worker's social and psychological needs.

There were other researchers who developed different theories and methods to help organize work, provide organizational structure, and determine superior–subordinate authority relationships. During World War II and later in the space program, the systems model was introduced and used. Ludwig von Bertalanffy, a biologist, introduced and defined the systems approach as the relationship among and interdependence of parts, emphasizing the flow of information, the work, and the inputs and outputs. His model is made up of four basic components: inputs, transformation, outputs, and feedback (see Figure 13–1).

Feedback is the information received from internal as well as external sources to assist the system in making needed changes that meet customer needs, reduce cost, and/or improve quality and increase productivity or morale of workers. It also provides information for evaluation and control.

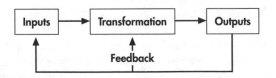

Figure 13–1 Basic systems model.

In the late 1890s and the early 1900s, workers and the work they were performing were changing. The invention of a variety of machines made mass production possible, and the demand for more goods at lower cost increased competition among most factories. As managers became more concerned with production, they tried to push and coerce workers by speeding up production lines and to increase daily quotas while employees were working the same hours with the same pay. Workers rebelled, and the union was born. Some of the managers realized that this was not the way to do things, and as a result efficiency experts were employed. Frequently these experts overlooked the human element and focused on increased production. Management and the experts also failed to realize that workers would be resentful and suspicious of outsiders who entered their area of work and told them how to do their jobs more efficiently without seeking input from them first.

TODAY'S WORKERS

As we approach the 21st century, the workplace and its workers are faced with some of the same turmoil as their predecessors. Managed care, customer demands, outside resource consultants, proliferation of information, computer programs, quality improvement methods, limited resources, patient-focused care, and competition have all increased the demand on management and workers to be more productive while providing quality and maintaining or reducing costs.

Labor cost accounts for 60% to 70% of an organization's resources. Therefore, reduction in labor expense is the first area targeted when cost reduction or increased productivity is discussed. There are numerous engineering techniques and quality improvements that have been utilized to determine labor production standards. Some methodologies that were used in the early part of this century are still applicable in today's high-paced environment. The same questions need to be answered now as then:

- Is there a quicker way to accomplish the task?
- Is the right person assigned to the task?
- Has the worker been trained to do the task?
- When is the best time to perform this task?
- Can this task be combined with others?
- Does this task need to be done at all?

STRATEGIES FOR IMPROVING PRODUCTIVITY

There is a current trend toward the use of industrial engineering techniques in the health care field. Restructuring focuses on changing the organizational structure and is global in scope. Rightsizing is normally implemented when the budgets or staffing patterns of all departments are cut by a certain percentage and it is left up to the leaders of each service to alter their systems accordingly. Reengineering, on the other hand, targets work processes. According to Kolssak (1995), the engineer who recently assisted in reengineering dietary processes at Rush Presbyterian–St. Luke's Medical Center, this concept can achieve greater cost reductions than others because it entails a total rethinking and radical redesign of the system. Some methodologies that are used for reengineering, such as job analysis and job redesign, are discussed in Chapter 3. The concept of work simplification is built into most of these techniques.

Reengineering Tasks through Work Simplification

Work simplification, or methods improvement, is a practical procedure that assists the supervisor in making the best use of labor, machines, and materials. The principle is to do more and better quality work with less effort and time. Work simplification increases the quality of production by improving job methods and reducing waste of time, energy, equipment, and materials. The steps used in the work simplification method are shown in Exhibit 13–1.

Step 1: Select the Job To Be Improved

The job that needs the most improvement may not be the most obvious. Therefore, a complete study of the overall operation will be needed. Look for time-consuming jobs, poor layout, unnecessary travel, hazardous conditions, and unnecessary paperwork. Seek input from the workers, and have discussions with the next level of management or administration.

Step 2: Break the Job Down in Writing

List all the details of the work to be accomplished. Observe employees as they perform their daily work, and explain to them what is being done while seeking their input. A useful tool in determining the chronological flow of work

---

Exhibit 13–1 Six Steps of Work Simplification

1. Select the job to be improved.
2. Break the job down in writing.
3. Question each detail and task.
4. Develop a better method.
5. Implement the new method.
6. Monitor, evaluate, and revise as needed.

is called a flow process chart, which is a graphic representation of an orderly, logical sequence of events, steps, or procedures that take place in a system. Five basic symbols are used to graph the flow; these are shown in Exhibit 13–2 (West, Wood, Harger, & Shugart, 1977).

Work sampling is another way to measure work. The work to be sampled is conducted randomly, and the number of observations must be large enough to ensure accuracy. Motion analysis and balancing studies can be used to improve a process and increase productivity. For example, one goal would be to improve a process by ensuring that work is distributed between the worker's hands so that both hands are being used simultaneously. Tools and materials should be located for easy accessibility and in such a way that the worker uses the best possible sequence of motion. The heights of work tables, shelves, and other pieces of equipment are judged to determine whether they are ergonomically sound so that they afford optimal worker comfort and positioning. Efforts can be made to cut down on the *picking up* and *moving of* tools and equipment; when everything is kept in its assigned place, increased productivity results. Balancing the work also ensures that no one employee is doing more work than another.

Step 3: Question Each Detail and Task

Once the flow is charted, each separate task should be questioned. Challenge the validity of each detail by asking the following:

- What is the purpose of the detail or task, and is this necessary? Does it add value? Can quality and expected outcome be obtained if it is deleted?

Exhibit 13–2 Symbols Used in a Flow Process Chart

Operation or main step in the process. Operations advance as the task is completed. Examples are slicing, portioning, wrapping, etc.

Transportation, which represents any movement encountered in the process, such as walking, carrying, etc.

Delays, which occur when conditions do not permit or require immediate performance in the next planned action.

Storage or holding, which occurs when something remains in one place, not being worked on in a regular process and awaiting further action at a later date.

Inspection, which occurs when an item is checked, verified, revised, or examined for quality or quantity and is not changed.

- Where is the best place or area to perform this detail or task? If it is necessary, is it being performed in the right place? If not, where should it be performed?
- When is the best time to do this detail or task? Is it being done at the right time? Should it be performed at another time? Could it be combined with another detail or task? Could it be done before or after another detail or task?
- Who should perform this detail or task? Is the right person performing it? Would it improve or increase efficiency if someone else did it?
- How should the detail or task be done? Should a different machine, tool, or material be used? Can the working environment be improved? Can workers cut down on the waste and wear of equipment? Can worker stress and fatigue be reduced? Can the detail or task be made safer?

Step 4: Develop a Better Method

The manager needs to answer the question: Is this detail or task necessary, and if it were eliminated, would this result in a loss or simply increase efficiency? If necessity is established, one can explore other sequences or combinations of tasks. Try to simplify the process further by using both hands, shortening transportation time, or using other efficient motions and tools. Discussions with employees are extremely helpful while one is developing new methods.

Developing productivity work and time standards takes time, skill, and knowledge. Usually, management systems engineers observe an average employee who is given the same working conditions as other employees. Tasks are broken down into a sequence as they are performed, and the work is timed with stopwatches. The observations are made at different times and on different days to determine a representative time for each task. Next, a performance rating is provided. Allowances for fatigue, personal needs, and interruptions are included as a measurable factor in the time standards.

Step 5: Implement the New Method

Continue to involve workers in the process. Provide them with information about exactly how the new methods will work and what the outcome of the new procedures will be. Explain and demonstrate how new methods are best applied. Seek their input. Ask questions and elicit feedback. Show how the new methods will improve their work, save time, decrease cost, and result in any other realistic improvements. Seek their cooperation. Try to eliminate fear by using trial runs before the new methods are actually implemented, and mutually work out any problems that surface. Give credit and recognition to all who participated in the project. Continue to provide information, and seek feedback from managers and administration. Check for weaknesses and areas that may have been overlooked. Admit shortcomings and failures. Seek acceptance and support.

Step 6: Monitor, Evaluate, and Revise as Needed

Once the new system has been introduced, make frequent observations to determine whether the new method is being followed as originally implemented. Check to ensure that no safety or sanitary regulations are violated. Graciously accept suggestions for revision. Continue to seek feedback from workers, managers, and administration.

Quality Improvement Teams

Quality improvement teams represent another approach for increasing productivity (Organizational Dynamics, 1990). The purpose of the interdisciplinary team is to incorporate quality improvement as an integral, ongoing part of every employee's job. Employees at all levels of the organization are provided with the knowledge and skills that are necessary for them to serve on a team and to strive continually for improvement. In many instances, improving the quality works to improve productivity as well. The teams work collaboratively.

Exhibit 13–3 outlines the activities of a quality improvement team. At each phase of the process, an output is determined, and the most appropriate tool for that phase is used. Written reports are a major component of this process. Additional information regarding quality improvement as well as the tools shown in Exhibit 13–3 can be found in Chapter 14.

Other Methods

There are still other methods that can be used to evaluate and improve productivity. They include work sampling, Gantt charting, and the Performance

---

Exhibit 13–3 Quality Improvement Team Activities

1. Identify the opportunity or need for a quality improvement process.
2. Identify the highest priority problems that need to be solved.
3. Analyze the problems utilizing various quality improvement tools (charts, checklists, diagrams, brainstorming, Pareto analyses, cause and effect diagrams, samplings, surveys, input/output models, etc.).
4. Develop realistic solutions.
5. Monitor and evaluate how the new solution works.

Evaluation Review Technique (PERT). Gantt charting entails the development of scheduling and progress charts that emphasize the work–time relationship that is necessary to meet a defined goal. PERT is a planning and coordinating tool that is used with large, complex undertakings that are nonrepetitive in nature and require integrated management of several projects. Many of these techniques can be completed by the department director and staff; others may need input from a management systems engineer.

MONITORING PRODUCTIVITY

As health care organizations and their food and nutrition service directors seek operational efficiencies and cost containment, productivity measurement and benchmarking with other institutions continue to be stressed. To elucidate productivity and benchmarking and the impact they have on the professionals in the field, some definitions are explored.

Productivity Defined

The Productivity Task Force of American Dietetic Association Members with Management Responsibility defines productivity as "The efficiency with which production or service activity converts inputs into outputs; often expressed as an output/input ratio, thereby integrating effectiveness, efficiency, and quality" (Halling, Lafferty, & Feller, 1986, pp. 1, 53). Gilbert (1990) states:

> A comprehensive definition of productivity encompasses more than how to increase work output in relation to the resources available to perform work. True productivity results from the staff working together efficiently to provide high quality services while forwarding the organization's goals and deriving personal and professional satisfaction from doing a job well. The quality of work does not have to suffer at the expense of productivity; quality is always an important consideration when analyzing a department's work. Productivity is an efficiency measurement related to production, a relationship between outputs (work accomplished or work load) and inputs (the amount of resources available to do the work). (p. 15)

Puckett and Miller (1988) define productivity as "the relationship of the amount of resources or services used to the amount of products or services produced, or the relationship between inputs and outputs. Productivity can be simply calculated by dividing the amount of input by the amount of output" (p. 94). Olsen and Meyer (1987) state that productivity concerns "the efficient utilization of human, equipment, and financial resources, and it is often expressed mathematically as the ratio of outputs to inputs" (p. 87). Spears (1995) defines productivity as "the ratio of outputs to inputs, or the ratio of goals to resources of the foodservice system. It can be increased by reducing inputs, by increasing outputs, or doing both at the same time" (p. 444).

The Systems Approach

To illustrate the systems approach (see Figure 13–1), Puckett (1995) used coleslaw as the output of the system. The inputs were identified as the *resources* available to produce this product. The *action* or *transformation* included the subsystems working in harmony to produce the output. Therefore, the *output* is the result of the *input* and *action* (or transformation) working in harmony to produce a *result* or *product*.

Chapter 1 illustrates the overall inputs and outputs for the food and nutrition care delivery system (see Figure 1–6). *Inputs* or resources are obtained from the community and include human resources, financial resources, materials, equipment, supplies, and information. *Transformations* include food service and nutrition intervention activities. The outputs are identified as nutrition care plans, nutrition education, nutrition support, and food services. These *outputs* represent both products and services that are provided for patients, employees, and other customers.

There is always a control on the system. Control refers to the plans, missions, values, goals, and objectives of the organization, which lay the framework for leaders to plan, direct, coordinate, and improve all processes involved in the transformation. Controls are also imposed from the outside in the form of external influences, such as rules, regulations, and laws; they also come from within, such as budgets and standardized menus. Controls are necessary to ensure that managers and employees utilize the inputs in an efficient and effective manner while meeting quality standards.

Feedback may be external or internal. It assists the system in making changes that are necessary so that goals can be met for customer satisfaction, cost reduction, productivity improvement, high employee morale, and so forth. Some typical methods of obtaining feedback are customer focus groups, plate waste analysis, and patient satisfaction surveys.

The literature documents a variety of methods that have been used to measure and monitor labor productivity. There is still a need for standardization because commonly accepted methods will help the industry reap sure benefits from comparison among facilities through benchmarking efforts.

Food Service Productivity

Productivity in food service is usually measured with respect to labor hours, although measurements that involve all inputs in relation to outputs are just as important. The most common method for measuring food service productivity is to divide the number of meals served during a specific period of time (outputs) by labor hours for the same time (inputs) to obtain meals per labor hour. Some practitioners use the opposite ratio, which reflects labor minutes per meal served.

In 1975, Kotschevar suggested that hospital food services could produce 5.5 meals per labor hour, nursing homes could produce 3.0 to 6.0 meals per labor hour, and large hospitals could produce 11.6 meals per labor hour. Coble (1975) noted that 11 to 12 employees are needed in a hospital food service department for every 100 beds. In 1988, Puckett and Miller suggested, "for a health care institution that provides three meals per day, 7 days a week, an average labor time of 14 minutes per meal can be used" (p. 46). This equates to 4.3 meals per labor hour. In 1980, Rose suggested that acute care facilities that use conventional food service systems could produce 3.5 meals per labor hour. Another standard that has been accepted by some food service consultants for use in large institutions assumes that 7,200 meals can be produced by each employee. This is all inclusive for every employee in the department, including all managers, clerical staff, and the like.

In 1989, Sneed and Henderson Kresse published average productivity levels for various types of food service operations (see Table 13–1). These authors caution those using the averages as follows:

> These productivity levels reflect industry averages and should serve only as a guide for determining staffing needs and evaluating performance. To control labor costs effectively, the manager should assess employee performance, identify methods for reducing labor costs, and monitor productivity over time. While it is useful to compare productivity levels of an operation to industry averages, it is critical to com-

---

Table 13–1 Average Productivity Levels for Various Food Service Operations

Food Service Operation	Meals per Labor Hour
Quick service restaurants	9.5
Luxury restaurant	1.4
Family restaurant	4.8
Cafeteria	5.5
Acute care facility	3.5
Extended care facility	5.0
School food service	13.0–15.0

Source: Reprinted from J. Sneed, K. Henderson Kresse, *Understanding Foodservice Financial Management,* © 1989, Aspen Publishers, Inc.

pare productivity levels for the operation over time. Because there are many factors that influence productivity, comparisons with other operations may mean little because of the differences in the operation. Therefore, it may be best to let an operation serve as its own comparison. In that way, deviations in productivity can be determined and improvement identified. (pp. 31–32)

One major trend in recent years has been toward patient-focused care, which has resulted in many of the traditional labor-intensive food service tasks being deployed to other services. This trend will have a great impact on total labor hours in the food service department. Therefore, pre-1990 averages and recommendations should only be used as a guide for facilities that continue to use the more traditional systems.

There are other approaches that can be taken for measuring productivity. Meals per patient day, for example, reflects the average number of meals that are served to patients each day. If this ratio increases over time while staffing remains constant, the department is increasing in productivity. Other common methods are as follows:

Meals per patient day = Total meals served per patient day ÷ Paid labor hours per patient day

Labor cost per patient day = Total payroll, including fringe benefits and other direct labor costs per patient day

Labor cost per meal served = Total labor cost per patient day ÷ Meals served per day

Total labor hours can be broken down to productive and nonproductive time. Productive time includes actual hours worked plus overtime. Nonproductive hours are hours paid but not worked, such as sick, vacation, holiday, and personal days. Total labor cost includes the salaries that are paid to workers for regular time, overtime, nonproductive time, and fringe benefits. This accounts for 10% to 38% of the total pay.

Some food service managers find the need to monitor other indicators of productivity, which may include the following (for those interested in tray line productivity, Chapter 10 includes a discussion of this topic):

- revenue produced per full-time equivalent (FTE) in the retail operation
- number of transactions performed per FTE assigned to the retail operation
- number of retail customers per cashier
- total number of FTEs per day versus budgeted FTEs per day
- total meals per productive work hour

- total meals per nonproductive work hour
- number of trays per minute

What Is a Meal?

Determining how to calculate a meal or meal equivalent has been an ongoing industry saga. There are no industry standards, even though large organizations such as the Voluntary Hospital Association (VHA) and MECON have established a uniform definition. The great diversity of formulas that are used creates confusion when administrators and food service directors try to compare their facilities with others, especially when results are used as a basis for productivity benchmarks, such as meals per labor hour or cost per meal. The lack of standardization is perhaps why administrators and financial officers tend not to take statistics based on meals too seriously when they evaluate the bottom line.

Most hospital administrators are content with knowing food, supply, and labor costs per admission or patient day. A dilemma has always existed for food service directors, however, because two hospitals with the same number of patient days can easily serve a different number of meals as a result of the nature of the services they offer to patients. A hospital with a number of surgical cases may have a large percentage of orders for nothing by mouth (NPO), whereas another with many long-term patients may serve more full meals per patient day. In addition, the same two hospitals are bound to have differences in the scope of nonpatient food services. Because of these factors, directors have always resisted cross-organizational comparisons of cost and productivity based on patient days alone. They have insisted on using more accurate measures of the actual work done by their departments based on actual meals served.

The Patient Meal

A patient meal has traditionally been defined as the food provided for an inpatient on a tray, excluding nourishments, tube feedings, and infant formulas. Nonpatient meals are cafeteria, catering, vending, and other food services provided for persons other than inpatients. These definitions were used in the American Hospital Association's Monitrend comparisons in the 1970s and 1980s until that system was discontinued; many directors still follow them, however.

One major controversy regarding the definition of a patient meal is whether supplemental nourishments should be included. Most directors who include them convert their total monthly raw food cost to meal equivalents. Others identify a ratio based on cost and allocate anywhere from two to six nourishments to one meal equivalent, depending upon the amount of food provided. Even though tube feedings were excluded from patient meal calculations in the past, it is now commonly thought that they should be included if the food and nutrition department purchases, issues, and delivers them.

Some facilities count actual patient meal trays delivered to patients' rooms, including late and guest meals, and count double portions as two meals. When this is done, a log should be kept for late trays so that they can be included in this count. Others use the midnight census, multiply this number by a factor of 2.5 to 2.8, and use the resulting figure. This shortcut method is not as accurate, and the basis for the multiplication factor should be regularly verified and updated. Still others establish a formula to determine how many nourishments, items of floor stock, and enteral formulas are provided. When nourishments and tube and infant feedings that are purchased and issued by the department are included, one can keep track of their raw food cost and divide this by the average cost of a patient meal to obtain a meal equivalent figure.

Nonpatient Food Services

An even greater variety of formulas is found for retail meals. Because cafeteria, catering, and vending services do not always provide full meals for customers, food service directors have traditionally striven to convert the overall volume of foods provided through these services to patient meal equivalents.

The most prevalent method for calculating meal equivalents is based upon sales, whereby the selling price of a sample noon meal is divided into total revenues and stipends. Many directors continue to select this sales-based method for the same reasons that it has been used historically and/or because of the lack of a more appropriate method. Many use the former American Hospital Association system and compute the selling price of a commonly used luncheon meal consisting of meat, starch, bread and butter, vegetable, soup or salad, beverage, and dessert. Results of this calculation can easily be skewed by the actual meal that is selected. If a low-priced meal is used, the number of meal equivalents will be inflated, food cost will appear to be low, and the productivity ratio (meals per labor hour) will be high. If, on the other hand, a high-priced meal is selected, fewer meal equivalents will result, the cost per meal will be high, and productivity will be low.

Sales-Based Formulas

In past years, not all food service directors understood just how much of their food, labor, and supply expenses should be allocated to patient and nonpatient cost centers. Many practiced "shoebox accounting," where all expenses and revenues were tossed in one large cost center that covered all services provided by the department. As a result, actual costs for cafeteria, catering, and vending services were not available, and total sales was the only basis for calculating meal equivalents. Even though some operations are still run like this, it is simply not acceptable, and one should devise a reliable method for allocating costs properly to patient and nonpatient services, even if administrators do not encourage this. Gone are the days when after-the-fact allocations can be made because they maximize reimbursement or look good on paper. This was never ethical and should not be practiced.

Many food service directors whose background is in the restaurant industry are familiar with the concept of an average check. They tend to consider a meal equivalent that is based upon sales volume divided by the number of actual customers. To determine the number of customers, records are kept for a specified period of time, and averages are calculated from them. It is necessary to include holidays and weekends. The average should be trended and reviewed at least annually. For example, this method could be used in a hospital that serves 1,856 customers in a day and has total cash sales of $5,200. The average check would be $2.80, and this would be the meal equivalent figure. Managers who use this formula then divide monthly sales by the meal equivalent figure to obtain the number of meals served.

Others have been more specific because they consider the fact that most customers do not consume an entire meal. For benchmarking purposes, the VHA has defined a nonpatient meal to consist of a boneless, skinless chicken breast (5 oz EP), whipped potatoes (1/2 cup), green beans (1/2 cup), white bread (1 slice), butter/margarine (1 pat), plain gelatin salad (3" × 3" square), pie (1/8 slice of a 10-inch pie), and coffee (1 cup). Other benchmarking plans use a similar "market basket" approach with slightly different food items. Participants submit raw market basket costs and selling prices of these foods and convert them to cafeteria meal equivalents by dividing total cafeteria sales by the selling price, which is weighted by the percentages of full and discounted meals that are sold. This sales-based method is mixed with a cost-based method for nourishments, catering, and other nonpatient services.

A committee of food service directors affiliated with the University Hospital Consortium worked with MECON associates to assist in defining a meal equivalent that would promote consistency in reporting benchmarking data. They established a meal equivalent to consist of the following items:

- 3 oz roast beef $1.95
- ½ cup mashed potatoes   0.54
- ½ cup green beans   0.52
- gelatin salad   0.50
- bread and butter   0.40

- apple pie   0.75
- beverage   0.40
- total selling price $5.06

These foods are commonly served in every institution and can be quickly calculated. To determine the meal equivalent, the selling price for each menu is totaled, resulting in the selling price of a meal equivalent. Utilizing total sales figures (minus taxes) divided by the meal equivalent amount, a meal equivalent figure can be achieved. Using the example above, for daily sales of $5,200, the meal equivalents would be 1,028 ($5,200 divided by $5.06). As can be seen in the results of this method compared with the average check formula, there is a difference of more than 800 meals. It is easy to see why it is difficult to determine just *what is a meal.*

In addition, even if the content of the sample meal is standardized, another uncontrolled variable of profit margin (or loss) continues to exist. It is indeed possible that two hospitals serving the same menu and volume of cafeteria food with different mark-up percentages would yield varying results. Also, if the sample meal is not equivalent to the hospital's average patient meal, additional inconsistencies occur. These problems have caused some directors to avoid the issue entirely, as did the American Society of Hospital Food Service Administrators (which includes only costs per patient days and revenues in its benchmarking program), or to look at other ways to define a meal.

Cost-Based Formulas

In contrast to past years, when separated cost centers were not commonly used, many directors now separate the actual costs of patient and nonpatient food services and even keep track of supplemental feedings and nourishment costs. This has opened the door to a simpler alternative method of determining patient meal equivalents that is devoid of the controversies related to the sales-based formulas. The cost-based method entails first calculating the average cost of a patient meal (raw food cost for patient meals divided by number of patient meals served). The resulting figure is divided into the raw food cost of all other categories from nourishments to cafeteria services. Figure 13–2 is a form for using this method.

One benefit of a cost-based system is that there is no need to tackle the problem of arbitrarily selecting a sample cafeteria meal because a sample meal is not required for these calculations. People cannot manipulate the data by using a sample meal in their formulas that will make them look good. In addition, because it is a cost-based system, the complications introduced by varying profit margins are eliminated. The method is consistent and simple to perform, and

	RFC	ME
A. Patient Meals		
1. Raw food cost (RFC) for patient trays (total patient food cost minus costs reported in Section B)	$_____	
2. Inpatient tray count + late trays		_____
3. Number of other patient-related trays (ER, outpatient, guest, etc.)		_____
4. Total patient trays (add A2 + A3)		_____
5. RFC per meal served (A1 divided by A4)	$_____	
B. Patients' Nourishments and Supplemental Feedings		
1. RFC for tube feedings and infant formulas if purchased and issued by food services	$_____	
2. RFC for commercial supplements	$_____	
3. RFC for other snacks and floor stock	$_____	
4. Add B1 + B2 + B3 and divide by A5 to get meal equivalents for nourishments and supplemental feedings		_____
C. Nonpatient Services		
1. RFC for foods issued to cafeteria	$_____	
2. RFC for foods issued for catering	$_____	
3. RFC for foods issued to fill facility operated vending machines	$_____	
4. RFC for other nonpatient services	$_____	
5. Add C1 + C2 + C3 + C4 and divide by A5 to get meal equivalents for nonpatient food services		_____
D. Total RFC	$_____	
E. Total patient meal equivalents served		_____
F. RFC per patient meal equivalent (copy from A5)	$_____	

Figure 13–2 Form for cost-based method for calculating patient meal equivalents. *Source:* Reprinted from R. Jackson, Defining a "Meal," *Hospital Food & Nutrition Focus,* Vol. 11, No. 12, insert, © 1995, Aspen Publishers, Inc.

all services are treated in the same manner. Most of all, the alternative cost-based method reflects what it is intended to do: identify patient meal equivalents by converting the foods that are not served on patient trays to a monetary figure that most closely represents the average patient meal. The major disadvantage of the system is that it is dependent upon the cost of the patient meal, which may vary from facility to facility.

Although no system is perfect, the industry is getting closer to improved standardized methods as a result of increased accountability for cost allocations, computerization, and the growing importance of benchmarking.

Labor Hours

Labor hours are commonly monitored by the payroll period, month, and year. Actual *paid* hours are used as the basis for productivity calculations because this reflects productive time. Managers may also wish to include comparisons of total labor hours, which reflects productive and nonproductive time as previously described.

An FTE is based on one employee who works on a full-time basis for a specific period of time (e.g., 2,080 hours per year). It does not reflect the total number of employees in a department because some workers may be employed on a part-time basis or may not work the number of standard hours that the institution identifies to be full time. Under normal circumstances, according to Sneed and Henderson Kresse (1989), one FTE equals 8 hours per day, 40 hours per week, 173.3 hours per month, or 2,080 hours per year. For positions that vary from these norms, alternative standards should be used for the purposes of budgeting and comparing actual paid hours with budgeted amounts. While one is establishing the number of FTEs needed in a department, relief time must be considered. One full-time employee, for example, may have 104 days per year off (52 × 2), 10 vacation days, 8 holidays, and 8 days of sick leave. Based upon this plan, the employee would actually work 235 days per year. Meals must be served three times a day, 365 days per year, however, so to provide coverage it will take 1.55 employees for each full-time position or three workers to cover every two full-time positions (365 days/235 days = 1.55).

To calculate labor hours, a specific time period needs to be established first (e.g., a week, month, or year). Actual hours paid for the same period can be obtained from payroll records or financial reports. Total labor hours are then divided by the FTE (40 hours) to identify the number of FTEs. Total labor hours can also be divided into the number of meal equivalents served to identify meals per labor hour.

Factors Affecting Food Service Productivity

As discussed, measuring food service productivity is no simple task. There are many variables that can explain the differences from one point in time to another in a given facility and the difference in productivity ratios when one institution is benchmarked against another. These variables include at least the following:

- methodology used to determine a meal and meal equivalent
- bed size
- occupancy rate
- type of food services offered
- type of purchasing, receiving, inventorying, issuing, production, assembly, and service systems used
- complexity of the menu and extent to which convenience foods are used
- number and types of modified menus
- off-site facilities
- branding/franchising
- value-added services
- sanitation duties assumed by food service employees
- use of automated systems and computers
- layout of department and facility
- transportation
- competencies and skill level of employees
- clerical duties performed
- on-site preparation of formulas
- age and working condition of equipment
- maintenance policies
- use of patient-focused work teams

Clinical Productivity

Monitoring Clinical Productivity

Addressing the topic of labor productivity for clinical nutrition services, Laramee (1995) states:

> When the issue of monitoring productivity to measure the output of clinical services is first presented to staff, it is often resisted. The common fear is that there is a hidden agenda such as trying to eliminate positions. Many will express the concern that by emphasizing productivity, quality of patient services will decline. Care providers often reject the "numbers" associated with productivity measurement as a lack of concern for the patient. They will argue that the time spent on keeping records cuts down on the time devoted to patient care. There will be a deep discomfort with the emphasis on cost issues, and some professional disappointment at having to deal with maintaining productiv-

ity goals. Many have a fear of being found out or judged to be inadequate performers. Recognizing the importance of productivity measurement and these issues prior to introducing productivity monitoring is paramount to success and a strategy to deal with staff concerns is necessary. (p. 4)

According to Laramee, it is important to make the following decisions before a system for monitoring clinical productivity is determined.

Determine staff to include. Will only the activities of registered dietitians be included, or will dietetic technicians also be asked to track activities? Are some tasks, such as menu or patient screening, questionnaire collection, and electronic scanning, completed by clerks, and if so, will these activities be included? Grant and DeHoog (1991) advise that each level of care be well defined so that staff can be assigned accordingly. For example, clinical dietitians are assigned to high-risk patients, dietetic technicians to moderate-risk patients, and dietary managers to low-risk patients.

Identify the system of measurement. Will a general approach be taken? Will the actual time spent in performing specific activities be measured, or will a weighted activity value (WAV) be used? Formulas for measuring techniques range from simple to detailed. Those who have limited resources and time for data collection and analysis may wish to use the more general approaches, such as the number of clinical staffhours per patient day. A general measure used by some administrators for benchmarking purposes is patient contacts per hour worked. Although lacking any meaningful measure of the length or type of each contact (i.e., screening, assessment, counseling, etc.), this measure can easily be standardized across institutions.

When the number of hours worked is calculated, only actual time on the job is included, not vacation, holiday, sick, and personal time. When general measurements are used, however, variations or changes in these factors can lead to fluctuations in productivity rates and cause a shift in how time is utilized. For example, a rise in admissions combined with a decline in length of stay may increase the time spent in screening, decreasing the length of time spent in monitoring care plans and indicating the need to add a diet technician and decrease staffing of registered dietitians. These concerns have led many to focus on the more detailed approach, where specific types of patient care activities are measured.

Some global ratios can be applied for clinical nutrition activities. They include calculations of total clinical hours per patient day, per patient admission, or per adjusted patient admission. These methods can be helpful in determining staffing patterns, especially when flexible scheduling is used. Chapter 3 describes this process.

While determining the exact clinical outputs to be monitored, it will be helpful for practitioners to review the classification system provided in Chapter 4, where dietitians' time is divided into direct, indirect, and nonpatient or administrative tasks. Exhibit 4–4 provides information and a sample form for how job analysis can be applied to clinical dietetics. Some alternative systems for measuring clinical productivity are shown in Exhibit 13–4.

Decide how data will be summarized. Will the data be calculated from the total time spent on each activity or from the total WAV for each activity? Most managers set a calculation based on a WAV system for ease of use by staff and for report preparation. The activities of the clinical staff are organized and reported in many different ways; there is no standard for the industry as yet.

One common method is to summarize periodically the data from the daily logs kept by staff members. For example, at Carolinas Medical Center in Charlotte, North Carolina, the actual time used for the following activities is reported by dietitians and summarized monthly:

- Direct patient care
  1. nutrition screening
  2. nutrition assessments
  3. follow-up contacts
  4. formal consults
  5. patient care meetings
  6. nutrition education
  7. documentation
  8. discharge planning
  9. postdischarge contacts
- Nondirect patient care
  1. recordkeeping
  2. meetings
  3. project time
  4. group class education
  5. continuing education
  6. student education

At this facility, assessments and care planning are also identified by type (e.g., tube feeding, total parenteral nutrition, etc.). Nutrition education is divided into group or individual sessions and whether it is formal, informal, or ordered at the last minute.

Exhibit 13–4 Alternative Methods for Measuring Clinical Productivity

---

Clinical labor hours per patient day

  Formula: Actual labor hours ÷ Number of patient days

  Example: 2 dietitians and 2 technicians work 600 hours in a month that has 7,000 patient days = 5.1 minutes per patient day

Patient contacts per labor hour worked

  Formula: Number of patient contacts ÷ Actual work hours

  Example: 2 dietitians and 2 technicians work 600 hours in a month screening 1,000 patients and providing 300 nutrition assessments or education sessions = 2.2 contacts per labor hour

Direct patient care hours per labor hour worked

  Formula: Labor hours for direct patient care ÷ Total labor hours

  Example: An outpatient dietitian works 136 hours in a month and completes 60 basic assessments/care plans (30 minutes each), 80 basic follow-ups (15 minutes each), and 120 basic nutrition education sessions (30 minutes each) = 125 ÷ 136 = 91.9%

Relative value units (RVUs)

  Time can also be measured in RVUs, such as 15 minutes being equal to one RVU. When this system is used, time spent in each clinical activity is recorded in the number of units closest to the amount of time allocated to each activity.

  Example: If 15 minutes = 1 RVU, a 45-minute basic assessment and care plan is equivalent to 3 RVUs.
  Total RVUs are added for each month, so the dietitian specified above completed 500 RVUs.

WAVs

  A WAV is a specific amount of time assigned to each activity, such as 45 minutes for a basic assessment and care plan. Actual time spent usually is not measured; rather, the number of patients for whom the activity is completed is measured. When used, time studies are extremely helpful in determining the appropriate type and average time for each activity to be included. WAVs per hour can also be calculated to help identify problems in individual performance.

  Example: A dietitian completes 160 basic assessments in a month, and this is weighted by 45 in totaling productive hours.

Notes: For labor hours worked, do not include vacation, holiday, sick, and personal time. Examples of patient contacts are screening, assessment, counseling, and patient education.

Source: Adapted from S.L. Laramee, Monitoring Productivity of the Clinical Staff, *Hospital Food and Nutrition Focus*, Vol. 11, No. 10, pp. 4–5, insert, © 1995, Aspen Publishers, Inc.

Relative value units (RVUs) can also be summarized. A system using RVUs from one benchmarking program ("Benchmarking Program," 1996) is outlined below. Because the care of high-risk patients often takes longer than that for others, direct patient care activities are identified as either basic or comprehensive. To determine RVUs for activities, the standardized times that are identified are used as weights for each activity. The time allocations in the example were derived from Grant and DeHoog (1991), DeHoog (1985), McManners and Barina (1984), Gates Smith, Konkle, and Semen (1991), and the Dietetic Staffing Committee (1982).

- **Nutrition screening:** The process of reviewing all newly admitted patients and those with changed medical conditions to determine risk status and need for further assessment and care (basic, 5 minutes; comprehensive, 10 minutes).
- **Nutrition assessment and care planning:** Evaluating data on nutrition status and providing a written plan that identifies what will be done to improve the nutritional status of patients (basic, 45 minutes; comprehensive, 60 minutes).
- **Follow-up:** Monitoring patient progress and documenting results in the medical record (basic, 15 minutes; comprehensive, 30 minutes).
- **Discharge planning:** Formulating and documenting a plan for nutrition care after discharge (basic, 15 minutes; comprehensive, 30 minutes).
- **Nutrition education:** Provision of diet instructions for patients and/or caregivers (basic, 30 minutes; comprehensive, 45 minutes).
- **Team consultation:** Conferring with other members of the health care team (basic, 15 minutes; comprehensive, 30 minutes).
- **Nutrient analysis:** Evaluation of 3-day nutrient intake and documenting nutrient consumption (45 minutes for all patients).

Dietitians log their daily activities, and data are summarized as shown in Figure 13–3. The definitions and time values given above are the basis for this summary. Averages can be taken from data that are collected monthly or even quarterly. This method eliminates the need to have the clinical staff count actual minutes for all daily activities because the RVUs are used as the measuring tool. It focuses on the outputs of the clinical nutrition function, and the goal is to have the highest possible percentage of time spent in activities that have the best potential for reimbursement. The final productivity ratio represents total RVUs per labor hour worked for inpatient and outpatient nutrition care.

Determine the methods for reporting. Will productivity data be reported weekly, monthly, or quarterly? Who will tabulate or calculate the information? Many managers ask staff to summarize their own individual reports and submit them on a weekly or monthly basis. Once productivity logs have been summarized over a period of time, perhaps 3 to 6 months, the consultant or manager can evaluate the record against the departmental and facility mission and goals (S. Escott-Stump, personal communication, 1995). For example, if goals have been set that direct patient care services are two thirds of paid time and indirect services are one third of paid time, it is possible to determine whether time has

Direct Patient Care Activities	Inpatient Clinical Care			Outpatient Clinical Care		
	Average RVUs per day	× Time Factor	= Time Allocation	Average RVUs per day	× Time Factor	= Time Allocation
Basic Nutrition Screening	_____	5 min.	_____	_____	5 min.	_____
Comprehensive Screening	_____	10 min.	_____	_____	10 min.	_____
Basic Assessments/ Care Plans	_____	45 min.	_____	_____	45 min.	_____
Comprehensive Assessments/Care Plans	_____	60 min.	_____	_____	60 min.	_____
Basic Follow-up	_____	15 min.	_____	_____	15 min.	_____
Comprehensive Follow-up	_____	30 min.	_____	_____	30 min.	_____
Basic Nutrition Education	_____	30 min.	_____	_____	30 min.	_____
Comprehensive Education	_____	45 min.	_____	_____	45 min.	_____
Team Consultation	_____	15 min.	_____	_____	15 min.	_____
3-Day Nutrient Analysis	_____	45 min.	_____	_____	45 min.	_____
Basic Discharge Plans	_____	15 min.	_____	_____	15 min.	_____
Comprehensive Discharge Plans	_____	30 min.	_____	_____	30 min.	_____
Total minutes allocated for direct patient care		_____				_____
Divided by 60 minutes		_____				_____
Total RVUs per day (1 RVU = 1 hour)		_____				_____
Divided by average hours worked per day for clinical staff during same period		_____				_____
Clinical productivity (RVUs per labor hour)		_____%				_____%

Figure 13–3 Quarterly summary of RVUs. *Source:* Reprinted from Benchmarking Program for Food and Nutrition Services, *Hospital Food & Nutrition Focus,* © 1996, Aspen Publishers, Inc.

been well spent. If the dietitian is spending too much time in basic services (such as menu processing, handling diet order changes, or conducting meal rounds), these tasks could be reassigned to technicians or dietetic managers. It might be feasible to revise the staffing pattern when the next opportunity arises, as with staff turnover or realignment.

Factors Affecting Clinical Productivity

Patient acuity is often cited as the major factor affecting labor productivity for clinical nutrition services. Although standardized methods for measuring productivity are useful for external benchmarking purposes, the establishment of criteria is difficult because of variations in patients' medical conditions. In the field of nursing, patient acuity is commonly used to develop staffing levels for nursing personnel. In 1985, Lutton et al. suggested the use of acuity levels in establishing dietitians' staffing levels as well. This was also recommended more recently by Ford and Fairchild (1990), who developed a classification system for monitoring clinical nutrition productivity.

Staffing and productivity levels have been studied in comparison with diagnosis-specific standards (S. Escott-Stump, personal communication, 1995). Although there are no definitive studies, it is likely that certain diagnoses and procedures will require more time by the dietitian (e.g., newly diagnosed diabetes, cystic fibrosis, gluten enteropathy, and extensive abdominal surgery with resection of the gastrointestinal tract). The time required for patient assessment, care plan development and implementation, counseling, and medical record documentation will vary according to the extent of disease involvement, patient awareness and knowledge level, and other variables. In addition, for cases where nutritional intake will be modified in several ways (such as cardiovascular diet orders for altered sodium, calories, fat, and fiber), the dietitian's role and time spent will be more involved than in a simple diet order for no concentrated sweets in a newly diagnosed elderly patient with mild diabetes. Similar time alterations will be noticed in regard to technician time in menu planning and processing as well as in tallying production orders for the food service personnel.

Other factors that affect the amount of labor hours needed for this function include the following:

- methodology used to determine the output of clinical work
- bed size
- occupancy rate
- type of nutrition services offered
- extent to which clinical staff are responsible for functions other than screening, assessment, care planning, nutrition consultation, and nutrition education
- complexity of the menu
- number and types of modified diets
- off-site and ambulatory care services
- accessibility of the medical record and patient database
- value-added services
- policies regarding nutrition support, formularies, and patient nourishments/supplements

- use of paraprofessionals to assist dietitians
- degree of involvement of clinical staff in various committees and managerial functions (e.g., quality improvement, risk management, etc.)
- cooperation and efficiency of communications with other members of the health care team
- use of automated systems and computers
- layout of the department and facility
- competencies and skill level of employees
- clerical duties performed
- use of patient-focused work teams

REIMBURSEMENT AND INCOME PRODUCING SERVICES

Productivity involves the relationship of inputs to outputs (see Figure 13–1). Although labor is important because it represents the single largest cost in most food service operations, viewing labor productivity alone can be limiting. As a result, the overall balance of inputs (labor, food, supplies, etc.) to outputs needs to be considered. This is most commonly done by calculating total cost per meal and per patient day and by comparing actual income with expenses. As described in Chapter 12, cost centers are commonly used for a realistic view of expenses. This can lead to identification of areas that are most promising for cost reduction. For specific recommendations regarding commercial food services, readers are referred to Chapter 12.

Figure 13–4 is a form used for analyzing and summarizing the income and expenses for food and nutrition services. From the data on this form, food service directors and clinical managers can generate a variety of productivity ratios, including those that follow. With the addition of other categories, such as FTEs, number of customers, patient discharges, and the like, the other indicators of productivity that are discussed in this chapter and Chapter 12 can also be included, and indirect expenses can be factored in as well.

- Food cost per meal served: patient, commercial, and total department
- Labor cost per meal served: patient, commercial, and total department
- Supply cost per meal served: patient, commercial, and total department
- Total direct cost per meal served: patient, commercial, and total department
- Meals served per patient day: patient, commercial, and total department
- Food cost per patient day: patient, commercial, and total department
- Labor cost per patient day: patient, commercial, and total department
- Supply cost per patient day: patient, commercial, and total department

Cost Center	Income and Expenses	Actual	Budgeted	YTD Variance

Patient Food Services	Total Direct Expenses
	    Labor Dollars (regular, overtime, benefits)
	    Food Expense
	    Supply Expense
	    Other Direct Expenses
	Total Meals Served
	Patient Days
		$_____	$_____	$_____

Commercial Food Services (Note: commercial and other services can be defined separately as needed)	Total Revenue: Cash Sales
	Total Direct Expenses
	    Labor Dollars (regular, overtime, benefits)
	    Food Expense
	    Supply Expense
	    Other Direct Expenses
	Net Gain/Loss (total revenue − total expenses)
	Total Meals Equivalents Served
		$_____	$_____	$_____

Inpatient Nutrition Care Services	Total Revenue
	Total Direct Expenses
	    Labor Dollars (regular, overtime, benefits)
	    Supply Expense
	    Other Direct Expenses
	Net Gain/Loss (total revenue − total expenses)
	RVUs
		$_____	$_____	$_____

Outpatient Nutrition Care Services	Total Revenue
	Total Direct Expenses
	    Labor Dollars (regular, overtime, benefits)
	    Supply Expense
	    Other Direct Expenses
	Net Gain/Loss (total revenue − total expenses)
	RVUs
	Admissions
		$_____	$_____	$_____

Figure 13–4 Monthly financial summary form.

- Total direct cost per patient day: patient, commercial, and total department
- Labor, supply, and other costs: inpatient nutrition care and ambulatory nutrition care
- Total direct cost per patient day: inpatient nutrition care and ambulatory nutrition care

- Total direct cost per admission: inpatient nutrition care
- Profit/loss: commercial food services, inpatient nutrition care, and ambulatory nutrition care
- Meals per labor hour: labor productivity for patient, commercial, and all department services
- RVUs per labor hour: labor productivity for inpatient and ambulatory nutrition care services

Just as in the case of commercial food services, the costs of clinical nutrition services can be monitored to determine whether the clinical nutrition unit is sustaining itself by providing reimbursed services. In 1985, Rose presented a method for analyzing the costs of outpatient nutrition services that included labor and other expenses such as telephone, mail, printing, and supplies. These costs can be routinely related to the income that a facility receives for nutrition intervention. In a retrospective study reported in 1992, Trimble found that coding for malnutrition could increase hospital reimbursement by $103,000 annually. Sayarath (1993) studied four diagnosis-related groups (DRGs) to track potential income for a 200-bed community hospital and estimated potential reimbursement to be in excess of $34,000 per year.

As noted in Chapter 1, dietitians have become proactive in recent years as they have learned to cost justify their services. Not only are they identifying cases of malnutrition, but they are seeking the typical "loser DRGs," those diagnoses or conditions that a facility consistently loses money on because of complications that result in longer lengths of stay than projected for reimbursement (Verderose, Smith, & Nagy-Nero, 1995). Figure 13–5 is a sample form used by dietitians to charge for their services. Close monitoring of charges and actual income to the facility is suggested so that the clinical nutrition manager can report income and expenses in a manner similar to that shown for the commercial food service operation.

It is clear from the trends discussed in Chapter 1 that managed care and preventive care will be very much a part of the future of the health care industry. Dietitians should not expect managed care organizations to knock on their doors and offer to pay for nutrition services. Nor should they wait for legislation to cover nutrition intervention and education. Verderose et al. (1995) suggest strategies for increased participation of dietitians in the decisions made by managed care organizations. They encourage dietitians to understand the managed care process, who the decision makers are, and which DRGs are most beneficial to target. Others advise dietitians to approach the decision makers with simple, concise facts on the cost benefits of nutrition intervention (Carey & Gillespie, 1995), protocols for nutrition services, staff qualifications, and cost estimates. Finally, it is recommended that dietitians offer to conduct a pilot that

☐ INPATIENT ☐ OUTPATIENT		
DATE_____ RD/DT/RN_____		
NUTRITION CONSULT		
Description	Task	Rev. Code
Mini		34600082
Brief		34600015
Limited		34600058
Intermediate		34600040
Extended		34600031
Comprehensive $		34600023
NUTRITION SUPPORT CONSULT		
Brief		28600046
Limited		28600089
Extended		28600062
Comprehensive $		28600054
AMBULATORY NUTRITION CONSULT		
Mini		28700032
Brief		28700041
Intermediate		28700083
Extended		28700067
Comprehensive $		28700059
Group Ed./Rtn.		287_____

Figure 13–5 Sample form for nutrition service charges. Courtesy Geisinger Medical Center, Danville, Pennsylvania.

includes protocols agreed upon by physicians and the managed care organization. The steps suggested for implementing a successful pilot are as follows:

1. Begin with patient care protocols that define a specific diagnosis, population, treatment, and expected outcome (Beyer et al., 1991).

2. Gain agreement from managed care physicians and the organization itself that the protocol is appropriate for their patients.

3. Develop and implement the system within the managed care organization and its physician networks to gain referral of patients who fit the protocols.

4. Develop and implement formal evaluation processes with specific outcomes and effectiveness measures.

5. Once the pilot has proved successful, work with the managed care organization to expand coverage to other diseases or a broader geographical area.

Several authors address the topic of obtaining reimbursement for nutrition services and monitoring costs of clinical nutrition services (Beyer et al., 1991; Gallagher-Allred, 1993; Sneed & Henderson Kresse, 1989; Verderose et al., 1995).

IMPROVING PRODUCTIVITY

There is a delicate balance between quality and productivity. Chapter 1 described how directors of food and nutrition services in general have done quite well compared with other departments in hospitals in containing costs since the DRGs were implemented in 1983 (see Table 1–4). As a result, administrators often look at food and nutrition departments as a source for additional cost reduction. It must be realized that the services they provide have a great impact on the perceived quality of health care services and that their costs represent a relatively small part of the facility's budget at the present time.

It is the responsibility of directors in the field to know the level of quality that is attained by the services they offer and to be able to project how quality will be affected if and when resources are decreased. Independent directors can learn a great deal from contracted food service management firms in this regard. If cost centers are used for financial accounting and accurate records are kept to identify the real costs of the various services that are offered, directors will be in a better position to present alternatives to administration when cost reduction is mandated. On the other hand, when administrators request additional programs that may improve the quality of customer services, directors should be able to present clearly and accurately the expected costs for such programs. With efficient use of the resources available, successful managers are able to do these things in the most cost-effective manner. The technique of value analysis presented in Chapter 12 can help directors work with their administrators in deciding the types and levels of services that can be afforded by the institution and should be offered to patients and other customers. Methods such as work analysis, job redesign, reengineering, flexible scheduling, and empowerment of teams can help directors continuously increase productivity.

BENCHMARKING

Benchmarking is the concept of setting goals based on knowing what has been achieved by others (Juran, 1992). It involves comparing and rating one institution's products and services against another's, which may be at the median or at the forefront. A variety of measures may be used, but all are concerned with inputs and outputs and note differences and likenesses. MECON, SunHealth, VHA, and others have developed these ratings and reporting systems. MECON has an exclusive focus on health care. According to Freund (1994), there are presently 350 MECON clients in 50 states. MECON PEER X is a service that provides performance information from a number of perspectives, ranging from worked hours per unit of service to total expense dollar per unit of service. VHA's system for benchmarking includes food service costs and productivity ratios. One professional organization, the American Society for Hospital Food Service Administrators, tracks overall cost per patient day and revenues. The Benchmarking Program for Food and Nutrition Services ("Benchmarking Program," 1996) provides methods for cross-organizational comparison of data regarding patient satisfaction, clinical performance, food service productivity, and clinical productivity.

According to Gift and Mosel (1994), "Health care benchmarking is the continual and collaborative discipline of measuring and comparing the results of key work processes with those of the best performers. It is learning how to adapt these best practices to achieve breakthrough process improvements and build healthier communities" (p. 5). They describe three different types of benchmarking:

1. internal benchmarking, or comparison of best practices within the organization (internal best)
2. competitive benchmarking, or comparison with the best performer in the health care market (competitive best)
3. functional benchmarking, or cross-industry comparison of the same or analogous processes (best in class)

Internal benchmarking is easy and the least expensive type of assessment. There are few intervening variables that can skew the comparison. Because the health care industry is highly competitive, however, and because the Joint Commission on Accreditation of Healthcare Organizations (Joint Commission) requires external comparisons as well, internal benchmarking is not enough.

The Joint Commission (1995) standards include four types of assessment: internal comparisons over time, comparisons with up-to-date practice guidelines and standards, comparisons with other organizations, and consideration of legal and regulatory requirements. The Joint Commission's agenda for change (1990) describes the establishment of the indicator monitoring system (IMSystem) for cross-organizational comparison of data. Once health care organizations participate, information will be sent on a quarterly basis via modem, tapes, or diskettes ("Indicator Software," 1993; "Joint Commission launches," 1994; "State hospital associations," 1993). Data will be analyzed by the Joint Commission, and results will enable comparison with national norms. The American Dietetic Association has been working with the Joint Commission to identify indicators that can be used to monitor the success of patient nutrition care (Kushner et al., 1994; Queen, Caldwell, & Balogun, 1993). Chapter 1 describes their participation and input thus far. Initially, financial data were included in the descriptions of the IMSystem, but this concept has not yet been implemented. To prepare for the time when participation in the IMSystem becomes manadatory, clinical nutrition managers and department directors can do the following (Jackson, 1994):

- Learn the facility's status with regard to participation in the voluntary IMSystem program for data collection. This will provide a suitable time frame for preparation.
- Stay abreast of the progress of the IMSystem testing results and the addition of performance indicators that relate to food and nutrition services by attending seminars and reading publications on this subject.
- Because other disciplines are already covered in existing indicators, become familiar with their activities and see how they are implementing them.
- Finally, as revisions in the quality improvement program are made, consider some of the nutrition care indicators proposed by the American Dietetic Association.

CONCLUSION

There is no simple answer to monitoring and increasing productivity. Although managers have many well-established techniques to do so, there is a need in the industry for standard methods so that more valid cross-organizational comparisons can be made.

In today's health care environment, it is key to success that the work and the worker are balanced and in harmony. Employees want input into the design of their jobs, empowerment, feedback, recognition, and the ability to communicate with management on issues that are important to them or may have an effect on their jobs. They want involvement, the opportunity to be accountable, and to be held responsible for the consequences. Workers have not changed much from the late 1890s and early 1900s; they still want to have their social and psychological needs met. There is an ongoing need to be more productive, but while doing so managers need to apply sound management techniques and the behavioral sciences to the work they perform.

REFERENCES

Benchmarking program for food and nutrition services. (1996). *Hospital Food and Nutrition Focus.*

Beyer, P.L., et al. (1991). *Reimbursement and insurance coverage for nutrition services.* Chicago: American Dietetic Association.

Carey, M., & Gillespie, S. (1995). Position of the American Dietetic Association: Cost-effectiveness of medical nutrition therapy. *Journal of the American Dietetic Association, 95,* 88–91.

Coble, M.C. (1975). *A guide to nutrition and food service for nursing homes and homes for the aged* (Rev. ed.). Washington, DC: U.S. Department of Health, Education, and Welfare.

DeHoog, S. (1985). Identifying patients at nutrition risk and determining clinical productivity: Essentials for an effective nutrition care program. *Journal of the American Dietetic Association, 85,* 1620–1622.

Dietetic Staffing Committee. (1982). *Clinical dietetic staffing kit.* Chicago: American Dietetic Association.

Ford, D.A., & Fairchild, M.M. (1990). Managing inpatient clinical nutrition services: A comprehensive program assures accountability for success. *Journal of the American Dietetic Association, 90,* 695–702.

Freund, L.E. (1994, September). *Identifying your strengths and weaknesses with benchmarking.* Presented at the annual meeting of Hospital Foodservice Managers, Palm Beach, Florida.

Gallagher-Allred, C. (1993). *Reimbursement success: Coverage and reimbursement for nutrition services.* Columbus, OH: Ross Laboratories.

Gates Smith, K., Konkle, K.R., & Semen, M. (1991). Charging for hospital-based nutrition services. In M.K. Fox (Ed.), *Reimbursement and insurance coverage for nutrition services* (pp. 35–60). Chicago: American Dietetic Association.

Gift, R.G., & Mosel, D. (1994). *Benchmarking in health care: A collaborative approach.* Chicago: American Hospital Publishing.

Gilbert, J.A. (1990). *Productivity management: A step-by-step guide for health care professionals.* Chicago: American Hospital Publishing.

Grant, A., & DeHoog, S. (1991). *Nutrition assessment and support.* Seattle: Authors.

Halling, J.F., Lafferty, L.L., & Feller, K.S. (Eds.). (1986). *Productivity management for nutrition care systems.* Chicago: American Dietetic Association.

Indicator software supports data submission. (1993, May/June). *Joint Commission Perspectives,* 11.

Joint Commission launches indicator monitoring system in 1994. (1994). *Joint Commission Perspectives,* 14–15.

Joint Commission on Accreditation of Healthcare Organizations. (1990). *The Joint Commission's agenda for change—Stimulating continual improvement in the quality of care.* Oakbrook Terrace, IL: Author.

Joint Commission on Accreditation of Healthcare Organizations. (1995). *1996 Accreditation manual for hospitals.* Oakbrook Terrace, IL: Author.

Juran, J.J. (1992). *Juran on quality by design: The new steps for planning quality into goods and services.* New York: Free Press.

Kolssak, L.A. (1995, October). *Launching a clinical nutrition practice model for the 21st century.* Presented at the annual convention of the American Dietetic Association, Chicago.

Kotschevar, L.H. (1975). *Food service for the extended care facility.* Boston: Cahners Books International.

Kushner, R.F., Ayello, E.A., Beyer, P.L., Skipper, A., Van Way, C.W., Young, E.A., & Balogun, L.B. (1994). National Coordinating Committee clinical indicators of nutrition. *Journal of the American Dietetic Association, 94,* 1168–1177.

Laramee, S.L. (1995). Monitoring productivity of the clinical staff. *Hospital Food and Nutrition Focus, 11,* 4–5, 10.

Lutton, S.E., et al. (1985). Levels of nutrition care for use in clinical decision making. *Journal of the American Dietetic Association, 85,* 849–852.

McManners, M.H., & Barina, S.A. (1984). Productivity in clinical dietetics. *Journal of the American Dietetic Association, 84,* 1035–1041.

Olsen, M.D., & Meyer, M.R. (1987). Current perspectives on productivity in food services and suggestions for the future. *School Food Service Research Review, 11*(2), 87–93.

Organizational Dynamics. (1990). *Quality action teams, health care version: Pocket guide.* Burlington, MA: Author.

Puckett, R.P. (1995). *Dietary manager training for pre-certification.* Gainesville: University of Florida Department of Independent Study by Correspondence.

Puckett, R.P., & Miller, B.B. (1988). *Food service manual for health care institutions.* Chicago: American Hospital Publishing.

Queen, P.M., Caldwell, M., & Balogun, L. (1993). Clinical indicators for oncology, cardiovascular, and surgical patients; report of the ADA Council on Practice Quality Assurance Committee. *Journal of the American Dietetic Association, 93,* 338–344.

Rose, J. (1980). Containing the labor cost of food service. *Hospitals, 54*(6), 94–98.

Rose, J. (1985). Pricing clinical services: Part 1. *Hospital Food and Nutrition Focus, 2,* 1, 5–6.

Sayarath, V.G. (1993). Nutrition screening for malnutrition: Potential economic impact at a community hospital. *Journal of the American Dietetic Association, 93,* 1440–1442.

Sneed, J., & Henderson Kresse, K. (1989). *Understanding food service financial management.* Gaithersburg, MD: Aspen.

Spears, M.C. (1995). *Foodservice organizations: A managerial and systems approach.* Englewood Cliffs, NJ: Prentice-Hall.

State hospital associations participate in "dialogue" on IMS. (1993, July/August). *Joint Commission Perspectives,* 6.

Trimble, J. (1992). Reimbursement enhancement in a New Jersey hospital: Coding for malnutrition in prospective payment systems. *Journal of the American Dietetic Association, 92,* 737–738.

Verderose, J.M., Smith, K.G., and Nagy-Nero, D.L. (1995, October). *Pitching proposals to MCOs.* Presented at the annual meeting of the American Dietetic Association, Chicago.

West, B.B., Wood, L., Harger, V., & Shugart, G. (1977). *Food service in institutions.* New York: Wiley.

Quality Improvement

Rita Jackson

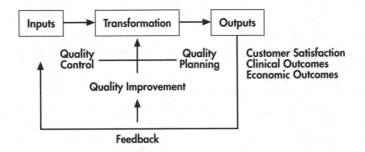

Food service directors and dietitians well remember the days when quality was measured subjectively. Their staff produced hundreds of meals each day and assessed as many patients as possible, and if only a few errors occurred in the course of a week, they and their administrators were well satisfied with the quality offered. If by chance a "Very Important Person" received as much as one soggy piece of toast, however, this became a historic event, and all of a sudden their jobs were on the line. This subjective view was not unique to food and nutrition services. For example, while describing how health care quality was perceived in the past, Wilkins (1995) says, "CEOs and CFOs were confident if they had a saint in their name, or if they were associated with a college or university." With a sigh of relief, many practitioners look back and are joyful that objective measures are now being used for a more balanced perspective of quality.

In the mid-1970s, the health care industry began to be stimulated by the nationwide trend toward quality improvement as a means to satisfy increased demands by consumers and regulatory agencies. A brief historical perspective regarding this trend is presented in Chapter 1 and elsewhere (Jackson, 1992; Joint Commission on Accreditation of Healthcare Organizations [Joint Commission], 1991a, 1992; Ruf, 1989; Shiller, Miller-Kovach, & Miller, 1994). This chapter provides an update on recent trends and important related concepts with special emphasis on methods to simplify the measurement of health care outcomes as quality improvement departments shrink and/or disappear as a result of restructuring and downsizing and because the practitioners who are left in the health care system do not have time to invest in sophisticated quality improvement systems. It also focuses on integrating quality improvement pro-

474

cesses in the operation of the department as well as on continuous learning because these are key to improvement.

QUALITY DEFINED

Juran (1989) provides a short but meaningful definition of quality: fitness for use. It is the extent to which products and services are designed to meet the needs and expectations of customers. In contrast, the 1996 standards of the Joint Commission provide the following operational definition of quality of care:

> The degree to which health services for individuals and populations increase the likelihood of desired health outcomes and are consistent with current professional knowledge. Dimensions of quality include the following: patient perspective issues, safety of the care environment, and accessibility, appropriateness, continuity, efficacy, efficiency, and timeliness of care. (Joint Commission, 1995, p. 270)

For accreditation, the Joint Commission requires a planned, systematic, facilitywide approach to process design and performance measurement, assessment, and improvement. The dimensions of quality that are presented in its definition can be easily incorporated into indicators that are planned to measure the quality of food and nutrition services.

Quality assessment and improvement are also mandated in federal, state, and local regulations, including those for hospitals, nursing homes, intermediate care facilities, homes for the developmentally disabled, and home care. When the Health Care Financing Administration enacted the Omnibus Budget Reconciliation Act of 1987, its regulations incorporated quality of care issues into the federal reimbursement provisions. This was a major advancement because the legislation encouraged quality improvement in the areas of resident's rights, quality of life, and the assessment and care of residents. Standards for the assessment and assurance of quality and for improving the competencies of direct care staff were also included. These regulations further motivated administrators and managers to view quality improvement as more than just another passing fad. The concept has now been applied for a long enough period of time in the industry to have changed people's vocabulary, how they view the quality of patient care, and the way they manage their departments.

Quality versus Quantity

"Folklore has it in America that quality and production are incompatible: that you cannot have both" (Scherkenbach, 1988, p. 18). Scherkenbach was a long-time student of W. Edward Deming who asked him to write a book which described Deming's *Fourteen Points.* He uses the example of a plant manager, who will typically say "it is either production or quality. It is his experience, if he pushes quality, he falls behind in production. If he pushes production, his quality suffers" (p. 18). This misconception is illustrated in Figure 14–1.

Deming's second point is "Adopt the new philosophy. We are in a new economic age, created by Japan. Western management must awaken to the challenge, must learn their responsibilities, and take on leadership for change." Instead of what he calls the "outmoded relationship" between quality and quantity that is illustrated, he says the following:

> Emphasis on improvement of the process however increases uniformity of output, reduces rework and mistakes, reduces waste of manpower, machine time, and materials and thus increases output with less effort and less cost. Other benefits of improved quality are lower costs, better competitive position, and happier people on the job, and more jobs, through better competitive position of the company. (p. 19)

Although it may take a while to convince employees that this is true, managers can implement the techniques suggested for work redesign, work simplification, and reengineering that have been suggested in preceding chapters to demonstrate the fact that it is quite possible to "work smarter, not harder" while improving the quality of food service and nutrition care. Of course, it is probably best to master these methods and exemplify their feasibility by applying them to the work of the manager first.

Several of the definitions for productivity given in Chapter 13 include the concept of quality. It is beneficial to managers if they avoid total preoccupation with efficiency and look at the tools for increasing it as a means to an end, not an end in itself. Lathrop (1993) discusses full-time equivalents and relative value

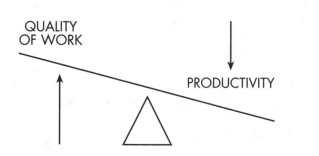

Figure 14–1 Misconception 1: Relationship between quality and productivity of work. *Source:* Reprinted with permission from W.W. Scherkenbach, *The Deming Route to Quality and Productivity: Road Maps and Roadblocks,* © 1988, Mercury Press.

units as benchmarking tools against other facilities but notes "these measures are limiting. In a sense, they measure only ends, not means" (p. 4).

Quality versus Cost

A second misconception regarding quality is that it costs more. Many practitioners have experienced situations that show them that the relationship shown in Figure 14–2 is not necessarily true. There are new kitchens scattered throughout the country that have state-of-the-art equipment, more than adequate numbers of highly credentialed staff members, and highly automated systems. Other, mostly smaller, facilities lack these things, but they often have the more essential characteristic that enables them to provide excellent care: dedicated leaders who use sound and creative management techniques to motivate employees to provide high-quality care to their patients.

THE USE OF QUALITY DATA

When quantitative methods are used to measure quality, it is easier for health care professionals to understand how their departments stand in relation to the goals of the organization. This enables them to develop plans that can be implemented to bring them closer to these goals. They can compare their results over

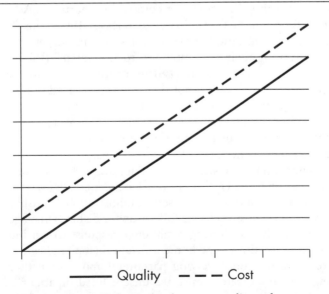

Figure 14–2 Misconception 2: Relationship between quality and cost.

time within the facility (internal benchmarking) or against results from other, similar facilities that use the same systems for measurement (external benchmarking). As described in Chapter 13, both internal and external benchmarking are required by the Joint Commission.

Internal Benchmarking

A baseline is established when an aspect of quality is first measured. Interdisciplinary teams then work to improve the organization's performance by learning about and applying new processes that have more positive outcomes so that the needs and expectations of patients and other customers are met. The system becomes customer driven, in that all major decisions in the organization are based upon results of quality measurement. As a result of this process, health care outcomes spiral upward as they continually improve. This not only pleases customers but establishes the financial security of the organization.

External Benchmarking

Because a health care facility cannot operate in a vacuum, standardized measurement of quality enables cross-organization comparisons to occur. As a part of its agenda for change, the Joint Commission (1990) developed the indicator monitoring system (IMSystem), whereby data from participating sites are transmitted and analyzed centrally for comparative purposes. According to the Joint Commission ("Joint Commission to release" 1994), this information is "intended to support facilities' internal efforts to improve performance and assist in demonstrating their accountability to the public" (Joint Commission, 1993, p. 14). A voluntary program has begun with hospitals first, and although the impact of the IMSystem has not yet been experienced in food service and nutrition departments, this is surely something to learn about in preparation for the time when it will become a part of the mandatory accreditation process.

Once the IMSystem is mandated, several indicators will relate to nutrition care. Currently, under the topic of medication usage, the routine activities of physicians, nurses, pharmacists, and dietitians are included. For example, one indicator focuses on patients with insulin-dependent diabetes who demonstrate self–blood glucose monitoring and self-administration of insulin before discharge or referral for postdischarge follow-up for diabetes management. Other indicators refer to the monitoring of patients' response to specific medications and adverse drug reactions. The home infusion therapy indicators include specific reference to patients receiving parenteral and enteral therapy. Among other things, these indicators measure unscheduled inpatient admissions to acute care, discontinued infusion before prescription completion, interruption of infusion therapy, prevention and surveillance of infection, adverse drug reactions, and client monitoring and intervention. Of special interest to dietitians is the indicator that measures home care clients receiving total parenteral nutrition or enteral therapy who have an identified weight goal and are achieving or maintaining a desired weight.

Public Accountability

Many states in the United States are now disclosing quality data to the public through a system of report cards, which grade hospitals with respect to specific, predefined indicators of quality such as average length of stay, average total charges, and mortality rates for the various medical services. Data are often adjusted for certain variables, such as the socioeconomic level of patients.

In addition, hospital performance reports are also made available to the general public by the Joint Commission for a fee. This is the first nationwide system for consumer information. According to Dr. Dennis O'Leary, President of the Joint Commission, "Our new policy fully accommodates the public interest, while preserving long-standing fairness and due process for health care organizations" ("Joint Commission to release," 1994, p. 7). By the end of 1996, it is expected that 11,000 accredited organizations will be covered by the Joint Commission's public disclosure policy. In addition to hospitals, nursing homes, home care agencies, mental health facilities, and ambulatory care centers are included in this program. The report that health care consumers receive shows the most recent accreditation scores for individual hospitals and compares them with aggregate results from other accredited hospitals.

When consumers make a general inquiry about hospitals, they receive a packet of information that contains a sample report with instructions for understanding it. They also receive a list of accredited facilities from which to select, along with a description of the Joint Commission and the accreditation process. If consumers decide to order a performance report, they receive information regarding the accreditation date and decision and the overall evaluation score, which is given on a scale from 0 to 100. As shown in Figure 14–3, the report compares scores with other hospital ranges and includes recommendations that were made by the Joint Commission for performance improvement. When reports are purchased, the Joint Commission will provide hospitals with the names and addresses of consumers so that direct correspondence can occur if the hospital so wishes.

INDICATORS OF QUALITY

With increased public attention on quality data, the important questions today are: How do we measure quality, and what do we measure? Indicators are used to assess quality. According to the Joint Commission (1995), indicators are

HOSPITAL PERFORMANCE REPORT

GENERAL HOSPITAL
1234 Main Street
Anywhere, IL 98765

Overall Accreditation Information

Accreditation Date: March 1, 19xx
Accreditation Decision: Accreditation with recommendations for improvement
Overall Evaluation Score: 80
Percent of Other Hospitals Surveyed That Received an Overall Evaluation Score Between
90–100   43%
80–89   51%
70–79   6%
60–69   0%
59 or lower   0%

	Performance Area Score	Percent of Other Hospitals Surveyed That Received a Score Between				
		90–100	80–89	70–79	60–69	59 or lower
AREAS EVALUATED						
Patient Care Functions						
Assessment of Patients	73	77	16	6	0	0
Medication Use	65	73	19	8	1	0
Patient Rights	75	21	—	13	—	66
Organizational Leadership and Management						
Organizational Leadership	88	36	24	21	9	10
Governing Body	100	48	—	22	—	30
Improving Organization Performance	75	74	15	6	4	1

Figure 14–3 Sample excerpt from the Joint Commission's hospital performance report. *Source:* © Joint Commission Perspectives. Oakbrook Terrace, IL: Joint Commission on Accreditation of Healthcare Organizations, 1994, p. 1. Reprinted with permission.

"the tools used to measure, over time, the performance of functions, processes, and outcomes of an organization" (p. 713).

Types of Indicators

Indicators are based on structure, process, or outcome. A structural standard is a statement that defines the organization's structural capacity to provide quality care, and it pertains to characteristics of the resources of health care providers, such as numbers and qualifications of staff (Joint Commission, 1991b). Although structure-based indicators are important, adequate staffing, plenty of space and equipment, and well-written procedures do not necessarily result in quality. A well-equipped site will not satisfy customers if procedures are not followed or resources are mismanaged. Therefore, measurements of the organization's structure are not always representative of the quality of patient care. Nevertheless, there are times when structure-based indicators may apply.

A process standard defines the organization's functional capacity to provide quality care (Joint Commission, 1991b), and it pertains to what is done directly or indirectly for patients, such as assessment and treatment planning. If staff members follow procedures, perhaps they can improve quality. The shortcoming of this approach is that it is predicated, of course, on the assumption that policies and procedures actually correlate with high-quality care.

Outcomes are the results of performance. They answer the question: Have the needs and expectations of patients really been met? Patients come to hospitals to regain their health. They also want to be treated cordially, and some wish to leave with the ability to prevent recurrence of their problems. The reason why the report cards disclosed in some states include length of stay and health care charges is that patients want all these things at a reasonable cost. Unlike the global indicators of quality used for report cards, the indicators used to measure quality of food service and nutrition care are not yet standardized. At the present time, it is left up to each individual institution to develop its own indicators of quality.

The examples in Exhibit 14–1 reflect how structure-, process-, and outcome-based indicators can be written to evaluate treatment of malnourished patients. The outcome approach is clearly most appropriate. Not only is it more patient

---

Exhibit 14–1 Examples of Three Different Indicators To Evaluate the Treatment of Malnourished Patients

---

Structure Indicator: Competency of professionals and evidence of policies and procedures that include screening, assessment, care planning, and nutrition education.

Process Indicator: Medical records containing documentation showing that protocols for screening, assessment, treatment, and education are followed by the health care team.

Outcome Indicator: Patients discharged with improved weight and/or prealbumin levels.

Outcome Indicator: Readmitted patients classified with moderate or high nutritional risk who exhibit one or more of the same problems noted during former hospital admissions.

focused, but fewer things have to be measured. This is not to say that all structure and process measurements should be abandoned; they can be used in cases where the direct evaluation of outcomes is not possible and when follow-up evaluation is needed to identify reasons why outcomes are poor.

Some practitioners use volume indicators to identify the number of patients or customers that are served, or to quantify other activities. Although this type of measurement may reflect availability of care, it does not necessarily reflect quality.

Selecting Indicators

To measure performance, the Joint Commission (1995) standards require that the following data on a hospital be collected (often simultaneously):

- processes and outcomes
- a comprehensive set of performance measures
- high-risk, high-volume, and problem-prone processes
- other sensors of performance
  1. patients' needs, expectations, and satisfaction
  2. results of infection control activities
  3. safety of the care environment
  4. utilization management and risk management findings

The Joint Commission recommends starting with the important health care functions as identified in its accreditation manual, such as patients' rights, assessment of patients, care of patients, patient education, and continuity of care. One can measure either the rates of compliance (i.e., the percentage of cases found to be desirable or acceptable) or sentinel events (which are more serious occurrences that require intensive assessment if only a single incident is found). For example, the process and outcome indicators shown in Exhibit 14–1 are rate based. An example of a sentinel event could be patients with undetected malnutrition, or an outbreak of foodborne illness, which would trigger immediate action on the part of the health care team if only one incident was found.

Progress toward Standard Indicators for Nutrition Care

Starting in 1989, the American Dietetic Association (ADA) has worked with the Joint Commission to identify indicators that can be used to monitor the success of patient nutrition care. Its first effort included specific indicators for oncology, surgery, and cardiovascular care that were carefully reviewed and tested in the field before recommendations were made to the Joint Commission. These indicators were sent to the Joint Commission for consideration in its standards (Queen, Caldwell, & Balogun, 1993). Field tests were completed and percentage compliance was reported for the hospitals involved in these tests.

One important outcome of testing was that data regarding patient weights were not commonly available in medical records, and the ADA presented this as a multidisciplinary issue to the Joint Commission. Since that time, the five additional clinical indicators shown in Exhibit 14–2 were developed by the National Coordinating Committee, which comprises the ADA and 10 other organizations representing dietitians, pharmacists, nurses, and physicians. These indicators have been released to the clinical nutrition community and hospital administrators for use as quality assessment tools (Hummell, Bloch, MacInnis, & Winkler, 1994). They have not yet been field tested, and their use and location in the standards have not yet been established.

MEASURING, ASSESSING, AND IMPROVING OUTCOMES

There are many systems available for monitoring and evaluating outcomes. They are thoroughly outlined in the literature and include the Deming cycle (plan-act-check-do) and the Joint Commission's 10-step model, among others (Jackson, 1992; Joint Commission, 1991a, 1992; Ruf, 1989; Shiller et al., 1994). Current Joint Commission standards show five stages for improving organizational performance: plan, design, measure, assess, and improve.

Juran's Trilogy®

Juran's Trilogy® is a simple scheme that was initially developed for manufacturing processes. It involves three stages: quality planning, quality control, and quality improvement (see Figure 14–4).

Quality Planning

According to Juran (1989), quality planning involves the following steps:

1. Determining who the customers are.
2. Determining what their needs are.
3. Developing product features that respond to customers' needs.
4. Developing processes that are able to produce the product features.
5. Transferring the plans to operating forces.

Exhibit 14–2 Recommended Clinical Indicators by the National Coordinating Committee

---

1. Assessment upon Admission
A nutrition screening and assessment are included in the medical record at least for patients with diabetes, gastrointestinal cancer, and trauma (comparative rate indicator).
Some related ICD-9-CM codes:

150–150.9	868.0	901.89
151–151.9	900.82	901.9
153–153.9	900.89	959.1
154.0	900.9	
250–250.8	901.82	

2. Reassessment after Admission
Patients with hospital stays longer than 5 to 7 days who are on NPO or clear liquid diet order and do not have nutrition support will be identified (comparative rate indicator).

3. Implementing and Monitoring Therapy
A nutrition assessment is included in the medical record of patients hospitalized for more than 7 days who at admission have an albumin level less than 3.0 g/dL, weight loss greater than 10% over the previous 3 months, or pressure (decubitus) ulcer(s) (comparative rate indicator).
Some related ICD-9-CM codes:

260	262	263.1
261	263.0	261.9
		707.0

4. Complications of Nutrition Therapy
Patients receiving specialized nutrition support are monitored for metabolic, mechanical, or infectious complications (sentinel event).
Some related ICD-9-CM codes:

275.3	790.6
507	998.2

5. Discharge Planning
A specific discharge plan is developed with and communicated to patients with myocardial infarction, renal disease, or neurologic disorders or those on specialized home nutrition support and their families (comparative rate indicator).
Some related ICD-9-CM codes:

298.2	437.9	593.9
342.9	582.0–582.4	787.2
410.0–410.9	584.5	791
434.9	585	

Source: Reprinted with permission from R.F. Kushner, et al., National Coordinating Committee Clinical Indicators of Nutrition Care, *Journal of the American Dietetic Association*, 94, pp. 1168–1177, © 1994.

The customers of the health care industry include individual patients or groups of patients, who put their purchasing decisions in the hands of others, and internal customers, who use the products and services that are provided by food service and nutrition departments (see Chapter 1 for an explanation of the vital few, useful many, internal, and external consumers).

After identifying the customers, one must learn about their needs and expectations. Juran (1989) suggests that the customer be asked questions such as:

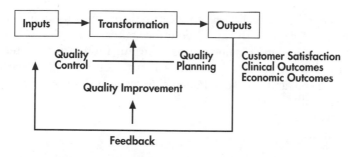

Figure 14-4 Model for quality improvement.

What benefit are you hoping to get from this product? He also suggests trying to distinguish between real and perceived needs. To learn about customers' needs, several methods can be used: One can be a customer, communicate with customers using market research studies, or simulate customers' use. Information will of course be collected in the language of the customer. Therefore, after data are collected, it should be translated into the producer's or "our" language, so that the technological characteristics of the goods or precise protocols for the services can be standardized. The company then adapts its production system to conform with established customer needs and expectations.

The major advantage of this customer-centered approach is that it assists practitioners in setting departmental priorities and organizing their work. It clearly puts everyone on the same track. There are no hidden agendas. Quality is clearly defined, and it is commonly accepted as important by administrators, managers, and employees alike. This represents a better approach than the methods used in the past.

One caution regarding the determination of customers' needs: Market surveys need to be updated routinely. In the words of Juran (1989), customers' needs are a moving *target*. They are not static. They constantly shift with technological, social, economic, and other market trends. As a result, quality improvement is not a closed system. It receives routine input from many other systems inside and outside the health care institution, and the many different types of customers of the health care system need to be considered (patients, family members, employees, and others).

Developing product features that respond to customers' needs and developing processes that are able to produce the product features may sound like tasks that apply only to the manufacturing setting, but in reality they have direct application to health care. Product features and the standards of quality are used to accurately describe the products and services that are offered. For food products, specific standards of quality are described in Chapters 8 and 10. Customers' perceptions of quality can be measured routinely using interviews and questionnaires. Chapters 10 and 12 describe standards for the service of food that can be measured in the same manner. For nutrition care, Chapters 4 and 5 describe the use of practice guidelines for determining how patients are screened, assessed, and educated. Patients' perceptions of these services can be measured as well.

Quality Control

Plans for products and services are reflected in the policies, procedures, standards, and methods that are used to manage the work of employees. As workers engage in producing products and services, the quality control mechanism continuously checks to identify errors and correct them. According to Juran's (1989) model, quality control entails the following steps:

1. Evaluate actual product performance.
2. Compare actual performance with performance goals.
3. Act on the difference.

As applied to food service, these are the routine activities that are normally performed by supervisors, such as checks of trays, temperatures, food quality, meal delivery times, sanitary conditions, and the like. Production activities are measured against the predefined standards that were set during the planning phase, and corrective measures are taken when errors are found.

Quality Improvement

Juran (1989) defines quality improvement as "the organized creation of beneficial change; the attainment of unprecedented levels of performance" (p. 21). It involves the following steps:

1. Establish the infrastructure.
2. Identify improvement projects.
3. Establish project teams.
4. Provide resources, such as training and motivation, so that teams can diagnose causes, stimulate remedies, and establish new controls to hold the gains.

A synonym for *quality improvement*, according to Juran (1989), is *breakthrough*. This is different from what he calls firefighting, which involves the quality control mechanisms described above. Firefighting is important, but it only acts to restore performance to the previous level.

The control chart in Figure 14–5 illustrates the relationship among quality planning, quality control, and quality improvement. It applies to production errors, or the rate of unacceptable meals produced in a food service department. When a major deviation occurs, quality improvement teams act to provide solutions, resources, training, motivation, and new controls that can establish a new norm that has a higher level of quality. The cycle then repeats itself as the quality planning function redesigns the product and/or processes so that the new level of quality can be achieved and maintained.

Measurement of Health Care Outcomes

Wilkins (1995) identifies three outcomes of the health care system: patient satisfaction, clinical outcomes, and economic outcomes. These are issues upon which consumers base their decisions, whether they be individual patients or groups of patients, who put their purchasing decisions in the hands of others. Despite popular belief, health care professionals do not always know what their patients expect, and this is why patient satisfaction is listed separately. Wilkins (1995) states that people make decisions based upon satisfaction and economics but usually do not have the "know-how" to evaluate all clinical outcomes. Providers of care and case managers employed by third party payers normally have this expertise.

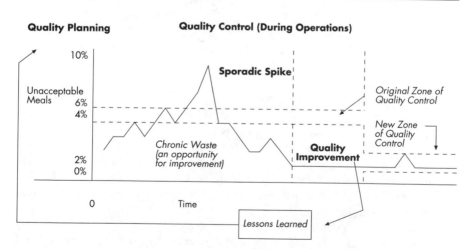

Figure 14–5 Control chart showing Juran's Trilogy®. *Source:* Adapted with permission from J.M. Juran, *Leadership for Quality: An Executive Handbook,* Copyright © 1989, The Juran Trilogy.

After a review of 75 reports in the medical literature, Gill and Feinstein (1994) concluded "Because quality of life is a uniquely personal perception, denoting the way that individual patients feel about their health status and/or nonmedical aspects of their lives, most measurements of quality of life in the medical literature seem to aim at the wrong target" (p. 624). They further stated "Unless greater emphasis is placed on the distinctive sentiments of patients, quality of life may continue to be measured with a psychometric statistical elegance that is accompanied by unsatisfactory face validity" (p. 624).

Professionals in all aspects of health care are redefining the term *quality*. In the nursing literature, Giordano (1994) described a poll of 139,830 surgical patients and concluded "Viewing patients as customers requires a significant shift in thinking that doesn't come easy for many health care professionals. When patients become customers, the traditional relationship between the 'dependent patient' and the 'all-knowing professional' takes on a customer/supplier nature" (p. 79).

Patient Satisfaction

Data regarding satisfaction can be obtained through interviews or written surveys. Structured interviews are most appropriate for patients who may have difficulty communicating in writing. Questionnaires can be administered while patients are receiving treatment or after discharge (see Figure 14–6). One advantage of questionnaires administered while patients are in the facility is that, if problems are identified, they can be corrected immediately, and the patient leaves the facility satisfied. Another advantage is that the department can design a questionnaire that best suits the situation at hand. An advantage of postdischarge questionnaires is that they are usually mailed out and tabulated by another department in the facility, which of course saves time in the department. Sample sizes are usually larger as well.

With less time at their disposal, directors of food and nutrition services might benefit by looking at a two-tiered approach to collecting data on patient satisfaction. If routine postdischarge monitoring is done centrally in the facility, detailed satisfaction surveys can be administered only when negative trends are detected or thresholds are crossed. This method, of course, assumes that a correlation can be established between the two methods (Jackson, 1995a). While one is considering such a method, it will be important to include measures of satisfaction for both clinical care and food services.

For validity and reliability of data and results, appropriate methods and sample sizes must be used. The Joint Commission does not stipulate standards for sample size. Becker (1991) reported that an acceptable sample size could be all patients, 5% of the cases, or 20 cases, whichever is larger. As the industry

Our goal in food and nutrition services is to provide quality meals that are within your diet order and quality nutrition services, including assessment and diet counseling. Please rate how we are doing. A person from food and nutrition services will visit you today and pick up this form.

Please circle the number for your evaluation of each statement:

	Very Poor	Poor	Fair	Good	Very Good
The likelihood of getting the food you checked off on the menu is	1	2	3	4	5
The quality of the food is	1	2	3	4	5
The taste of your food is	1	2	3	4	5
The variety of foods you are offered is	1	2	3	4	5
The amount of food you are served is	1	2	3	4	5
The temperature of the food (cold foods cold, hot foods hot) is	1	2	3	4	5
The time that your meals are delivered is	1	2	3	4	5
The courtesy of the person delivering your tray is	1	2	3	4	5
The attention given you by Food & Nutrition Services is	1	2	3	4	5
The explanations you receive about your diet, if you are on a special diet, are	1	2	3	4	5
Your overall satisfaction with your food is	1	2	3	4	5

What type of diet are you receiving? _____

Please indicate the person filling out this form:
❏ patient ❏ family member ❏ other _____
(fill in)

During this admission, how many patient meals have you been served:
❏ 0 ❏ 1–4 ❏ 5–10 ❏ 11+

Additional comments:

Figure 14–6 Sample patient satisfaction questionnaire. Courtesy of the Department of Food and Nutrition Services, Rush-Presbyterian, St. Luke's Medical Center, Chicago, Illinois.

becomes more sophisticated in its measurement techniques, it is expected that statistical significance will become increasingly important (Jackson, 1992; Shiller et al., 1994).

Figure 14–7 shows a patient questionnaire with questions that can be related to the components of quality suggested by the Joint Commission (Jackson, 1995a). The first two questions relate to efficacy, and the second two relate to appropriateness of care. Availability of care is reflected in questions 5 and 6, timeliness is reflected in 7 and 8, continuity in 11 and 12, food safety in 13 and 14, and respect and caring in 15 and 16.

Clinical Outcomes

Clinical pathways are an excellent vehicle for the measurement and evaluation of clinical outcomes. Chapter 4 and other references describe and illustrate the use of these pathways (Jackson, 1992, 1995b; Joint Commission, 1991a, 1992; Ruf, 1989; Shiller et al., 1994).

Outcomes assessment is easy to perform in the long-term care setting, where factors such as albumin, weight, and glucose levels can be monitored over time. For the acute care setting, postdischarge data may have to be collected. This can be done via clinical records or by making follow-up telephone calls to former patients. With increased use of integrated health care systems and computerized medical records, ongoing data collection and follow-up are very possible. Exhibit 14–3 describes a vision of a future in which the monitoring of patient care quality will be much easier than it is today. To assist dietitians in identifying and measuring clinical, functional, and behavioral outcomes, The American Dietetic Association also publishes a guide which helps practitioners set protocols for specific disease states (Medical Nutrition Therapy, 1996).

The following example emphasizes the underlying principles that apply to the development of clinical indicators. This indicator includes an evaluation of clinical outcomes as well as patient involvement in the design of the nutrition care plan for obese patients with uncontrolled diabetes mellitus. It is a rate-based, outcome-oriented indicator that includes components of patient care continuity, effectiveness, appropriateness, and patient satisfaction, each of which can be objectively measured:

> Patients discharged with controlled glucose and decreased weight who were able to prevent readmission for the same problems after receiving satisfactory nutrition therapy, education, and long-term support that were tailored to meet their expressed needs.

While revising the quality improvement program, one can alter performance indicators to reflect patients' perceived needs and have a more outcome-oriented focus. For example, at Olin E. Teague Veteran's Center in Temple,

What Do You Think About Our Food and Nutrition Services?

In an effort to provide you with appetizing and nourishing meals and further improve our nutrition services, we ask you to take a few moments to fill out this questionnaire. It will be collected from you today. If you have any questions regarding your diet, please ask to see a dietitian or call extension 624. Our staff is anxious to serve you in the best possible manner during your hospital stay.

Thank you.

Name _____

Room _____

Diet _____

Level _____

Days Since Admission _____

				How can we improve?
1. The foods I received meet my personal needs and expectations	❏ Always	❏ Usually	❏ Sometimes ❏ Never	_____
2. If I required a dietitian's help to improve food intake or to tailor the diet to meet my therapeutic needs, this was done	❏ Very Well	❏ Well	❏ Fairly Well ❏ Poorly	_____
3. On the menu I select from, I find the variety of foods to be	❏ Very Good	❏ Good	❏ Fair	❏ Poor _____
4. The portion sizes for foods on my tray are adequate	❏ Always	❏ Usually	❏ Sometimes ❏ Never	_____
5. I receive exactly what I order on my trays	❏ Always	❏ Usually	❏ Sometimes ❏ Never	_____
6. Someone is available to answer any dietary questions I have	❏ Always	❏ Usually	❏ Sometimes ❏ Never	_____
7. Meals are served at times when I feel the most like eating	❏ Always	❏ Usually	❏ Sometimes ❏ Never	_____
8. I have been able to receive between meal snacks when I want	❏ Always	❏ Usually	❏ Sometimes ❏ Never	_____
9. The appearance of trays and serviceware is neat and attractive	❏ Always	❏ Usually	❏ Sometimes ❏ Never	_____
10. I find the taste of the foods to be	❏ Very Good	❏ Good	❏ Fair	❏ Poor _____
11. If I require assistance with meals, it is provided when needed	❏ Always	❏ Usually	❏ Sometimes ❏ Never	_____
12. If ever I have a food-related problem, someone quickly responds	❏ Always	❏ Usually	❏ Sometimes ❏ Never	_____
13. Hot foods such as soups, entrees, and coffee are hot enough	❏ Always	❏ Usually	❏ Sometimes ❏ Never	_____
14. Cold foods such as juice, milk and desserts are cold enough	❏ Always	❏ Usually	❏ Sometimes ❏ Never	_____
15. The attitude of the personnel serving my tray has been	❏ Very Good	❏ Good	❏ Fair	❏ Poor _____
16. Someone visited me routinely to see how well I liked my diet	❏ Daily	❏ Most Days ❏ Some Days ❏ Never	_____
17. My overall opinion of quality of Food & Nutrition Service is	❏ Very Good	❏ Good	❏ Fair	❏ Poor _____

We would appreciate any further suggestions as to how we can better serve you. Please write additional comments below. You may also list foods you would like to see on our menu or employees from Food & Nutrition Services that have been most memorable.

_____

_____

_____

Figure 14–7 Sample patient satisfaction questionnaire reflecting the Joint Commission's components of care. *Source:* Reprinted from Benchmarking Program for Food and Nutrition Services, *Hospital Food & Nutrition Focus,* © 1996, Aspen Publishers, Inc.

Exhibit 14–3 The Computerized Medical Record of the Future

Christina Biesemeier is the Clinical Nutrition Manager at St. Luke's Hospital in Kansas City, Missouri, where she sits on various committees that define computer requirements for the hospital and its health care documentation system. "It has been estimated," says Biesemeier, "that dietitians dedicate approximately 32% of their time to documentation." Dietitians document in the medical record and frequently write in the nursing Kardex, nutrition Kardex or binder, separate nutrition files, and one or more computer programs. Even within the medical records, several locations often require documentation such as progress notes, flow sheets, clinical pathways, calorie counts, care plans, and discharge planning records.

Biesemeier has an exciting vision of the future for clinical dietitians. A big part of this picture involves the computerized medical record. Many, if not all, of the following conveniences will be available to professionals, so that they will be able to spend more time in direct patient care activities. Here are her thoughts:

There will be "point of care" access to medical information and documentation. That "point of care" may be in a variety of places from the hospital bedside to the home. Nutrition data elements will be in the patient minimum data base sets, just as they are now for nursing professionals. We will have subsets of desired data as Gates (1992) suggested for specific patient populations. Prior to caring for patients, we will have all the information we need and be able to scan the record for an overview while having the ability to focus more closely on the areas where we need more information.

At our disposal will be the ability to link to patients' family records as well as to other nutrition care providers along the continuum of care such as WIC or other community-based programs. This will give us access to patient history data, past nutrition related encounters, and education processes.

Nutrition screening will occur at predefined intervals so we will not have to determine each time it will happen. This will occur when people are in the hospital, when they are outpatients, at home, or elsewhere. We will set the intervals to make sure it occurs and the data will be evaluated based upon the standards that we set. Our "at risk" patients will be identified for us and we will be notified with beepers or through a "risk list" given to us when we log on each day. Automatic interventions can occur until we can get to each patient, and this is OK because we will have expanded our scope of practice to initiating those interventions and to authorizing them.

Our nutrition assessment data will be readily available. We will identify what we want as baseline data from the computerized medical record. Our calculations will be completed for us and results will be automatically compared to the norms. When there are problems identified, we will be alerted. For reference, we will have the standards of practice available on screen. Initiation of care protocols will occur for high risk therapy via explosion orders. User friendly order screens and accuracy checks on orders will occur for individualization based on parameters such as age, size, and sex. Interactions will be noted and we will be alerted to them.

Linkages will be available to our computerized equipment so that if there are pumps used to infuse TPN or enteral nutrition formulas we will be able to see the data. Other similar data, such as glucose monitoring results, will automatically be downloaded into the medical record for immediate use by the system for screening and our consideration. Reassessment will occur at times that we define, and data will be gathered for us.

We shall be able to format information for specific users in order to have a more simplified format for our staff. And, we will be able to automatically contact physicians with our recommendations and quickly learn if they have been implemented. Data such as weights, blood levels, protein and calorie intakes will be trended for us. Our diet manuals, tutorials, and

continues

Exhibit 14–3 continued

patient education information will be on line; and we will have the ability to print them in any language.

Discharge planning reminders will signal us to make plans that will automatically go to the next provider of care. In the acute care settings, there will be immediate access to information needed for follow-up so we will know if our plans worked or not. This feedback will enable us to improve our practice. If there is a need to see someone for outpatient follow-ups, an automatic linkage with the scheduling system will be available as a part of the medical record system.

Dietitians will be able to do superior outcomes research because they will have the availability of a nutrition data base and data analysis which will incorporate a common data dictionary. All of the tools we need will be there, right at our fingertips.

Source: Reprinted from R. Jackson, Computerized Medical Records: A Look at the Future, *Hospital Food & Nutrition Focus*, Vol. 12, No. 8, pp. 6–7, © 1996, Aspen Publishers, Inc.

Texas, routine 100% compliance was found with an indicator that measures the process of providing patient education for food–drug interactions (D. Bashara, personal communication, 1995). This indicator is now being revised to determine whether patients really learn and practice the precautions that are taught in the hospital. The revised indicator will focus on newly admitted patients with specific food–drug interactions, starting with insulin, oral diabetic agents, monoamine oxidase inhibitors, and coumadin. Records from previous hospital stays will be checked. If it is found that previous food–drug instruction was given, its effectiveness will be judged after cases with unrelated variables are excluded. Factors such as patient response to education and date of previous instruction will help establish effectiveness curves, and results should help improve retention and application of information that patients receive.

Economic Outcomes

Economic outcomes can be measured by collecting data on the costs of care. This is typically done by focusing on specific disease states to discover the processes that contain costs. Dietitians have been involved in cost justifying their services for quite some time now. For example, in 1995 the ADA issued documentation of per case savings for selected diseases and conditions for which medical nutrition therapy is appropriate. Data were derived from a study of 2,392 cases, and the results were as follows:

- cancer $10,535
- heart disease   9,134
- type I diabetes   9,049

- type II diabetes   1,994
- gestational diabetes   10,088
- kidney disease   18,467
- tube and intravenous feeding 7,051
- high cholesterol   2,709
- hypertension   4,075

Further examples of studies that can be conducted at various facilities are provided in Chapters 4 and 13.

Model for Assessing Quality Data

Many directors and dietitians today have more quality data than they know what to do with. The Joint Commission (1995) requires a systematic process to assess collected data to determine whether performance improvement is needed. Intensive assessment and corrective action need to be initiated under certain circumstances when undesirable variation in performance occurs, but not for all types of results. The circumstances that must trigger intensive assessment for nutrition care functions are:

- sentinel events, including significant adverse drug reactions
- patterns or trends
- significant undesirable variation from the performance of other organizations
- significant undesirable variation from recognized standards

For sentinel events, one incident should trigger intensive assessment. For other indicators (rate based), intensive assessment should occur when threshold levels are crossed. If threshold levels are not crossed but negative patterns or trends are seen, intensive assessment should occur to halt possible destructive tendencies.

Figure 14–8 shows a model that may help one visualize the actions one can take while assessing quality data and deciding whether corrective action is indicated. In this model, it is assumed that recognized professional standards are used as minimal criteria for monitoring purposes and that the selected threshold levels are aligned with the performance of other organizations. Most practitioners do this anyway because it makes it easier to justify programs and analyze results. It is also important to realize that information for sources other than the quality improvement system can be meaningful enough to trigger intensive assessment and corrective action.

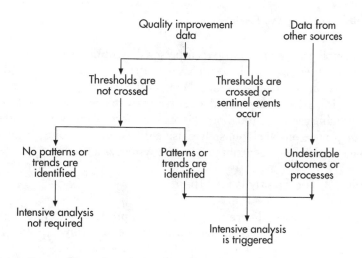

Figure 14–8 Determining the need for intensive assessment of quality improvement data. *Source:* Reprinted from R. Jackson, Model for Assessing Quality Data, *Hospital Food & Nutrition Focus*, Vol. 11, No. 9, p. 8, © 1995, Aspen Publishers, Inc.

THE LEARNING ORGANIZATION

Senge (1990) states that learning disabilities "are tragic in children, especially when they go undetected. They are no less tragic in organizations where they also go largely undetected. . . . Because of them, few corporations live even half as long as a person—most die before they reach the age of forty" (p. 18). There is no doubt that there has been a recent increase in corporate mortality in the health care field. Can some of this be attributed to learning disabilities?

Because training is key to quality improvement, leaders are responsible for looking at training for change as one of the most effective tools they have to demonstrate success. The importance of training is obvious: It often makes the difference between a department that remains stagnant over the years and one that continues to improve. This leads to the question: Just how effective are the department's training efforts?

Senge (1990) describes seven conditions that inhibit the ability to be a learning organization. He states that it is no accident that organizations learn poorly. The way they are designed, the way they are managed, the way jobs are defined, and the way people are taught to think tend to create fundamental learning disabilities. The first step in correcting this problem is to recognize and understand the types of corporate learning disabilities that exist in the work environment.

Condition 1: I Am My Position

Loyal employees often confuse their personal identities with their jobs. When this happens, there is too much emphasis on the assigned tasks at hand and too little on how one's job fits into the scheme of the whole system and its goals for patient service. Staff members tend to relate poorly to one another, and they establish little "monarchies" throughout the organization. Blaming frequently occurs, and some professionals seldom stray outside the boundaries of their job description to make significant contributions to the system as a whole.

Condition 2: The Enemy Is Out There

Senge (1990) states "There is in each of us a propensity to find someone or something outside ourselves to blame when things go wrong" (p. 19). This gets in the way of learning and growth of the organization. Turfism, which is described in Chapter 1, is often related to this problem. Interdisciplinary training techniques can work to correct this problem. Also, because employees often emulate the attitudes of their superiors, leaders should be cautious about the example they provide.

This syndrome can be corrected as soon as staff members realize that all disciplines are a part of the patient care team and share the same goals. Meetings involving persons from other disciplines can be held; most of all, the attitudes that are exhibited by administrative and managerial personnel can act as good examples of a positive interdisciplinary approach. To get a group out of the defensive mode, a trainer can admit that causes for problems may stem from others outside the department and that these are also being addressed but, for the current time, the department is focusing on what its employees can do personally to help improve patient satisfaction.

Condition 3: The Illusion of Taking Charge

Rather than waiting for situations to get out of hand, managers are often encouraged to be less reactive and more assertive and proactive. Without proper role models and guidance, some of these managers use aggressive behavior instead. They begin to fight "the enemy out there," they end up offending instead of taking charge, and they tend to utilize authoritarian leadership styles. This results in an environment that is not conducive to learning. "All too often proactiveness is reactiveness in disguise. True proactiveness comes from seeing how we contribute to our own problems. It is a product of our way of thinking, not our emotional state" (Senge, 1990, p. 21).

Condition 4: Fixation on Events

Many directors of food and nutrition services are victims of this phenomenon, and/or they practice it themselves. A typical case was presented at the beginning of this chapter, the piece of soggy toast being served to a VIP. If the director followed the boss' example, and approached the production manager with the job threat based on an isolated incident, in turn, the manager might approach the cook in the same manner. Everyone assumes a defensive posture, and a poor climate for learning is established. This preoccupation with events is similar to treating disease symptoms without really understanding their underlying cause. If the event reflects a serious disease that has taken a long time to develop, one needs to recognize this and focus attention in the proper direction. Fixation on events tends to foster an unsystematic evaluation of patient services, which cannot uncover real opportunities for improvement in quality.

Condition 5: The Parable of the Boiled Frog

Because people are programmed to react to sudden events, subtle changes in the environment go unnoticed for long periods of time and become, as a result, most destructive. Senge's (1990) parable is described below.

> If you place a frog in a pot of boiling water, it will immediately try to scramble out. But if you place the frog in room temperature water, and don't scare him, he'll stay put. Now, if the pot sits on a heat source, and if you gradually turn up the temperature, something very interesting happens. As the temperature rises from 70°F to 80°F, the frog will do nothing. In fact, he will show every sign of enjoying himself. As the temperature gradually increases, the frog will become groggier and groggier, until he is unable to climb out of the pot. Though there is nothing restraining him, the frog will sit there and boil. Why? Because the frog's internal apparatus for sensing threats to survival is geared to sudden changes in his environment, not to slow, gradual changes. (p. 22)

This is clearly illustrated when professionals change job settings. It is easy to identify problems when one first enters the new setting; they are obvious to outsiders. The longer one stays, however, the more difficult it is to identify subtle negative trends. This is why the Joint Commission requires that action be taken when negative trends are noticed as well as when quality scores cross threshold levels.

Condition 6: The Illusion of Learning from Experience

According to the ADA ("Position," 1993), academic preparation in dietetics or food and nutrition without management competence is not sufficient for successful direction of health care food and nutrition services. Many people say that experience is the best teacher. Unfortunately, people do not always experience the outcomes of their most important decisions and learn the proper lessons from them, or they do not choose to recognize the negative effects of their actions because pride gets in the way of the ability to learn from past decisions. For example, look at the number of good managers in the food and nutrition field who have convinced their administrators to invest thousands of dollars on high-technology equipment and systems that are meant to control costs. Do all these systems work? Have they actually saved the amount of money that was projected? Not all of them. It is hard for one to admit failure and even to recognize some of the flaws in one's own designs. Unbiased evaluation techniques will enable one to look back objectively and assess the success of one's decisions. Without these techniques in place, it is impossible to learn the truth from past experiences.

Condition 7: The Myth of the Management Team

Senge (1990) notes that groups want to keep up the image of cohesiveness and therefore tend to squelch disagreement among their members. Solutions to problems are merely watered-down compromises that everyone can live with, or they reflect the opinion of the strongest member of the group. Also, team members often tend to put more emphasis on protecting their turf, taking defensive postures, or laying blame on each other rather than working honestly together to resolve a problem. These tactics result in poor decisions and a management team that breaks down easily under pressure. In the words of Argyris (1990), such teams demonstrate skilled incompetence; they are groups of professionally qualified persons who are incredibly proficient at keeping themselves from learning.

Before group learning and growth can occur, members need to admit that they do not have all the answers and take an honest, humble approach to problem solving. The group succeeds when people listen to each other and build upon one another's ideas. Through collective inquiry, the final solution that evolves is better than what any one team member could have developed on his or her own. This process fosters group commitment and improved learning ability.

CUSTOMER-DRIVEN PROCESSES

Quality data help administrators and department directors to set priorities. As they react to results, changes can be made in the services that are offered and

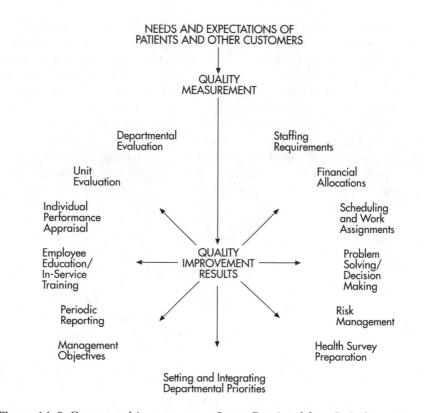

NEEDS AND EXPECTATIONS OF
PATIENTS AND OTHER CUSTOMERS

QUALITY
MEASUREMENT

Departmental
Evaluation

Staffing
Requirements

Unit
Evaluation

Financial
Allocations

Individual
Performance
Appraisal

Scheduling
and Work
Assignments

Employee
Education/
In-Service
Training

QUALITY
IMPROVEMENT
RESULTS

Problem
Solving/
Decision
Making

Periodic
Reporting

Risk
Management

Management
Objectives

Health Survey
Preparation

Setting and Integrating
Departmental Priorities

Figure 14–9 Customer-driven processes. *Source:* Reprinted from R. Jackson, *Continuous Quality Improvement for Nutrition Care,* © 1992, American Nutri-Tech.

the processes that are used in a continuous effort to improve quality scores. When handled correctly, the results of quality assessment can improve the way all activities are performed in the department. Figure 14–9 shows some of the processes that can be altered as a result of quality improvement results.

Performance Appraisal

For departmental evaluation, it is clear that the overall quality of patient care is reflected in the results of the quality improvement program. The departmental director can objectively answer the question: How well are we doing? This can be done in qualitative as well as quantitative terms. For example, instead of saying "the patients seem to accept the meal service because we get few complaints," one can more clearly evaluate this acceptance and say "92% of the patients report the meal services to be acceptable, and major problems appear to be in the areas of hot food temperature (75%) and menu variety (80%)." Such a statement is more valuable in identifying the processes that need improvement and learning the extent to which overall standards for meal acceptability are being met. Instead of saying "the dietitians do a good job in assessing the nutritional status of patients," one can say "85% of the patients in the facility are receiving a nutritional assessment within 72 hours of admission, and 90% of these assessments meet all the criteria for quality nutritional care. The major problems appear for patients admitted on weekends (62%) and in some dietitians' ability to deal with drug–nutrient interactions properly (78%)." This type of statement gives a clear picture of the services provided by the dietitians and identifies specific opportunities for increasing the level of patient care.

An effective quality improvement system has indicators, criteria, and methods that are commonly accepted by the administration, related disciplines, the quality improvement committee, a panel of experts, and departmental personnel. Therefore, arbitrary comments or personal opinions based on isolated incidents are excluded because all agree on the way quality nutritional care is measured and evaluated. As a result, there are no questions about how the department should be evaluated for its overall efforts to provide good care.

If a quality improvement program is designed with accountability in mind, the different units or teams can be evaluated separately as well. In this manner, the success that a unit has in increasing its scores after reacting to solve problems is used for the evaluation of the performance of that unit. By integrating accountability into the program, the director of the department is able to identify specific dietary units that need improvement and support. Without such accountability, it becomes difficult to identify the source of problems and, of course, ways to correct them. Accountability also enables the director to analyze results objectively in terms of the success of each departmental function and to delegate the job of problem solving to the person(s) in charge of each function.

Just as accountability for each dietary unit is built into the quality improvement processes, so can accountability by individuals within each unit. The outcome of reviews can reflect the success of all unit managers when quality evaluation is divided into separate departmental functions. If the clinical nutrition manager is able to improve significantly the quality of nutrition care by increasing scores in nutrition assessment and nutrition education, it can be assumed that this individual is effectively managing the quality provided by his or her unit. Because this person's primary job is to provide high-quality nutrition care within the budget allocated, the foundation for the annual performance appraisal is obtained from two objective sources: quality improvement and cost analysis.

In addition, annual performance appraisals normally require input regarding the employee's major accomplishments during the past year, and quality improvement results provide qualitative and quantitative data that can be incorporated directly into the employee evaluation. Performance appraisals should encourage improvement for the upcoming year. Again, information is readily available in the documentation from annual trends, plans for corrective action, and detailed reports of specific standards in need of improvement. The data have been collected and analyzed in an objective manner, so that the performance appraisal is free of subjective opinions. An added benefit for the employee is that he or she is familiar with the exact basis for evaluation scores, and there are no surprises at the end of the year because input on the same basic criteria has been received on a continuous basis throughout the year via the quality improvement results. The individual can also clearly see how he or she can improve performance and is able to focus directly and immediately on the scores that are in need of correction. Therefore, the individual has all the information necessary to achieve better appraisals in the future without having to guess at what is expected of him or her.

Individuals or teams can be rewarded for their contributions. Such a plan fosters motivation for all to do a better job in meeting facilitywide standards for quality care, and it rewards the workforce as a whole for good performance. Benefits of this include the placement of subtle peer pressure on marginal workers to do a better job. If any individual employee is rated poorly, caution must be exercised to ensure that poor performance is not due to inadequacies in the system itself. It is estimated that greater than 90% of the problems found in health care today are due to problems in processes and methods themselves, not people or other resources used by the system (O'Leary, 1992). The Joint Commission encourages that the sources of variation in specific processes and outcomes be sought within all contributory organizational processes as well as in the activities of individuals, and it has specific guidelines to handle cases when practitioners' performance is deficient.

All too often, performance appraisals are based upon how friendly or cooperative employees are or on easily observed criteria such as attendance and reporting to work on time. These aspects are important, but they should not predominate. The real issue is whether the employee is fulfilling the job function in contributing quality patient care. When this aspect is ignored for evaluation purposes, the director of the service promotes the situation where many employees receive excellent and good ratings while the overall department still fails to achieve its goals for patient care. Everyone thinks that he or she is doing a good job, but the patients do not receive good care. This type of situation is definitely undesirable, and more objective and accountable means are in order.

Just as the unit managers can be made accountable by using quality improvement results as input for performance appraisals, so can their respective supervisors and subordinates. For example, suppose results show that 85% of the patients receive nutritional assessments within 72 hours of admission and that

90% of the assessments meet all the criteria for quality care. If this quality review had been designed so that each staff dietitian had his or her charts reviewed separately, a score could be generated for each individual so that variation within the group could be determined and addressed. The performance appraisal of the clinical nutrition manager would include the overall average of these scores for his or her group of subordinates, reflecting all charts reviewed over the past year. The individual dietitians' performance appraisals would reflect their own personal contribution compared with the group average or goal. This could help identify individual strengths, weaknesses, and needs for training. This same concept can apply to cafeteria supervisors, catering managers, production managers or supervisors, cooks, tray assembly supervisors, and so on.

Team effort is of the utmost importance, so that the manner in which individuals are evaluated is critical. The person doing performance appraisals needs to emphasize each person's contribution to the team and the overall outcome of the team's effort. Rewards for group success therefore play a significant role. According to Deming, "Merit rating rewards people [who] do well in the system. It does not reward attempts to improve the system" (Walton, 1990, p. 221). This is why concepts such as profit sharing have been found to be most desirable. They instill accountability for employees' contribution toward the team effort and organizational goals.

Employee Training

Because the results of a quality assessment indicate areas that need correction, and one method of correcting employee performance is through training, a framework is available for planning the department's training schedule. Not all corrective action includes the need for training, but quite often criteria for quality patient care are not met because employees do not know or do not follow departmental standards while performing their jobs. To reinforce these standards, training is useful as long as appropriate follow-up is provided to ensure that the poor work habits are discontinued and acceptable ones are implemented on a continuous basis.

Some departments offering dietetic services have creative and effective inservice training programs, whereas others have training schedules that look the same from year to year, with similar topics repeated and others neglected regardless of the department's real needs. Also, perceived problems are frequently addressed rather than actual problems (i.e., those from the patient's point of view). When an effective program is used, the results are easily used to create a meaningful and more successful employee training program. Individuals or groups of employees in the department receive information about the results, and they proceed to learn how they can directly influence patient care by improving their knowledge and work habits. In addition, the department is not overwhelmed with the continual provision of classes in areas where performance is already satisfactory. Training is given in topics that have low or decreasing scores. Priorities for training need to be based on quality in an effort to promote a continuous upward trend in all results. Exhibit 14–4 shows the characteristics of an effective training program.

It may be necessary to train and retrain in a specific topic until favorable results are found. Also, one may even have to *train the trainer* so that he or she is more capable of communicating in an effective way. All too often, employees approach an inservice training class with the same mind set they have when they watch a soap opera on television: They are entertained by the departure from their normal work routine and often go back to work unmotivated and unchanged by the experience. The training program and the trainer need to be accountable; employees should automatically return to work motivated and able to do a better job. Because follow-up is an essential part of training, the topic should be effectively presented, whenever possible, by the person with direct line responsibility for the group of employees trained. Often, when a person from outside the immediate work environment, such as a training dieti-

Exhibit 14–4 Characteristics of an Effective Training Program

- Addresses specific patient needs (those of high priority first) and relates to the results of the quality measurement.
- Translates information into a change in employee work behavior immediately and continuously after the training is given.
- Is followed up by on-the-job observation and correction, if needed, for specific employees.
- Covers all employees in the intended group, not just those who happen to attend the class or be on duty when classes are given.
- Motivates employees to do a better job.
- Improves the competency level of employees.
- Accurately covers needed information in short time intervals for optimal retention.
- Is presented at the level of employees' understanding.
- Provides individualized instruction for those in need rather than repetitive classes for the majority of employees who have already incorporated the principles into their work.
- Includes the immediate supervisor for the group of employees as the trainer, or at least as an active participant.
- Promotes accountability in all persons trained.
- Is scheduled at the most convenient time around employees' tasks to avoid stress on the job and during training.
- Results in high-quality care and is followed by an increase in quality scores for the topic that is presented.

tian or consultant, does the training, this person is not available for follow-up, and a change in work habits does not occur.

To increase the competency level of employees, the Joint Commission encourages training when opportunities to improve patient care are identified through quality improvement evaluations. This training can be done on site or outside the organization. Methods for identifying and increasing the competency level of staff members are presented in the last section of Chapter 4.

Routine Reporting

Most department directors and unit managers are required to submit monthly reports of activities and progress made to administration. It is quite easy to assemble, analyze, and report financial data because the objective formulas for this aspect of the service are understood and commonly accepted by all. It is also easy to present a listing of activities during a specified period of time, and this is frequently included in periodic reports as well. But have the financial resources and activities resulted in high-quality patient care? Has the department met its overall goals and contributed to facilitywide objectives during the period? These are the real questions that need to be answered in such reports, and they are not always addressed. One is not able to document the progress in the level of quality care unless an effective quality improvement program is in place. Also, the output of this program provides clear and indisputable evidence of progress that has been made.

Professionals in dietetic services have little free time on their hands, and they seem to be constantly involved in a multitude of projects and activities. Just how these activities contribute to patient care is of the utmost importance to administration so that justification of departmental costs can be made. Are the department staff spinning their wheels, or do the selected activities really enhance patient care? Continuous quality improvement allows managers and dietitians to chart or graph past and present results in quantitative terms, similar to the way departmental costs are presented. As a result, the reports to administration clearly reveal how the department uses its budgeted allotment to meet institutional objectives.

Management Objectives

Many health care facilities employ techniques of management by objectives. Administrators call for specific departmental objectives each year with timetables for attaining these objectives. The objectives set by individual department heads should conform to facilitywide objectives. Methods for achieving these goals are normally outlined with descriptions of resources to be utilized and measurable outcomes that are expected.

Because the primary goal is to provide high-quality food services and nutrition care, and because most management objectives fall within this realm, quality improvement is a convenient mechanism for identifying objectives that should be included and for determining the present status of the department with regard to each specific management objective selected. High-priority issues revealed through quality improvement efforts should be addressed. The methods used to collect and analyze data for quality improvement can be used to measure progress as the timetable is implemented as well as the outcome of departmental efforts. Without acceptable methods for quantifying results, it is difficult to identify whether the objectives have really been met.

Staffing Requirements

The job of the director of food service and nutrition care is to allocate appropriate resources to each departmental function so that positive outcomes will result. People are the primary resource in the department, and there are times when staffing patterns, tables of organization, job descriptions, and employee competencies are found to be insufficient to meet the goals of the department. Often, problems occur in areas that are not properly staffed or organized. For example, it may be found, from quality results, that too few patients receive timely nutrition screening and assessments. Further investigation into the matter may reveal that dietitians are properly trained and proficient at the care they presently give but that they are too few in number to cover the entire patient population in need of their care. To require increased productivity in staff that are performing sufficiently may decrease the quality of their work. Another action may be warranted, such as the allocation of more personnel resources.

Perhaps another unit in the department is meeting all its objectives with some time to spare, or perhaps its function is not directly related to patient care. If so, justification exists for reallocating personnel or positions to resolve the problem. One might have to change the staffing pattern or redesign jobs to alleviate the problem. After this is done, one should expect quality scores in timeliness of nutrition screening and assessments to increase as a result.

When employees are to be transferred or reassigned, they can be given the opportunity to apply for newly established positions. It is often said that what an employee has done in the past is the best indicator of what he or she will do in the future. Although there is a great deal of merit in this concept, it must be used in combination with other approaches for successful restructuring to occur. Some precautions to take while screening potential candidates are as follows:

- Realize that the new job requirements may be different from the new employees' past experiences and that their motivation and flexibility are important factors to consider.

- The fact that an employee has excelled in one set of tasks in the past does not necessarily mean that he or she will succeed in another set of tasks in the future.

- While screening in-house transfers, be aware of the fact that some department heads have been known to "dump" their poor performers on other departments and keep the most satisfactory employees to themselves. Carefully review annual performance evaluations, disciplinary actions, and all files related to an employee. Confront any issues that are questionable.

- When past achievements are reviewed, remember that careful verification of the facts is always necessary to avoid errors of memory, exaggeration, deliberate falsification, and repression of unpleasant failures.

- Learn the value of networking with colleagues within and outside the facility who are familiar with the actual work of candidates. The labor laws have a tendency to limit the amount of information available from personnel departments, but written or verbal communications that include accurate details about true work performance are often obtainable.

- Describe the new position to those who are familiar with the candidate's work, and solicit information as to whether they think the person will succeed and be happy in the new role.

There are four basic tools used to select the right candidates for new positions in the department: the application form, the reference check, skill testing, and the personal interview. If these activities are undertaken in this sequence, a great deal of time can be saved.

The application form is used to collect the facts. When properly structured, it reveals more than the resume, especially for applicants who are selective about what they choose to report. It also lays the foundation for the other three methods of selection. Reference checks should be completed before time-consuming skill tests and interviews are done. One major reason for this is that information reported by potential candidates must be verified for accuracy first. Unfortunately, some people "stretch the truth" when they fill out application forms and submit resumes. No one wants to invite trouble, so if a problem is discovered during the initial stages of selection, time can be saved by screening out undesirable applicants before more time and energy are invested.

A second reason for doing reference checks at this point is so that the candidate's positive and negative characteristics can be identified. This helps identify the skills that need to be tested and focuses the topic of conversation for the interview. While checking references, one should try to speak personally to past immediate supervisors of all potential candidates. Managers at high levels may not be familiar with the day-to-day activities, achievements, or problems of employees. Workers who are transferring from another department may have had past performance evaluations that are available, but these do not always reflect the true characteristics of employees, and their validity is highly dependent upon the competency of the person who completes them. Not all reference checks will be positive, and it is possible that an applicant will have a negative reference that he or she does not deserve. While reviewing the answers to standardized questions that are asked during personal discussions with past immediate supervisors, one should always be aware of possible personality conflicts and unfair judgments. This is why one must try to see the overall picture. One or two isolated incidents may not be important, but when a common theme of problems is seen it is worthy of consideration.

Skill testing can range from the simple tasks of reading and writing to computer literacy. For dietitians and dietetic technicians, the performance of a nutritional assessment based upon a case study is helpful. Ideas are presented in Exhibit 4–15. For cooks and other food production personnel, Chapter 3 presents standard protocols; one can ask potential candidates about common techniques or even require that they follow a standardized recipe to ascertain their skill level.

Personal interviews enable a manager to observe aspects of an individual that cannot be conveyed on the application form or gathered from reference checks. Interviews should occur after those two procedures because work history and reference checks provide the basis for discussion during an interview. When skillfully conducted, interviews provide important information. They help both the candidate and the interviewer to determine collaboratively whether there is a good match. Any anticipated problems based on data collected before this point should be openly discussed as the two persons try to predict the potential for success on the new job.

Financial Allocations

Just as the allocation of personnel needs to be planned and modified to ensure enhancement in the quality of care given to patients, so do financial allocations. The departmental director normally makes budget requests on an annual basis and needs to have justification for changes in cost center allotments or budgetary increases. Quality improvement results provide this justification as it is related to patient care. The results help reveal those departmental functions and cost centers that are in need of reallocation of funds or increased financing and show how the quality of care can be improved when budgets are approved. Purchases of food, equipment, and supplies therefore can be justified in terms of how the allocation will enhance patient care, and it will be up to the department staff to ensure that there is indeed a positive outcome after the investment is made.

Scheduling and Work Assignments

Directors are responsible for seeing that employees are scheduled on shifts and days that best contribute to optimal patient care and that each employee on duty properly performs a series of preplanned tasks. When productivity statistics are compared, a variance is often seen from facility to facility. Unsatisfactory quality scores can be corrected by analyzing schedules and work assignments, and justification for changes in terms of patient care can be made to administrators and employees alike. Even in unionized departments, management retains the right to schedule and assign employees according to the needs of the facility, and it behooves managers to exercise this right because they are responsible for enhancing the level of patient care.

Problem Solving and Decision Making

The primary goal of quality improvement is to identify problems and opportunities to increase the quality of patient care. During the course of a day's work, managers and dietitians see or hear reports of many problems, and it is sometimes difficult to discern whether they are just isolated incidents or common problems that require in-depth attention. Their perceptions and those received from others may not truly represent the actual situations because subjective opinions often enter into the picture in a subtle way. Quality improvement assists managers and dietitians in identifying problems in an objective manner without leaving problem identification to chance. It also provides a framework for learning the scope of the problem and the extent to which standards are being met in patient care. If one ascertains through quality improvement efforts that 1% of the patient population experiences one problem and 20% experiences another problem, more emphasis can be put on the problem that has a greater scope, assuming that both have the same degree of risk.

Most directors can quickly write a list of all the problems related to their departments and suggest several potential solutions for each. If an effective program is in place, the exact extent of noncompliance is known for each problem, and priorities are easily identified. Decisions can then be made solely on the basis of the severity of problems and within the constraints of available resources. Quality improvement encourages more structure and accountability in problem solving and decision making. Every problem has many solutions, and the task of decision making is logically and objectively to select the one solution that has the most potential to achieve improved results in the future.

Risk Management

The focus of risk management is protecting the financial assets of the facility and its human resources and preventing injury to patients, visitors, and property. Like quality improvement, it is based on increasing the quality of care through ongoing monitoring in an effort to prevent incidents and losses to the facility. Therefore, many activities of risk management overlap those of quality improvement. The major differences between these two programs is that risk managers deal more with legal and insurance activities, in that they review and report on incidents, whereas quality improvement searches for trends or patterns of nonconformance and opportunities for increasing the level of patient care. The Joint Commission requires operational linkages between the risk management functions related to the clinical aspects of patient care and safety and quality assessment and improvement. The director of food and nutrition services may be required to submit responses to the risk management staff regarding specific incidents that occur in the facility. It will also be helpful if the director is informed of high-risk cases before they are investigated by the risk management staff.

Preparation for Health Surveys

The purpose of quality improvement is to monitor and identify the extent to which high standards of care are followed for patient service. This is the same purpose of a health care survey, whether it be performed by local, state, federal, or Joint Commission inspection teams. If managers have a quality improvement plan that reflects the criteria and standards specified in health codes, the areas of noncompliance will surface on a regular basis, and plans for correction of the problems identified are continuously in place. One will know, at any point in time, potential citations for violations that the facility might receive if a survey should occur. Also, the focus is directed less toward last-minute preparation for a health survey and more toward continual improvements to the system so that all criteria for proper care are met at all times.

Incorporation of code regulations in quality reviews surely increases the amount of time and energy required to develop the program for dietetic services, but once this is done the benefits are great. Instead of undertaking last-minute preparation, the departmental staff is always ready for a survey. Patients and staff alike benefit from this change in attitude.

Setting Departmental Priorities

It is easy to fall into the situation where it seems as if one's time and attention are being pulled in 100 different directions. If managers empower employees and delegate their problem-solving tasks, the time of their staff members may be found to be diverted into as many directions. At the end of the day, staff say "We were busy all day, but what did we really accomplish?" Why not set a manageable number of priorities, based on patient care, that provide a foundation for all these functions so that the functions can mesh together? Instead of going in 100 different directions without accomplishing much in terms of quality patient care, why not go in 10 or 15 directions and integrate these priorities with other departmental functions so that resources can be pooled to show definite success as a result of a more concentrated effort? There is also a valid rationale for not being able to devote much time and energy to activities that do not resolve patient-related problems or enhance patient care. Some things may just have to sit on the back burner for a while until more critical issues are resolved. This rationale helps dietitians and managers screen out unimportant activities and concentrate more on the departmental goals and objectives set for high-quality patient care.

Quality improvement does not have to monopolize a practitioner's time. It can help integrate all food service and nutrition activities into one patient-directed function. Once this type of patient-focused system is established, it benefits everyone: managers, employees, patients, other customers, and the institution.

REFERENCES

American Dietetic Association. (1995). *Per case savings for selected diseases/conditions in which medical nutrition therapy is appropriate*. Chicago: Author.

Argyris, C. (1990). *Overcoming organizational defenses: Facilitating organizational learning*. Boston: Allyn & Bacon.

Becker, D.S. (1991, October). *Development of a quality assurance/quality improvement program for your facility*. Presented at the annual meeting of the American Dietetic Association, Dallas, TX.

Gates, G. (1992). Clinical reasoning: An essential component of dietetic practice. *Topics in Clinical Nutrition, 7*, 74–80.

Gill, T.M., & Feinstein, A.R. (1994). A critical appraisal of the quality of quality-of-life measurements. *JAMA, 272*, 619–626.

Giordano, B.P. (1994). Nineties-style nursing: Offering customer service. *Nursing 94, 7*, 79.

Hummell, A.C., Bloch, A.S., MacInnis, P., & Winkler, M.F. (1994). *Clinical indicator workbook for nutrition care systems*. Chicago: American Dietetic Association.

Jackson, R. (1992). *Continuous quality improvement for nutrition care*. Amelia Island, FL: American Nutri-Tech.

Jackson, R. (1995a). Measuring patient satisfaction. *Hospital Food and Nutrition Focus, 11*, 7–8.

Jackson, R. (1995b). The search for outcome indicators. *Hospital Food and Nutrition Focus, 11*, 4–5.

Joint Commission on Accreditation of Healthcare Organizations. (1990). *The Joint Commission's agenda for change—Stimulating continual improvement in the quality of care*. Oakbrook Terrace, IL: Author.

Joint Commission on Accreditation of Healthcare Organizations. (1991a). *An introduction to quality improvement in health care*. Oakbrook Terrace, IL: Author.

Joint Commission on Accreditation of Healthcare Organizations. (1991b). *Primer on indicator development and application: Measuring quality in health care*. Oakbrook Terrace, IL: Author.

Joint Commission on Accreditation of Healthcare Organizations. (1992). *Using quality improvement tools in a health care setting*. Oakbrook Terrace, IL: Author.

Joint Commission on Accreditation of Healthcare Organizations. (1993). *Joint Commission launches indicator monitoring system in 1994*. Oakbrook Terrace, IL: Author.

Joint Commission on Accreditation of Healthcare Organizations. (1995). *1996 Accreditation manual for hospitals*. Oakbrook Terrace, IL: Author.

Joint Commission to release organizational-specific performance information. (1994). *Joint Commission Perspectives, 14*(5), 1, 6–7.

Juran, J.M. (1989). *Juran on leadership for quality: An executive handbook*. New York: Free Press.

Lathrop, J.P. (1993). *Restructuring health care. The patient focused paradigm*. San Francisco: Jossey-Bass.

Medical Nutrition Therapy Across the Continuum of Care. (1996). Chicago: The American Dietetic Association.

O'Leary, D.S. (1992). Agenda for change fosters CQI concepts. *Joint Commission Perspectives, 12*, 1, 6.

Position of the American Dietetic Association: Management of health care food and nutrition services. (1993). *Journal of the American Dietetic Association, 93*, 914–915.

Queen, P.M., Caldwell, M., & Balogun, L. (1993). Clinical indicators for oncology, cardiovascular, and surgical patients: Report of the ADA Council on Practice Quality Assurance Committee. *Journal of the American Dietetic Association, 93*, 338–344.

Ruf, K. (1989). *Quality control, quality assurance manual for food and nutrition services*. Gaithersburg, MD: Aspen.

Scherkenbach, W.W. (1988). *The Deming route to quality and productivity: Road maps and roadblocks*. Rockville, MD: Mercury.

Senge, P.M. (1990). *The fifth discipline, the art and practice of the learning organization*. New York: Doubleday Currency.

Shiller, M.R., Miller-Kovach, K., & Miller, M.A. (1994). *Total quality management for hospital nutrition services*. Gaithersburg, MD: Aspen.

Walton, M. (1990). *Deming management at work*. New York: Putnam's Sons.

Wilkins, R.G. (1995, October). *Outcome assessment: Your role in documenting the value of medical nutrition therapy*. Presented at the annual meeting of the American Dietetic Association, Chicago, IL.

The Changing U.S. Health Care System

C. Nick Wilson

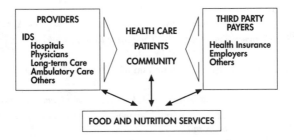

After having read all the chapters in this book about industry trends and how practitioners can succeed in today's challenging health care environment, the reader might well ask: What does all this mean for the future? Where is health care in the United States going in the next century, and what are the dynamic forces that are driving the health care system of this country?

There is so much energy being focused on health care in the United States, but at the same time there appears to be little progress in solving the country's major health care problems. Some doubt whether the *Healthy People 2000* (U.S. Department of Health and Human Services, 1990) objectives will be met. Food and nutrition services seem to be dragged along wherever the health care industry goes with little direction on assimilating into the health care team. Food and nutrition services may have minimal focus on the major trends evolving in America that could affect their services.

This chapter introduces some ideas that may explain these things and reiterates the basic dynamics that are driving the U.S. health care system so that the reader can better understand the central forces that are directing the future of health care in the United States. If the integrated delivery system (IDS) is to be the future, just where does food and nutrition fit in the scheme, and what can professionals do now to prepare to meet future challenges?

RISING HEALTH CARE COSTS

Chapter 1 describes the critical factors and influences that have contributed to the rising cost of health care, which represented 13.9% of the gross domestic product (GDP) in 1993. The major factors include the following:

- rising expectations of the value of health care services
- inflation
- population increases
- increase in the number of elderly, especially those older than 85
- technological advances
- government requirements affecting policies and procedures
- unions
- lack of competitive forces in the health care system to increase efficiency and productivity in the delivery of services

Inflation has had an effect on the cost of goods and services that the health care industry must purchase for daily activities. Population increases, particularly among the elderly (who require more extensive care), and costly technological advances have contributed to rising costs as well. Malpractice and the resulting practice of "defensive" medicine play a major role. Government policies and regulations at all levels are reflected in costs; good examples are Medicare, Medicaid, and worker's compensation insurance. The overspecialization of health care professionals, including physicians and other health care employees, is a contributory factor, as is employer-sponsored health care, which shields employees from the burden of health care costs. American society has supported each of these separate developments. They were not isolated policies, nor were they events that just happened to be forced upon the population. On the other hand, they all were, and continue to be, important social advances that were important at the time. Some continue to affect the growth of health care in general and rising health care costs.

The failures of our society, however, may be traced to a lack of integrated health care that would, on the part of providers to some degree, furnish leadership and control of these individual developments and changes in the health care system. Furthermore, governments need to be a part of the health care equation, if for no other reason than that they provide more than 60% of the funding for the system. Additionally, employers need to be a part of the system because they play an integral part in providing some level of health care benefits to their employees. Tied to the employers is the health care insurance industry, which has married with the employers to force more of the risk of caring for individuals and groups in society onto the providers. Last, individual patients and other customers need to be involved as a more active part of the growing health, wellness, and promotion/prevention paradigm that ebbs and flows toward integration of the health system. Figure 15–1 demonstrates the relationship among these entities.

It is inviting to blame rising health care costs on a particular segment of society, such as physicians, hospitals, or the federal government. Depending on

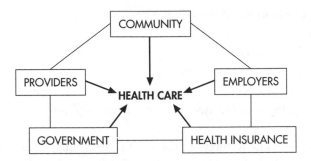

Figure 15–1 Integrated health care: A coordinated effort.

one's viewpoint, business could be the blame, or the health insurance industry, or the unions, or even the legal profession. All these sectors of society have had a part in the rise in costs. Rightly so, for each has a desire to effect changes in the health care system to ensure that we as a nation of people have access to health care, that it be reasonable in cost, and that the quality that we have become accustomed to and want remains. In summary, we all have contributed to rising health care costs.

Even though many have contributed, there is a growing concern over the health care delivery system in general because the health care component of the GDP commands an ever-growing share of the nation's productive capacity. How much more of the GDP health care will consume is anybody's guess. More important, it must be asked how much more can or should be allocated to the health care industry? Health care professionals and those in research may argue for more. Business argues that the continual push of inflationary health care costs is affecting the competitive position locally and abroad. If this scenario continues, we may lose jobs to foreign markets, thus pushing more of the population into uninsured health care roles. Government says that it will no longer tolerate the double-the-inflation rate of growth in health care costs because the public indicates that it does not want to spend more discretionary dollars on taxes to support those who do not have health insurance. The time has come for the health care system itself to hold down health care costs. It is also time for individual groups within the industry to meet this challenge. This, of course, includes the food service and nutrition professionals.

THE IDS

Until recently, the physician has been the central purchasing agent for health care services upon which the general population has relied. The current shift is from the physician to third party payers, managed care organizations, and the government, the last of which has assumed a greater and greater role in the purchase of health care services. For example, the rise in health care costs seemed to slow down in the mid-1980s as a result of government efforts to adopt stronger prospective payment schemes. Specifically, the adoption of the Medicare diagnosis-related groups (DRGs) method of reimbursement ushered in other prospective payment plans, including the resource-based relative value system (RBRVS), a DRG system of payment for physicians, and the development of capitated reimbursement mainly from the commercial health insurance industry. These types of payment plans affected how hospitals were to be paid in the future, and organizations responded just as it was predicted that they would. With the incentive to decrease inpatient care as a result of DRGs, hospitals have moved their patients to other settings where less restricted payment plans are in existence. This is much like a balloon: Squeeze it in one place, and it will expand in another place.

To maximize the revenues of the entire system, hospitals embarked on a system of purchasing the providers who were to be the major players in the change to more ambulatory and outpatient care services. Hospitals have been for so long the major focus of health care that they did not want to lose the power and influence that they had built up over the years. They did not want to lose that influence over the health care system to other hospital competitors, to physicians, or to the health insurance industry.

As a result, they began purchasing physician practices and are continuing to do so in a rapid pace. They purchase other hospitals to expand their market share. Some hospitals have been closed so that the population served will have to go to the central hospital. They form physician–hospital organizations to merge the major health care providers further into a system of seamless care for the market that each serves. If a patient needs one or all health services, the new IDS is available to provide total care almost under one roof.

With the IDS, there must be a broad band of health and other services available to the population that is purchasing health services. Those services may be defined as "cradle to grave," a seamless array of services available with which the major purchasers can contract. There must be acute care services. Long-term care services are a must. Home care is not a privilege anymore. The list can be exhaustive if we are truly looking at the IDS as the future health care system for the United States.

This sounds almost too good to be true. The hospitals form an integrated, full-service, health care system to control the delivery of health care in their service area. It was much like this until Columbia/HCA joined the health care race to capture the health care market in many areas around the country. In effect, Columbia/HCA moved into an area and then, in a focused, businesslike manner, reduced costs, contracted with local health insurance organizations, or directly contracted with local businesses to provide accessible (seamless) health care services, quality that could be measured, and care at a cost that could be guaranteed over time, sometimes lower than that of the competitors in some areas.

From the macro point of view, this meant that health care organizations in a market area not only had an IDS but also had to be competitive with accessibility, price, and quality. Again, some local health care organizations lost control of their ability to deliver a broad base of services to their communities. Those that have not responded well to the changes in reimbursement from the governments (particularly the federal government and DRGs), the movement to the IDS, and the pressure to affiliate with other providers and employers have found themselves in a poor competitive position. They have high cost, limited accessibility to all services, and quality that is not measurable in the community. For some, this has meant closure of their hospitals. To others, it has meant being sold to or swallowed up by another system.

Today's hospital is only one part of the system of delivering care to the community. If more of the services are to be provided in the outpatient or ambulatory setting, this means that fewer patients will actually be hospitalized. This factor has had, and will continue to have, an impact on food service and nutrition care because the patient mix is now more intense than in the past, and the average length of stay of 8 days has been cut in half from what it was just 5 years ago. Dietitians will have less time to develop a nutritional relationship with patients. No sooner will the patient's assessment and treatment plan be complete than the patient will be discharged without comprehensive consultation to maximize the healing process outside the hospital.

THE 21ST CENTURY

The era of shifting the financial risk of caring for patients is now here, and the transition to a managed care environment is accelerating rapidly. With 72% of the working population enrolled in some form of managed care, this transformation is well past the midpoint. Health reform continues almost unabated, restructuring the health care system. This process began with the development of health maintenance organizations in the 1970s, the adoption of DRG prospective payment systems in the 1980s, and the emergence of managed care in the 1990s. By the 21st century, a new pattern of health care delivery, financing, information system networks, and incentives for providers to change will reform and reshape the health care system. The roles of patients as consumers, providers, payers, and regulators will change dramatically from the way they are seen today.

Health Care Expenditures

In the past, health care expenditures grew each year at nearly twice the inflation rate. As the 41 million uninsured are captured under some form of Medicaid or health security program, health insurance premiums and the prices paid for health care will rise to just above the overall inflation rate. Continued pressure from managed care and the insistence that consumers pay more out-of-pocket copayments will drive costs down.

Responsibility for Self-Care

More consumers will assume responsibility for their own health. If they do not accomplish this, or at least move toward some healthy goal, they will end up paying more of their health insurance premiums out of their paychecks or through higher deductibles and copayments. Already those who smoke pay higher life insurance premiums. This will transfer over to health insurance premiums.

Physician Dependence

Physicians will move formally to join with the IDS, and more of them will work for salaries within these organizations. An increasing number of physicians will be associated with multispecialty groups or large single-specialty groups. These groups will form the basis for regaining control in the physician–patient relationships that they feel has been undermined by the managed care industry and moving to form management groups to negotiate as a sub-IDS with the managed care industry. This will be the foundation for taking on capitation and risk-sharing contracts with managed care organizations or employers through direct contracting methods.

Government Purchasers

The federal and state governments, through Medicare and Medicaid, will continue to be players in health reform. They will use market mechanisms by moving to contract with IDSs that use accessibility, quality, and cost considerations in the negotiation process. Low-cost, high-quality, accessible IDSs will receive the contracts to care for government beneficiaries. No longer will a Medicare beneficiary be able to choose where he or she will go for care. No longer will he or she go where his or her physician is affiliated. The beneficiary will go to the IDS that has the contract to provide the care. Otherwise, the beneficiary will pay more to have the privilege to go where he or she wants to receive care.

The Health Insurance Industry

Those that can compete, will. Instead of hundreds of health insurance companies vying for contracts, several large IDSs will align with employers and health insurance organizations that have joined the managed care plans.

Per Member per Month

The per member per month (PMPM) method of payment for services will emerge: This is capitation. Even with its drawbacks, PMPM will draw the public into it and force the public to understand the necessity of responsibility for self-care. A wellness and health promotion policy will emerge based on the capitation method of payment.

The Healthy 21st Century

Because all the players will be grouped into several large IDSs in a region, each region will develop its own health care objectives to tie the continuum of care to healthy lifestyles and behaviors for that region. In this way, the providers can remain in control of the process but involve governments, the health insurance industry, employers, and patients.

The Clinical Executive

More physicians and other clinicians will assume positions of leadership within the IDSs. If there is a merger between administration and clinicians to affect health behavior in the continuum of care, more clinicians can assume positions of power. No longer will financing and reimbursement be separate from clinical care; the two will fold together under the capitation umbrella.

Health Care Networks

The mergers and acquisitions of the 1990s will pale when compared to the growth of the networks, consolidations, and the overall restructuring of the health care delivery systems that will take place. Whether these arrangements are formal (IDSs) or informal (group purchasing arrangements, possibly organized by several IDSs), this growth will include joint ventures that encompass governments, IDSs, the health insurance industry, physicians, and employers in the effort to coordinate health care delivery services that are accessible and provide measurable quality at an acceptably low cost.

THE IMPACT ON HEALTH SERVICES

The impact of these changes on the health care system is causing a revolution in the way health care services are designed and delivered. The rise in the cost of health care has driven the federal and state governments and corporate America to adopt more restrictive payment plans with health care providers. With fewer tax dollars and profits squeezed by these growing health care costs, these three organizational bodies have made strong efforts to contain their expenditures.

Medicare has adopted the DRG method of reimbursement for hospitals. It has adopted the RBRVS system to constrict physician payments. Medicaid has moved to health maintenance organizations and managed care to hold down payments.

Employers have not sat on the sidelines watching their profits diminish at the expense of rising health care costs. Working with third party health insurance companies, many employers are trying to reduce benefit packages that were seen as overly generous in the past. On the other hand, employers have moved to increase employee cost sharing for health insurance benefits and for health services. This has resulted in more employees having increased deductibles and copayments, which has driven down the total health insurance bill that the employer receives each year from the health insurance carrier.

Additionally, employers have revisited the health promotion/wellness plans that were begun in the last decade but may not have been adopted because they did not affect the bottom line. The thrust of these programs is to teach employees about lifestyle changes that can alter poor health behavior. If these programs are not successful, then the employee will be taxed by the health insurance/life insurance companies to pay higher premiums for continuing the lifestyle that is deemed a risk by the insurer.

Along with Medicare and Medicaid, employers are adopting stringent utilization review methods to monitor health processes and outcomes. If the health insurance industry can adopt a list of health outcome measures for the providers in a community, the health insurance industry can move patients to the most cost-efficient provider who can provide an acceptable level of quality health care.

Throughout the United States, particular employers can exercise greater influence over health providers. They can influence the health care marketplace because they have greater numbers of employees (see Chapter 1). The health providers want to maintain or increase their market share and therefore will enter into direct contracting for health insurance with such companies to "lock up" the employer and the employees at competitive prices.

IMPACT ON PROVIDERS

With the major payers taking actions to control their expenditures, health care providers at all levels have taken notice and responded to these activities, particularly hospitals and physicians. There are only three ways to maintain or increase profits: reduce costs, raise prices, or increase volume.

Health care providers have responded as the incentives placed before them have dictated. With the inability to raise prices because of the contracts imposed by health maintenance organizations and managed care and the inability to increase the number of inpatient admissions because of increased utilization review practices, health care providers have moved to reduce their operating costs and to increase their revenues from other sources, particularly from ambulatory care settings.

No health care organization has escaped reengineering, downsizing, or rightsizing of its staff. Providers have been placed in the position of having to manage their operations more carefully or face financial or cash flow problems. They have linked with other providers through physician–hospital organizations, mergers, and acquisitions, all with the intent of moving closer to the IDS.

To cut costs, health care organizations have upgraded their information technology to assist management in identifying costs more readily and monitoring variances of actual to budgeted expenditures more closely, especially with regard to variable costs that are dependent on patient days. The department head who relied on technical skills in the past has had to adapt to these changes by acquiring new skills in financial management, negotiation, communication, and computer applications.

By adopting these new skills, food service and nutrition professionals can make better, more informed decisions to meet the goals and objectives of their departments and parent organizations. In the past, their decisions may have been limited to issues concerning quality, nutrition care, food production, and delivery. These same decisions are present today, but efficient utilization of all resources (food, personnel, supplies, space, energy, etc.) becomes of paramount importance if the organization is to survive and succeed.

As the hospital or parent organization is placed under more pressure to be a business, so is the food and nutrition service of that organization required to act more as a business itself. With a competitive marketplace vying for a smaller piece of the "patient pie," hospitals must be more conscious of their resource consumption and utilize resources more efficiently. For food and nutrition services, the same holds true. They are competing within the organization for fewer discretionary dollars, and if they cannot cost justify their existence and demonstrate efficiency, fewer dollars will come their way. Therefore, while hospitals have undertaken more aggressive marketing strategies to inform customers about their services, food and nutrition departments must market their services to maintain their own share of the marketplace. As can be seen, these approaches to the operation of the department require additional sets of skills that were not commonplace a few years ago.

ACCOUNTABILITY

In the future, health care organizations will be paid for keeping people healthy. This is the incentive under managed care and capitation. Underlying this is the transfer of the financial risk to the providers, who, if they accept that risk, must develop the risk management contracts to care for patients. This is a proactive strategy that incorporates a healthy outcome as a measure of the IDS's success.

The high-risk patients, possibly including the chronically ill, aged, and Medicare populations, will be moved to a case management approach under managed care. Additionally, all groups will be aggressively monitored for healthy behaviors and lifestyles. The future will entail an employer group, government group (Medicare, Medicaid, or worker's compensation), or health insurance group that demands extensive patient outcome reporting and monitors long-term health status. The industry is moving to manage health care delivery, accessibility, quality, and cost on at least a regional scale in a manner that was not commonly thought of during the 20th century.

IMPACT ON FOOD AND NUTRITION SERVICES

In the past, food and nutrition services may have acted much as an island in the stream. Whatever was requested or required from administrations, physicians, or accrediting groups was met with the idea that food and nutrition folded into the system by focusing on inpatient activities. Today, that same focus remains important to the overall delivery of health care. With the health care system moving more to the ambulatory setting, however, the focus of the department will have to change to meet the future missions of the parent organization.

If there is more of a demand for food and nutrition services to participate in the IDS, then these services must meet the demands of the system. The IDS is being formed first to survive and second to provide a continuum of services under one organizational roof. This means that departments will be more accountable for their services in the future. They, too, must be more businesslike in their operation.

Not only must food and nutrition services be accessible, but customer demands for high quality must be met. In conjunction with accessibility and quality, cost of services must be monitored and controlled. Food and nutrition services therefore can expect more emphasis in the future on the following issues.

Outcomes Measurements

There will be more emphasis placed on outcomes of food and nutrition services in terms of their impact on the health of the population. Chapter 14 describes some of the efforts that have already been made toward this goal.

Financial Benchmarking

The department will be measured more on the basis of its financial outcomes. It must be able to justify itself financially. To do so, it will have to participate in internal and external benchmarking so that financial results can be tracked over time within the organization and compared with those of other comparable providers of food and nutrition service. Large IDSs will find this much easier to accomplish. For isolated rural hospitals, obtaining comparative figures and data may not be possible, and such organizations may be at a relative disadvantage in not knowing where they stand and how well they are doing in the delivery of their services. Several options for this effort are presented in Chapter 13.

Quality Maintenance

In the face of external and internal pressures to cut costs and maintain and expand services, the quality of services cannot be compromised. Efforts must be made to reach out to more customers with food and nutrition services to ensure that feedback is gathered to measure the quality of services. Physicians, vendors, patients, employees, satellite facilities, and others will be important sources of data. Results will be used to implement new quality initiatives. They will become public in nature. Chapter 14 offers a system for ensuring continuous improvement of the quality of patient care.

IDS Focus, Not Just Hospital Focus

By necessity, food and nutrition services will move away from traditional settings. They will be drawn more into the real mission of the IDS and have more point-of-care contact time with patients and other customers wherever they are found in the community. Consulting and follow-up services in long-term care facilities along with home care initiatives will be commonplace. Patients will be followed throughout the continuum of care (see Exhibit 14–3). There will be more of a focus on effective nutrition education and prevention to alter and change dietary behavior patterns and to encourage more responsibility on the part of patients.

The IDS wants to be in a position of being responsible for the health care of its served population. However, the IDS and health care delivery system in general do not want to be blamed for or responsible for the cost of providing care to those who exhibit poor behavioral and unhealthy lifestyles. The high cost of health care may be in part to those who do not wear motorcycle helmets and then ask the health care system to care for them, at a great cost to society and the providers. The high cost of health care can be traced in part to the smoking habits, the drug habits, the poor eating habits, and other lifestyles that arrive at the health system's doors to be cured.

Charging for Services

Food and nutrition service will be a revenue-producing center in the next century. In the past, the cost of these activities was covered through the patient's room charges. This will change after the year 2000. Not only will all consultation services have a service charge, but basic services also will be charged. When the customer orders a service, a bill will be sent.

Therefore, more emphasis will be placed on accounting for the cost of food and nutrition services than ever before. If a specific service costs too much, it may not be ordered, especially if the outcome is not what is expected from that service. If it is not ordered, then it will be discarded. As described in Chapter 12, a greater emphasis on the marketing of food services to the community and to other customers served by food service will be seen. With a decrease in inpatient days, hospital food and nutrition departments will continue to shrink unless revenue can be generated to justify operating costs. Figure 13–4 provides a simple system for tracking costs and comparing them with revenues so that a more businesslike approach to profit and loss can be implemented by practitioners. As attempts are made to expand the market, professionals need to realize that they will be competing with others, just as their organizations will be doing.

SKILLS REQUIRED IN THE FUTURE

From the foregoing discussion, it is apparent that food and nutrition service professionals will have to adapt to the changing health care environment if they are to lead their profession into the next century on sound footing. The most critical skills that will be needed for success include the following:

- computer skills
- statistical analysis
- communication skills

- entrepreneurial outlook
- financial management
- critical analysis
- strategic planning
- negotiation
- motivation

Computer Skills

No longer will a sharp pencil solve the myriad problems facing food and nutrition service professionals. To analyze variances in the budget, to identify the impact of resource spending on the department's budget, and to track other expenditures, only a computer can assist managers in meeting the goals and objectives of the organization.

Computers and data technology should be used as educational and training tools as well as for meal planning and inventory control. Organizations in the IDS or related networks will have mountains of information available for use, in addition to the computerized medical record. Food service and nutrition leaders must create knowledge bases, and profitably eliminate barriers. They also need to be brought together through an open management system that encourages collaboration and cooperation among professionals in a variety of settings. If problems occur, the goal will be to work together to develop alternatives and solutions. The benefits of high-technological communications in food and nutrition service can be maximized. The more paperwork that can be eliminated, the better.

Statistical Analysis

Practitioners will need to use statistical methods more in the next century than ever before. Those with statistical analysis skills will be in a better position to analyze the mountains of data quickly. The purpose of statistical methods is to allow one to use observations made of a subset to understand the whole. Before professionals can appreciate the specific statistical methods used in health research to accomplish this goal, they will need to acquire or brush up on the basic statistical procedures in health research. The ability to select an appropriate method of analysis and to interpret the results will be beneficial to all.

Communication Skills

As stressed in Chapter 2, good writing and speaking skills will enhance the ability of food service and nutrition professionals to relate well with top managers in their organizations. Understanding and being able to communicate with financial managers will enhance the relationship between these two diverse areas. There is no time to deal with unclear messages. One must "get it right the first time" and be in a position to move quickly on new ideas as needed.

Entrepreneurial Outlook

Food service and nutrition professionals need to work more closely with others to develop joint ventures that can be undertaken both to attract new business to their department and parent organization and to strengthen ties with those outside the department. A perfect example of this can be seen in Exhibit 7–3.

Financial Management

It is clear that the developing health care system is being driven by financial incentives for the most part. Because of this, practitioners will have to be in a better position to understand financial management issues, problems, and solutions. Food service and nutrition professionals will be in a position to answer a myriad of questions concerning the business side of health care delivery. Cost/ benefit analysis, breakeven analysis, and financial ratio analysis are but a few of the management accounting techniques that they will use in developing a financial and accounting base.

Critical Analysis

To move into the next century on a sound footing, food service and nutrition professionals will be accepted not only for their skills in the areas described above but also for their ability to critically analyze thoughts, processes, the structure of the organization, and outcome measures that are quantifiable. Variance analysis skills will become of paramount importance for a successful professional to survive and perhaps thrive.

Strategic Planning

Not only will the parent organization have a mission, a vision, and goals and objectives, but food service and nutrition professionals will have to develop the skills described in Chapter 3 to organize their own department's mission, vision, goals, and objectives. These will have to link up with and mirror the organization's set of strategic planning goals. Administrators will depend upon the food service and nutrition staff to define future goals and objectives and to develop a strategy to meet them.

Negotiation

The ability to negotiate will be a skill that food service and nutrition professionals will need to develop. If one lacks this skill, valued resources may be lost to one's organization. It will be hard to do more or the same with less, but that is what looms over the next year's budget. Doing more or the same with *much* less may place the organization in peril. If failure occurs, there is always someone else waiting in the wings to take the organization's place and move to improve what it started. Sharp negotiation skills will enable practitioners to place themselves in a strong position so that they can finish what they start.

Motivation

Individual organizations are not alone as they face the challenges of the future. They are all in the same boat in this era of limited resources and constricted reimbursement. Employees often feel that they are the only boat in the water, however. Managers will benefit by learning the motivation skills necessary to move food services and nutrition forward, to make them accessible, to be cost conscious, and to maintain and improve the quality of services provided to patients, families, employees, and visitors.

REFERENCE

U.S. Department of Health and Human Services. (1990). *Healthy people 2000: National health promotion and disease prevention objectives.* Washington, D.C.: Public Health Service.

Index

A

Accountability
in future, 521
public, 479, *480*
staff, 502–506
Accreditation of hospitals, 42. *See also*
Joint Commission
Acquired immunodeficiency syndrome,
196, *197–198*
Acquisitions in health care industry, 40
Acute Physiology and Chronic Health
Evaluation, 257
Administration on Aging, 50
Advance medical directives, 189–190,
255–265
physicians' adherence to, 265
Advertising, 285–286. *See also* Marketing
food services
Agenda for Change, 41, 149, 471
Allergies to foods, 190
Alternative food production systems,
330–351, *331*, 422t
classification schemes for, 330–331
comparative costs of, 335–338
food, 335
labor, 336–337
supplies, 337–338
energy use by, 341–343
equipment for, 340–341
food quality and, 344, 375
food safety and, 345–346
impact on menu, 343–344
ingredient control for, 339–340
meal assembly and delivery options for,
355–356, *356–358*

product flow in, 330
production scheduling for, 338–339
references for case studies on, *376*
selection process for, 334, 347–351,
350
skill level of labor required for, 338
types of, 331–334
assembly-serve (convenience)
systems, 333, *334*
centralized rethermalization process,
333, 347
chilling/chilled storage process, 346–
347
commissary systems, 332, 334
conventional systems, 332, *332*, 333
cook-chill systems, 33, 332–334, *333*
cook-freeze systems, 33, 332
ready food systems, 332
sous vide systems, 332
American Dietetic Association, 25, 30,
38–39, 63–64, 168, 195, 211, 247–248,
482–483, 490
number of members of, 30
Standards of Education, 208, *209–210*
American Hospital Association, 195
American Society for Healthcare Food
Service Administration, 25–26
American Society for Hospital Food
Service Administrators, 470
American Society for Parenteral and
Enteral Nutrition, 25
Americans with Disabilities Act of 1990,
13
Anisakiasis infection, 395t
Anthropometric measurements, 178
Ascaria lumbricoides infection, 395t

Note: Page numbers in *italics* denote figures and exhibits; those followed by "t" denote
tables.

About the Author

Rita Jackson, PhD, RD, began her career in the restaurant industry, after which she worked in health care for more than 20 years as a supervisor, clinical dietitian, director of food and nutrition services, educator, and consultant for hospitals, nursing homes, homes for the developmentally disabled, and correctional facilities. Positions as director included Glenridge Hospital, Seaview Hospital, and St. Luke's Medical Center, all in New York State. Dr. Jackson has lectured for many groups across the country and has taught graduate and undergraduate courses in food service management, clinical nutrition, and quality improvement at Rutgers University, New York University, and the University of Florida. Her doctoral research in nutrition and dietetics at New York University focused on hospital food service systems. Dr. Jackson's publications include topics in nutrition and food service management with special emphasis on quality improvement and nutrient conservation in institutional settings. Currently, she is a Visiting Assistant Professor and the MSH/AP4 Director at the University of North Florida. Dr. Jackson is also the Editor of *Health Care Food & Nutrition Focus.*